THE CHANNEL DIVERGENCES

DEEPER PATHWAYS OF THE WEB

REVISED EDITION

MIKI SHIMA, OMD   CHARLES CHACE

BLUE POPPY PRESS • BOULDER, COLORADO

Published by:

BLUE POPPY PRESS
A Division of Blue Poppy Enterprises, Inc.
5441 Western Ave., #2
BOULDER, CO 80301

First Edition, May, 2001
Revised Edition, July 2002
ISBN 1-891845-15-2

COPYRIGHT 2001 © Charles Chace and Miki Shima

All rights reserved. No part of this book may be reproduced, stored in a retrieval system, transcribed in any form or by any means, electronic, mechanical, photocopy, recording, or any other means, or translated into any language without the prior written permission of the publisher.

The information in this book is given in good faith. However, the translators and the publishers cannot be held responsible for any error or omission. Nor can they be held in any way responsible for treatment given on the basis of information contained in this book. The publishers make this information available to English language readers for scholarly and research purposes only.

The publishers do not advocate nor endorse self-medication by laypersons. Chinese medicine is a professional medicine. Laypersons interested in availing themselves of the treatments described in this book should seek out a qualified professional practitioner of Chinese medicine.

COMP Designation: Original work based on a standard translational terminology

Printed at Johnson Printing, Boulder, CO

Graphics & Design by Frank J. Crawford
Cover design by Frank J. Crawford

10 9 8 7 6 5 4 3 2

Dedication

To my dad, my sister, Diana, my three children for their love and support.
— *Miki Shima*

To Monika, for the love and support that allowed this book to happen.
—*Charles Chace*

Acknowledgements

We would like to thank the following individuals for their invaluable help with this project.

Huang Ying-jun, Dan Bensky, Steve Birch, Joseph Helms, Sean Marshall, Guilio Piccozzi, Sylvia Pelcz, Michael Young, Butch Levy, Monika Chace, Nigel Wiseman, Bob Felt, Honora Wolfe, Frank J. Crawford, Jason Blalock, and Naga.

Table of Contents

	Author's Preface	VII
1.	Characteristics of the Channel Divergences	1
2.	The Nature of the Channel Divergences	41
3.	Channel Divergence Diagnostics	55
4.	Channel Divergence Therapeutics	65
5.	Tadashi Irie's Channel Divergence Treatment Style	77
6.	Kodo Seki's Channel Divergence Strategies	101
7.	Shigeji Naomoto's Biorhythmic Channel Divergence Pairings	124
8.	Miki Shima's Approach to Channel Divergence Therapy	137

Appendices

1.	Integrated Treatment Strategies, Treatment Formulary	201
2.	Extraordinary Vessel Pulses	219
3.	Auxiliary Diagnostic Methods	227
4.	Auxiliary Treatment Methods	231
5.	Ear Acupuncture Strategies: The Hibiki Method	235
6.	Tadashi Irie's Confluence-based Herbal Formulas	239
7.	Channel Divergence Hole Pairings	245
8.	Tadashi Irie's Magnet Specifications	247
9.	Electro-Acupuncture Devices	249
10.	Omura's Bi-digital O-ring Test	251

Bibliography	255
Index	261

Authors' Preface

There are those who know heaven and know humanity. Those who know heaven know that heaven gives one life. Whoever knows humanity uses knowing to nurture what cannot be known. They run out the string of their years and do not find it cut off in the middle. This is the fullest knowledge. And yet, though this is so, there is a problem. Knowledge waits on certainty, but certainty is never quite certain.
Zhuang Zi, Chapter 6, "The Great Ancestral Teacher"

Nie Que asked for instruction in the Dao from Pi Yi. "If you'll just straighten your form and concentrate your gaze," Pi Yi said, "you'll get to heavenly harmony. If you'll just put a hold on your knowing and concentrate on one good guess, the spirit will come to live with you, the power of virtue will beautify you, and you'll come to inhabit the Dao.
Zhuang Zi, Chapter 22, "Knowing Wandered North"

The channel divergences (*jing bie*) are one of the most enigmatic facets of the Chinese channel and network vessel system. They first appear within the Chinese medical literature in Chapter 11, *Jing Bie* "On the Channel Divergences" of the *Ling Shu (Divine Pivot)* compiled during the Warring States period (403 BCE - 221 BCE). Also known as the divergent meridians or distinct meridians, their trajectories and usually some conjecture concerning their function are discussed in nearly every basic textbook of acupuncture. Although the channel divergences are intriguing, they tend to fade from most Western acupuncturists' consciousness soon after being introduced. This is due to the fact that few Western acupuncturists have any idea of what to do with the channel divergences in actual clinical practice. Nevertheless, the compilers of the *Nei Jing* (*Inner Classic*) obviously believed the channel divergences were an essential component of the channel system. Otherwise, why

VIII The Channel Divergences

would they have included them? The channel divergences nag at us along with all the other bits of information in the *Nei Jing* that don't quite fit, demanding that we attempt to understand them.

In reviewing the modern Chinese medical literature on the channel divergences, one is left with the impression that their primary function is as a theoretical safety-net which serves to explain how the main channels influence areas not directly traversed by their main trajectories. Ellis, Wiseman, and Boss, in *Fundamentals of Chinese Acupuncture*, epitomize this perspective in their unequivocal statement: "The importance of the channel divergences is primarily theoretical."[1] While being given the lip service that is their due based on their inclusion in the *locus classicus* of Chinese medicine, the *Inner Classic*, there is little or no discussion of how to actually use these pathways in clinical practice.

Unfortunately, although the *Divine Pivot* provides us with a rough idea of the trajectories of the channel divergences, the *Inner Classic* also gives us few clues as to how to make them work in clinical practice.[2] Be that as it may, a number of modern investigators have pieced together whatever sparse information on the channel divergences does exist in the Chinese literature to develop treatment strategies of profound clinical efficacy. These modern investigators' approaches to the use of the channel divergences are often mutually contradictory. In addition, it is also sometimes difficult to understand why or how some of these supposed channel divergences techniques do, in fact, treat these pathways. Nevertheless, there are a number of contemporary acupuncturists who believe they are treating the channel divergences and who produce consistently impressive clinical results using these techniques. In this book, we examine these various contemporary approaches each on their own terms. When all is said and done, we believe that the channel divergences are valuable maps for efficacious acupuncture therapy. Indeed, the present authors believe that the channel divergences are among the most profoundly useful conceptual tools we have encountered in our practice of acupuncture, and, as such, we believe they deserve further exploration.

Therefore, the purpose of this book is to present a variety of approaches to understanding and using the channel divergences. We begin with some of the basic assumptions, both Asian and European, that have been made regarding the channel divergences and proceed to an examination of the source literature. Virtually all of the writings we have seen regarding the channel divergences are in some way incomplete or not totally satisfactory. French sources often present innovative ideas as if they were a matter of historical fact. They also tend to be short on clinical application. On the other hand, many Japanese channel divergence authors are so focused on clinical efficacy, they omit theoretical explanations entirely. Instead, these Japanese authors tend to proceed directly to therapy, leaving it to others to figure out the conceptual whys and wherefores for what they are doing.

Since there are few consensual rules regarding the contemporary clinical use of the channel divergences, each of us must make our own inferences. Because it is the *locus classicus* of the channel divergences in the Chinese medical literature, we begin this book by reviewing in some depth those passages from Chapter 11 of the *Divine Pivot* which first introduced these 12 pathways to all succeeding generations of acupuncturists. In a very real sense, these 12 terse passages are the only common ground we have concerning the channel divergences, and, without understanding what they do and do not say, it is impossible to make sense of anyone else's clinical application of these pathways. This introduction to the channel divergences is then followed by a discussion of some of the diagnostic methods used to evaluate the state of these pathways, after which we present a review of some of the ideas concerning the channel divergences found in the English and French language literature.

However, it is the Japanese-based channel divergences therapies culminating in Shima's own work that form the core of the book. The acupuncturists discussed in this section of this book are among the most influential developers of channel divergence therapies in Japan. In particular, Tadashi Irie and Kodo Seki were very influential in Shima's own development as a channel divergence specialist. Shima Sensei trained directly under both these masters and now has more than 20 years experience using the channel divergences in clinical practice.

In presenting all these styles, we hope to establish for the reader some sense of continuity in the development of channel divergences treatments while at the same time illustrating the great diversity of thought they have inspired. However, while we examine each style treatment critically, it is not our intent to rank one style of practice as superior to another. This is despite the fact that we explore the treatment style of one of the present authors (Shima) in the greatest depth. We would also like to make it clear that we have a great deal more personal experience with the Japanese-based styles than with the Chinese or European strategies contained in this book. When all is said and done, each style we describe herein does seem to work to a greater or lesser extent. We leave it to the reader to determine the methodology or combination of methodologies that best suits his or her personal needs and interests.

THE JAPANESE TOPOLOGICAL ACUPUNCTURE SOCIETY

The channel divergence investigators, Tadashi Irie, Kodo Seki, and Shigeji Naomoto, were all part of a circle of acupuncturists centered around Yoshio Manaka called the Japanese Topological Acupuncture Society. These practitioners were actively involved in expanding the theoretical boundaries of the acupuncture model and more fully utilizing the entire channel system. The development of the channel divergences was part of this larger goal. In the process, the members of the Japanese Topological Acupuncture Society came up with some very arcane diagnostic and treatment methods, and, over time, they developed a consensual set of assumptions and terminology regarding the acupuncture system. More importantly, they gravitated toward the use of diagnostic and treatment methodologies that were often unique to the Topological Acupuncture Society. For instance, the use of ion-pumping (IP) cords was so commonplace for those in the Topological Acupuncture Society that a fairly standardized system of notation was used when referring to IP treatments. Those unfamiliar with this modality are often at a loss to make sense of it. While ion-pumping cords have now made their way into the mainstream of acupuncture practice in the West, much of the other esoterica of the Topological Acupuncture Society has not appeared in the English language. It is, therefore, difficult to accurately reflect the treatment strategies of Irie, Seki, and Naomoto without describing some of these ancillary diagnostic and treatment techniques.

In their efforts to push the envelope of the acupuncture model, the members of the Topological Acupuncture Society clearly went out of their way to come up with new and ever more arcane diagnostic procedures. In addition, in the process of establishing their own distinctive treatment styles, each of these acupuncturists was strongly motivated to be innovative. Many of these techniques are fascinating and they must be understood if we are to grasp the intent of Irie and his peers. Nevertheless, in the interest of maintaining the focus of our work on the channel divergences, we have placed explanations for such methodologies in appendices in the back of the book. Some of the diagnostic approaches used by the acupuncturists presented in this book may strike the reader as somewhat divorced from their own day-to-day clinical reality. However, we believe that presentation of these techniques is essential for a complete understanding of the overall treatment strategies employed by the channel divergence specialists we discuss.

THE METHODOLOGY USED IN THE CREATION OF THIS BOOK

The terminology used for the translation of Chinese medical terms in this book is adopted from Wiseman and Feng's *A Practical Dictionary of Chinese Medicine* except in those cases where the Japanese use of a term conveys a fundamentally different meaning than its Chinese counterpart. In such cases, we have simply resorted to a transliteration of the Japanese term and footnoted the standard Chinese corollary. In a number of cases, we have included both the English and their original Chinese terms rendered in Pinyin in parentheses when we felt that this would promote further clarity for our readers. Acupuncture point identifications used in the book are based on the World Health Organization (WHO) *Standard Acupuncture Point Nomenclature*. Acupuncture points are first identified by the Pinyin romanization of their Chinese name in italic with each syllable capitalized. This is followed by the standard channel and point number notation in parentheses. However, Lu = LU, St = ST, Sp = SP, Ht = HT, Bl = BL, Ki = KI, Per = PC, TB = SJ, Liv = LV, GV = DU, and CV = REN.

Although the terms "master" and "couple" holes, *i.e.*, the paired meeting points of the extraordinary vessels, are modern innovations, they are useful in organizing and explaining treatment strategies.[3] Most channel divergence treatments similarly use paired acupuncture holes. However, no terminological standard has yet been agreed upon for referring to these pairs. For the purposes of the present work, we refer to the acupuncture holes on the head and neck pertaining to the channel divergences as "master holes," because the use of these holes is typical of many styles of channel divergence treatment. The use of these holes is, typically, the defining feature of a channel divergence treatment. These master holes must then be paired with one or more transport (*shu*), source (*yuan*), or network (*luo*) holes on the extremities to specifically treat the channel divergences as opposed to simply treating the main channel on which they are located. This is similar to using both *Nei Guan* (Per 6) and *Gong Sun* (Sp 4) to access either the *yin wei* or *chong mai* vessels. We refer to these latter holes as "access" holes because these are the points via which the channel divergences are initially accessed.

The first time premodern references appear in this book, they are identified by their Chinese or Japanese title in Roman letters followed by a translation of their title in parentheses. Subsequent references then only use their translated title in italics. Chapter cites include both their chapter number and a translation of the chapter title in quotation marks. Subsequent chapter cites only use the chapter numbers. For instance, *Ling Shu (Divine Pivot)*, Chapter 5, "On the Roots & Nodes" becomes the *Divine Pivot*, Chapter 5 in subsequent cites.

Readers will observe that the electro-acupuncture treatment methods in this book follow the common convention of assigning positive and negative poles to acupuncture points as a means of designating the direction of electrical current. Those familiar with the physics of electricity, particularly as it functions in AC current, will note that this is not a completely accurate reflection of what is occurring between the two leads of an electro acupuncture device. Since the acupuncturists profiled in the present work are undoubtedly aware of the fundamental laws of physics, it is clear that the assignment of positive and negative leads must be understood as nothing more than functional designations that facilitate optimal clinical outcomes. As we will see again, and again, emphasis is less on theory than on what yields an effective result.

Miki Shima, OMD
Corte Madera, CA

Charles Chace
Boulder, CO

XII The Channel Divergences

ENDNOTES

[1] Ellis, Wiseman & Boss: 40
[2] The validity of cross needling (*miu ci*) from Chapter 63 of the *Divine Pivot* as a channel divergence treatment strategy will be discussed in Chapter 2 of the present work.
[3] In Chinese, the main points used to treat the extraordinary vessels are simply called the meeting points (*hui xue*) or occasionally the meeting points (*he xue*).

1

CHARACTERISTICS OF THE 12 CHANNEL DIVERGENCES

One of the primary characteristics of the channel divergences (*jing bie*) is the divergence of opinions regarding them. A great deal of the commentary pertaining to the channel divergence system, including much of what has been said concerning their clinical application, has been advanced as a matter of fact, when, in fact, these observations are purely conjectural. There are a number of mutually exclusive propositions circulating in the literature regarding the channel divergences, each with a variety of different clinical implications. Therefore, it is essential for us to clarify the areas of common scholarly agreement concerning the channel divergences and those areas where there is substantial dissent. The following characteristics of the channel divergence system are all generally agreed upon.

All sources concur that the 12 channel divergences begin shallowly and then enter deeply into the body before ultimately surfacing again at or near their end points. With the exception of the hand *shao yang* channel divergence, all the channel divergences separate (*li*) from their root channel somewhere on the four extremities where they then enter (*ru*) deeply into the body. They finally emerge (*chu*) shallowly onto the exterior of the body.

In the course of the present discussion, it will become evident that those investigators who have looked at the channel divergences in any depth have all given careful consideration to the words used to describe their trajectories. A clear understanding of these terms is essential to a proper understanding of the channel divergences themselves, and we will discuss each of them in depth in subsequent chapters. For the time being, however, an initial image of the channel divergences travelling from the surface deeply into the core of the body and then re-emerging shallowly is sufficient.

2 The Channel Divergences

Once the channel divergences separate from their associated main channel, both the yin and yang channels of the divergence pairs then travel through the interior of the body. From here they ultimately re-enter the paired yang channel in the region of the head and neck. This intermingling of the trajectories of the yin-yang channel divergence pairs is the origin of the term the "six confluences (*liu he*)." In this book, we will refer to the yin-yang channel divergence pairings as "confluence pairs."

Over the course of its trajectory through the interior of the body, the yin channel of a confluence pair intersects with its paired yang channel divergence. For its part, the yang channel divergence homes to the network vessels of its related viscus and bowel along with its same-named main channel. In many cases it is the yang channel divergence that connects most directly with the viscera and bowels. However, because the yin channel of a confluence divergence unites with its yang pair, the yin channels are believed to influence and are influenced by the same regions as the yang channel of a confluence pair.

Hence, the channel divergences fulfill an essential role in connecting the main channel pathways with the interior of the body. This function is expressed in a number of ways. The 12 channel divergences enhance the interior-exterior relationships between yin-yang channel pairs. The main channel of the hand *yang ming* large intestine, for instance, is conceptualized as being distinctly more exterior than its pair, the hand *tai yin* lung channel. Nevertheless, one of the ways in which they are united is via the sixth confluence, the large intestine and lung channel divergences. The channel divergences also provide a direct link between the viscera at the core, and the main channels on the exterior of the body. Thus, the interior-exterior relationship is reinforced on both the level of the channels themselves and on the level of the channels and the viscera.

With the exception of the hand *tai yang* channel divergence, all of the other 11 channel divergences spread to the head and face. This enhances the relationship between the 12 main channels and the head and face and helps to explain how acupuncture holes on channels with no direct contact with the face can have an effect there. For instance *Lie Que* (Lu 7) is well known as having a significant influence on the head and particularly the face, yet the trajectory of the main lung channel goes nowhere near this region of the body. This influence can be explained by means of the lung channel's confluence pair relationship with the channel divergence of the large intestine channel which terminates roughly at *Cheng Qi* (St 1). Chapter 4 of the *Ling Shu* (*Divine Pivot*), "On the Disease Presentation of Evil Qi [vis-à-vis] the Viscera & Bowels," states: "The 12 channel vessels, the 365 network vessels, and the qi and blood all ascend to the face and travel to the empty orifices." The existence of an auxiliary system such as the channel divergence system is necessary to make sense of this statement. In addition to the theoretical framework this system of pathways provides for explaining the importance of the acupuncture holes on the face, the channel divergence system also helps us to understand how the distal influences of scalp and face acupuncture[1] and ear acupuncture[2] exert such a profound influence on the rest of the body.

Generally speaking, the trajectories of the 12 channel divergences supplement the trajectories of the 12 main channels. For instance, the acupuncture holes *Cheng Shan* (Bl 57) and *Cheng Jin* (Bl 56) on the urinary bladder channel are known to be empirically effective for treating rectal problems. While the trajectory of the foot *tai yang* urinary bladder channel does not traverse the anus, the trajectory of the foot *tai yang* channel divergence "diverges to enter the anus," thereby explaining the clinical efficacy of the above mentioned holes. Another example involves the trajectory of the foot *shao yin* channel divergence which is understood as "emerging to home to the *dai* vessel." While there is no direct main channel relationship between the kidney channel and *dai* vessel, this channel divergence connection helps explain the intimate relationship of the kidneys to gynecological problems. In addition, the influence of the kidneys in regulating bodily function as a whole is at least partially based on their relationship to the *dai* vessel, the horizontal trajectory of which encircles and regulates all of the other channels in the body.

ON THE RELATIONSHIP OF THE CHANNEL DIVERGENCES TO THE HEART

In the absence of any consistent pattern of relationships regarding the trajectories of the channel divergences as a whole, many commentators have taken the few explicit statements associated with their trajectories and then simply inferred similar relationships for other channels. One such area of inference concerns the trajectory of the channel divergences through the heart. Despite the fact that only five channel divergences are described as doing so, most commentators agree that all of the channel divergences travel through the heart. This assumption is based on the descriptions of the channel divergences' trajectories described in Chapter 11 of the *Divine Pivot*, "On the Channel Divergences". The *Divine Pivot* describes the trajectories of the channel divergences as follows:

> The foot *tai yang* channel divergence "returns to the heart to enter and dissipate there (*dang xin ru san*)."

> The foot *shao yang* channel divergence "ascends to the liver to link with the heart (*shang gan guan xin*)."

> The foot *yang ming* channel divergence "communicates with the heart above (*tong xin yu shang*)."

> The hand *tai yang* channel divergence "enters the axilla and travels to the heart (*ru ye zu xin*)."

> The hand *shao yang* channel divergence "enters the supraclavicular fossa and descends, travelling through the triple burner to dissipate within the chest (*ru que pen xia zu san jiao san yu xiong zhong*)."

4　The Channel Divergences

Some communication with the heart is immediately apparent in the first four statements associated with the channel divergences of the foot *tai yang*, foot *shao yang*, foot *yang ming*, and the hand *tai yang*. In the fifth description concerning the channel divergence of the hand *shao yang*, the phrase, "within the chest," is understood as falling within the scope of the heart as well. Interestingly, it is because of the yin channel divergences' confluence with the trajectories of their yang-paired channels through the interior of the body that all of the yin channel divergences may be understood as connecting with the heart. (See chart 1-A)

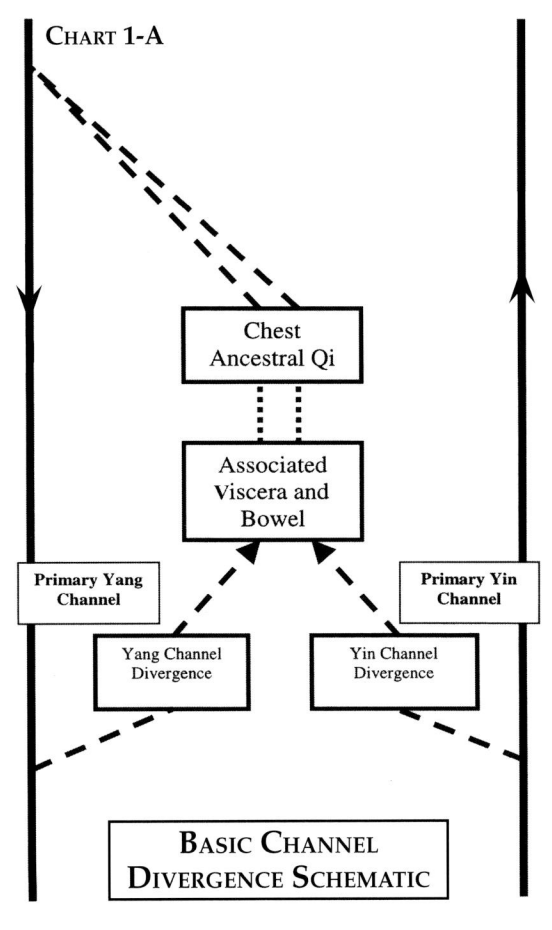

CHART 1-A

Chest Ancestral Qi

Associated Viscera and Bowel

Primary Yang Channel

Primary Yin Channel

Yang Channel Divergence

Yin Channel Divergence

BASIC CHANNEL DIVERGENCE SCHEMATIC

As we delve more deeply into the study of these channels, it becomes clear that the channel divergences clarify some of the more enigmatic issues concerning the Chinese channel and network vessel system. Consider the well known statement from the *Inner Classic* that, "The heart is the sovereign ruler, . . . and is the prime ruler of the five viscera and six bowels." Taken on its own, we might conclude that this is simply a general statement concerning the pervasiveness of the spirit in the human body or something equally as vague. However, if we understand the trajectories of the channel divergences, we begin to see at least one way of how the heart actually exerts its sovereign rule.

The French acupuncture investigator, Jean Marc Kespi, has taken the position that the *Divine Pivot* passages pertaining to the channel divergences do not refer to the heart at all. Rather, they refer to the solar plexus (*coeur solaire*) and the throat (*gorge*). In Kespi's scheme, the foot channel divergences pass through the solar plexus and the hand channel divergences pass through the throat. According to Kespi:

> Each channel divergence diverges from its main channel at a major joint of the extremities (except the hand *Shao Yang*). It then penetrates deep into the trunk where it resonates with all the impact points of the element to which it corresponds and organs to which it belongs. Next, each channel always passes through a channel energy zone, *i.e.*, the "heart" in the case of foot channel divergences and the "throat" in the case of arm divergences.

The "heart" here is not the heart-organ; moreover, the texts specifically state that the "heart-organ" is for the channels that go through it. Here, the "heart" is "solar," which means the center of the "solar plexus." What this means is that all the channel divergences of the foot pass always through the channel energetic zone underneath the diaphragm and then rise to the head. Thus we understand why Nugyen Van Nghi says that all the channel divergences go through the heart except "those of the metal element" (*i.e.*, the hand *Tai Yin* and hand *Yang Ming*). In addition, he says that the foot divergences transit through the "heart-solar plexus" as do the hand *Shao Yin* and *Tai Yang* (center-source of life). He also says that the hand *Jue Yin* and *Shao Yang* resonate at the "heart-organ" and that the hand *Tai Yin* and *Yang Ming* do not respond to one another.

There is no question that the passing (of confluences) through the heart is comparable to "consciousness." In either case, we cannot limit our understanding to the heart-center or to the heart-organ.

The hand channel divergences go through the "throat" which we have already defined as an energetic crossroad located over the clavicles, underneath the maxillary bones, and in front of the cervical vertebrae. The "throat" like the "heart" is, therefore, a channel energetic zone through which the hand channel divergences pass before rising to the head.[3] (See graphic 1-B)

A model wherein the foot channel divergences pass through the heart and the hand channel divergences pass through the throat creates a neat dichotomy but raises more questions than it answers. What are the clinical ramifications of these two "energy zones?" An energy zone in the throat, while potentially formidable, does not necessarily convey the same spirit resonances as that of the heart. In addition, the foot channel divergences clearly pass through the throat "energy center" as well as the heart "energy center." While Kespi's notion of the heart as the solar plexus is innovative, it does little to clarify the fundamental issues concerning the trajectories of the channel divergences through the chest.

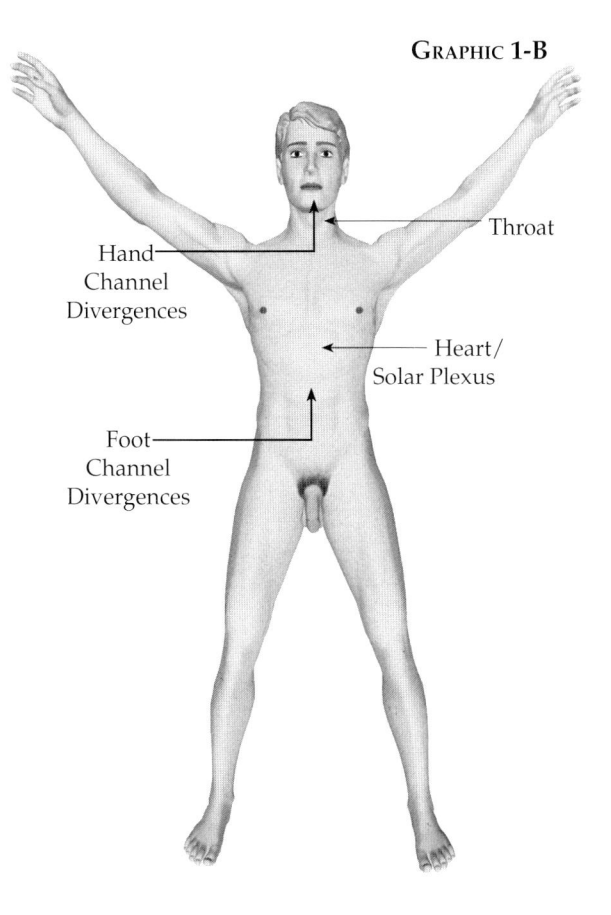

GRAPHIC 1-B

The Channel Divergences
Trajectories

The first differences of opinion in the surviving literature on the channel divergences concern the trajectories of the channel divergences themselves. If there is one thing that is clear when examining these trajectories, it is that the classical Chinese literature leaves much open to interpretation. We need only consider the trajectory of the first channel divergence described in the *Divine Pivot* to appreciate the extent of ambiguity surrounding the trajectories of the channel divergences. The primary foot *tai yang* bladder channel divergence is described as diverging at the popliteal fossa (*guo*). Based on this description, one might think that the channel divergence itself does not exist distal to the popliteal fossa. Indeed, most modern descriptions and illustrations of this channel divergence show it originating at the popliteal fossa. Nevertheless, at least two modern practitioners of channel divergences therapy, Kodo Seki[4] and Tadashi Irie,[5] see the channel divergence as running parallel to the main bladder channel at least as far distal as the source hole, *Jing Gu* (Bl 64). While this may simply be a convenient conceptual tool, it is, nonetheless, a clinical reality insofar as it seems to produce effective therapeutic outcomes. (See chart 1-C)

CHART 1-C

Chest Ancestral Qi

Associated Viscera and Bowel

Primary Yang Channel — Primary Yin Channel

Yang Channel Divergence *Zheng* — Yin Channel Divergence *Zheng*

Divergence *Bie*

UB 40 — Ki 10
UB 58 — Ki 4
UB 64 — Ki 3

Functional Channel Divergence Pathways

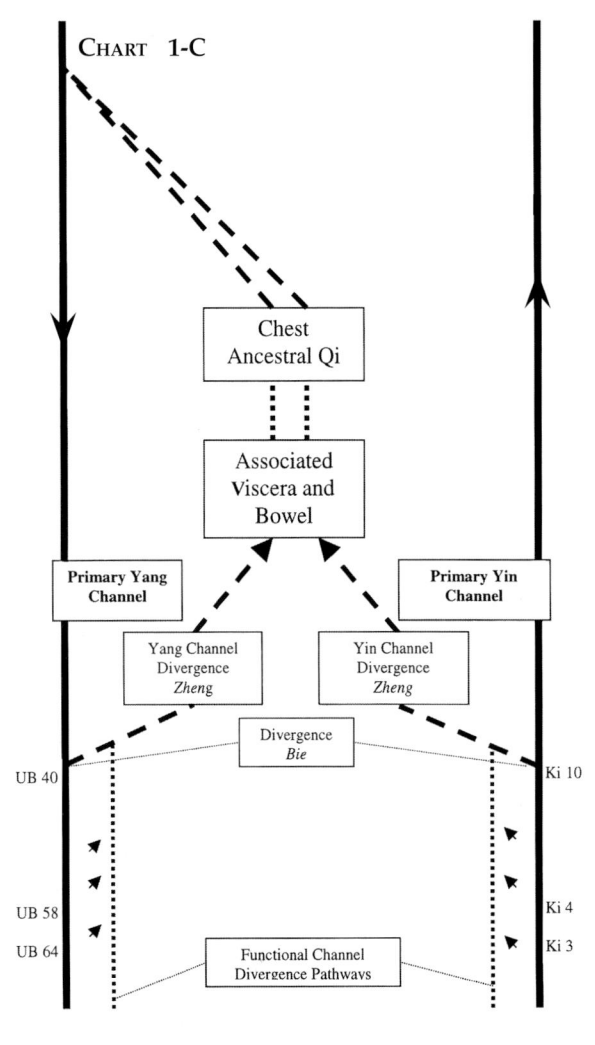

FUNCTIONAL TRAJECTORIES OF THE CHANNEL DIVERGENCES DISTAL TO THEIR POINT OF DIVERGENCE FROM THE MAIN CHANNEL

Regardless of where the channel divergence actually begins, one thing is certain, the trajectories of all channel divergences travel proximally from the extremities. If we assume for the present that qi flows in the direction of the stated trajectories, this means that, on the leg yang channels and hand yin channels, the qi in the channel divergences is moving in a manner contrary to the direction of flow in their associated main channels. This results in the circulation of the channel divergences running roughly in tandem with the circulation of the channel sinews and the network vessels through which defensive (*wei*) qi flows. This makes sense in light of the fact that some sources contend that the defensive qi flows in the channel divergences as well. According to this scheme of things, the defensive qi need only flow in one direction, from distal to proximal, regardless of the depth of its flow.

Another point that is unclear is precisely where on the foot *tai yang* urinary bladder channel the channel divergence actually separates. Most researchers presume that it is at the acupuncture hole *Wei Zhong* (Bl 40). We are, nonetheless, faced with the question of why the authors of the *Divine Pivot* were not more specific. One possible explanation is that the authors wished to imply that the channel divergence separates in the area of the popliteal fossa. This separation may occur at the specific acupuncture hole Bl 40, or it may not. In that case, it is up to the physician to determine the precise location. Similarly, the authors of the *Divine Pivot* are equally vague as to where the majority of the channel divergences terminate. Indeed, the descriptions of the trajectories of virtually all the channel divergences are characterized by their passage through anatomical areas as opposed to specific acupuncture holes.

The *Divine Pivot* states that a direct branch of the urinary bladder channel divergence travels along the paravertebral sinews to emerge at the nape of the neck and then returns home to the *tai yang* channel. The nape of the neck is a relatively large area. However, the most common interpretation is that the nape of the neck specifically means *Tian Zhu* (Bl 10). This is a logical interpretation, since Bl 10 lies on the urinary bladder channel on the nape of the neck. In addition, it is a window of the sky hole, which means that it regulates the circulation of the qi into and out of the head, an influence consistent with our overall understanding of the channel divergences. However, Tadashi Irie believes the confluence hole of the *tai yang* channel divergence is *Da Shu* (Bl 11). This is based largely on this hole's superior clinical effectiveness. This choice of holes has subsequently been adopted by most channel divergences practitioners in Japan. A probable contributing factor leading to Irie's choice of Bl 11 as a master hole is that it is also the meeting hole of the bones, giving it a decidedly kidney water related function. It is also interesting that Bl 11 is a meeting hole of the penetrating vessel (*chong mai*), thus forging a union between the deepest of the channel divergences and the deepest of the extraordinary vessels.

The trajectory of the bladder channel divergence is then described as continuing from the neck to return home to the *tai yang* channel (*fu shu hu tai yang*). There is a general consensus that "returning home" means that this channel divergence terminates at the beginning of the *tai yang* channel, hence at *Jing Ming* (Bl 1). However, this is largely conjecture. Clearly, a certain amount of interpretation is in order if one is to make any clinical use of this information.

8 The Channel Divergences

One of the central issues concerning the channel divergences involves the meaning of two of the key terms used in the description of their trajectories, *zheng* and *bie*. Although there is no definitive consensus on this question, the most common interpretations are outlined below. The most straightforward interpretation is to simply read *zheng* as "primary," ostensibly referring to the primary channel from which the *bie*, channel divergence, diverges or separates. (See chart 1-D) This results in a logically consistent reading, and the renderings of the channel divergence passages translated by Bensky and O'Connor in *Acupuncture, A Comprehensive Text*, and Ni in *Navigating the Channels of Traditional Chinese Medicine* appear to reflect this viewpoint.[6] The modern Chinese acupuncture text, *Zhong Guo Zhen Jiu Da Quan* (*A Comprehensive Encyclopedia of Chinese Acupuncture and Moxibustion*), takes this position as well. This encyclopedia's gloss of the trajectories of the channel divergences reads as follows:

> Once the 12 channel divergences have diverged or exited (*bie chu*) from the primary channel of the same name . . . they travel to enter the interior of the body, ultimately reaching the head and neck where they enter and reunite with the same named yang channel (if it is a yang channel divergence) or its interior exterior pair (if it is a yin channel divergence).[7]

In this interpretation, the "primary" (*zheng*) is the "primary channel of the same name (*tong ming zheng jing*)" or one of the 12 main channels.

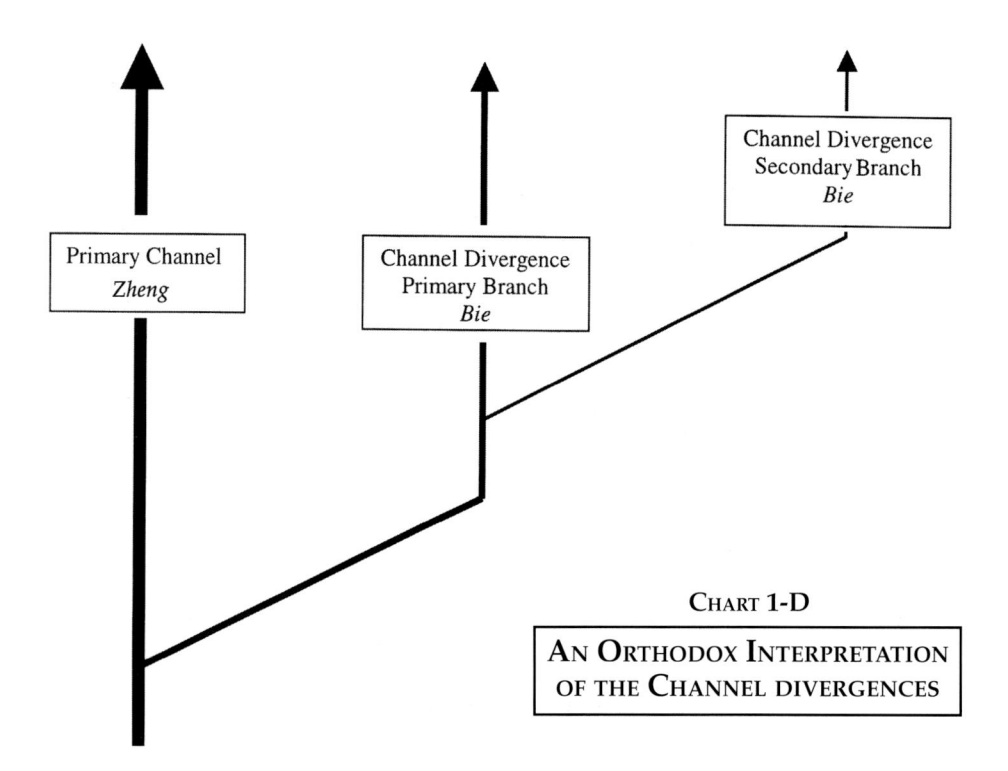

CHART 1-D

AN ORTHODOX INTERPRETATION OF THE CHANNEL DIVERGENCES

Some commentators follow the *Tai Su* (*Great Treatise*) interpretation of the *Inner Classic* and read *zheng* as pertaining specifically to the six yang channel divergences which reunite with their associated yang channels. (See chart 1-E)

> The 12 major channels also have primary and divergent (channels). The primary (channels) mean those divergences from the six major yang channels that travel to unite with their bowel channels. The divergences means those divergences from the six major yin channels that also travel to unite with their associated bowel channels but not with their primary channels. Hence the name "divergent (channels)."[8]

In this sense, the *zheng* are the primary pathways of the channel divergences. The *bie*, on the other hand, pertain to the yin channel divergences that diverge from their associated yin channel but do not reunite with them. While such an interpretation reinforces the supremacy of the yang channel in each pair, it makes little sense when subjected to grammatical scrutiny.

Another interpretation advanced by the eminent Japanese scholar Yasuzo Shibazaki is to read *zheng* as the first or primary branching of the channel divergence from the main channel. In this reading, *zheng* is essentially synonymous with the core trajectory of the channel divergence. Following this interpretation, *bie* has two meanings. First, it may refer to any branching between channels, whether it be

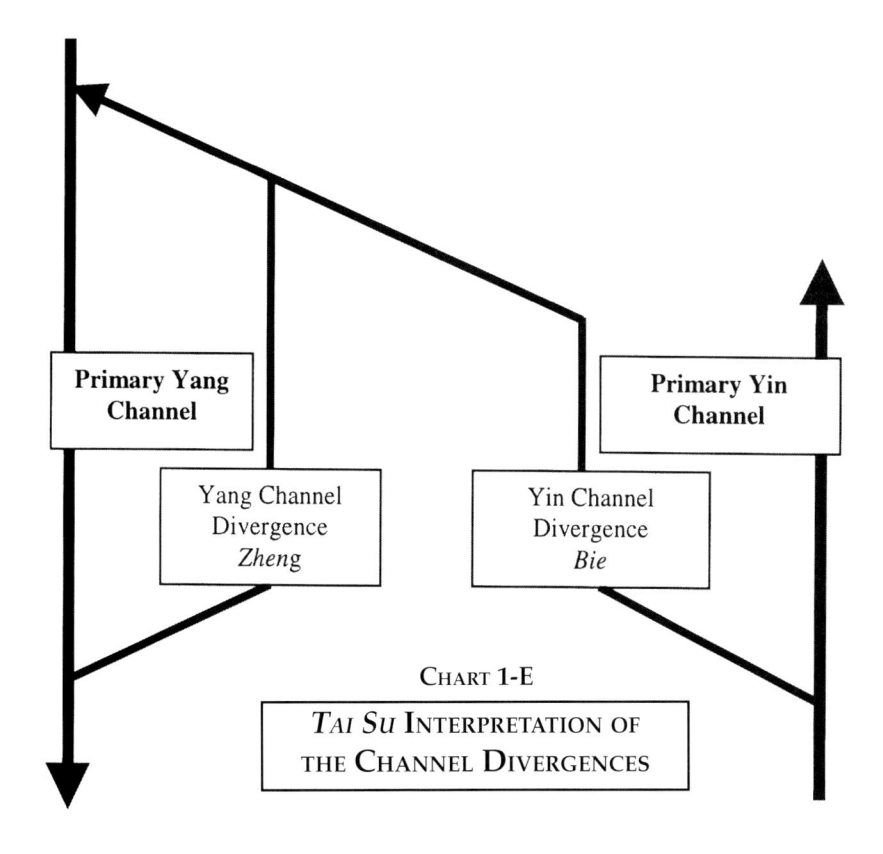

CHART 1-E

TAI SU INTERPRETATION OF THE CHANNEL DIVERGENCES

a *zheng bie*-ing or diverging from the main channel or a secondary facet of the channel divergences system branching off from the *zheng*. Second, these secondary facets of the channel divergences system may themselves be referred to as *bie*.[9,10] In other words, the word *bie* may operate as both a verb and a noun. The Japanese linguist, Akiyasu Todo, is also of the opinion that the syntax of the text supports this interpretation.[11] (See chart 1-F)

To this already bewildering mix of interpretations, Tadashi Irie has added a model of the channel divergences' trajectories that includes tertiary branches connecting each channel divergence to the paravertebral muscles.[12] This model is an extrapolation on his reading of the first confluence which he believes contains three separate branches, one of which connects the divergence to the paravertebrals.[13] In addition, it conforms nicely to Shibazaki's interpretation of the *bie* as secondary divergences. This interpretation was subsequently adopted by Seki. A network of "dendritic" communication between all of the channel divergences and the spine effectively serves to establish a direct link with the governing vessel. Such a link also implies an indirect communication with the *ren* and *chong* vessels, the functional core of the extraordinary vessel system (*qi jing ba mai*).

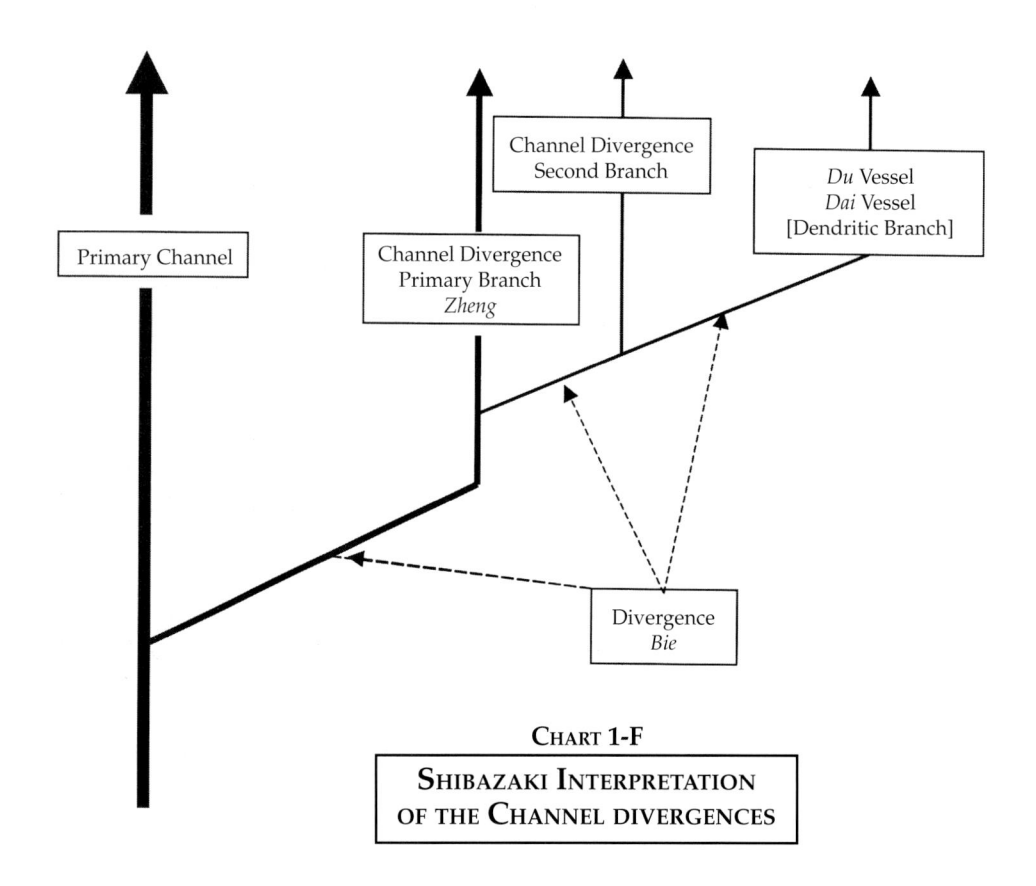

CHART 1-F

SHIBAZAKI INTERPRETATION OF THE CHANNEL DIVERGENCES

The clinical implications for such a relationship between the channel divergences and the extraordinary vessels are profound, and we will explore these further in subsequent chapters. However, regardless of which interpretation one prefers, every investigator who has tried to actually use the channel divergences in clinical practice has artificially imposed some degree of consistency on the channel divergences system. This consistency may be explicitly stated, but, more often than not, it is evidenced only in the uniformity of the treatment strategies each practitioner has developed. All of the other channels and network vessels within the Chinese channel and network system seem to exhibit reasonable consistency in terms of their trajectories. For instance, the trajectories of the main channels begin on the trunk for the hand yin channels and the toes for the foot yin, while the trajectories of the main yang channels begin on the fingers for the hand yang and the head for the foot yang. Furthermore, the channel sinews and the network vessels all begin on the fingers or toes and their qi invariably flows from distal to proximal. Variability such as this is not a problem if the channel divergences are conceptualized as adjunctive channels filling in the therapeutic gaps in the overall structure of the main channels. However, it is clear to the present authors that the channel divergences system is at least potentially much more than this, and, as such, warrants a consistent structure in its trajectories.

Much is left unstated in classical Chinese medical literature, its authors typically assuming a great deal on the part of their readers. It is very likely that the original *Divine Pivot* authors assumed that their readers would base their notions of the channel divergences as a whole on the pattern they established in the first confluence. Following this assumption, one would presume that the channel divergence of the foot *shao yang* gallbladder separates from the main channel at the uniting hole and follows the pathway of the main channel. Thus nothing need be explicitly stated until the channel "curves around the upper thigh and enters the region of the pubic hair where it unites with the *jue yin*." Thus, acupuncturists attempting to understand the channel divergences system have sometimes resorted to applying a characteristic that is clearly described on one of the channel divergences to another channel divergence with a more ambiguous trajectory. In a number of instances, certain characteristics of the channel divergences may be understood as composites derived from the descriptions of the channel divergences taken as a whole. This is particularly the case where the trajectories of the channel divergences traverse the heart. In fact, only five of the 12 channel divergences explicitly contact the heart.

Given the dearth of information regarding the channel divergences, it behooves us to thoroughly explore the material that is available. The terminology used to describe the channel divergences is, perhaps, the most direct means of beginning to understand these pathways. Below we discuss each of the words we believe provides potential insight into the nature of the channel divergences. These terms may be summarized as follows:

Term	Pinyin	Meaning
Primary (channel divergence)	Zheng	The main pathway of the channel divergences
Main (channel)	Jing tong ming	One of the 12 main channels from which the divergences emanate
Direct (branch of the CD)	Zhi	The same as the primary
Enters	Ru	Where the channel divergence plunges deeply, below the major channel, into the body
Strikes	Dang	The channel divergence simply contacts the heart
Contacts	Tong	The channel divergence contacts and flows into the heart
Penetrates	Guan	The strong penetration of the heart
Homes	Shu	The channel divergence travels to its associated viscera or bowel
Communicating	San	Dissipating or diffusing within a specific region

正, *zheng,* derives from an image of an army marching ahead and, therefore, evokes a strong connotation of straightness.[14] Foot *tai yang*'s *zheng* 足太阳之正 is not only the main or primary channel of the *tai yang,* it is any straight or direct facet of the channel system. It is also the main pathway of the channel divergence.

别, *bie,* pictures a knife slicing or severing a joint or bone of an animal. It is appropriate then that the channel divergences often *bie* at large joints or articulations, as in the foot *tai yang* diverging and entering the center of the popliteal fossa 别入于腘中.[15]

直, *zhi,* evokes the strongest sense of straightness, perhaps even more than *zheng*. *Zhi* is not only direct, it is distinctly straight.[19] This character originally represented an eye, evoking a directness of vision and spirit (*shen*). A straight branch of the channel divergence of the foot *tai yang* travels "straight up along the paravertebrals to the nape," 直者从脊上出于项.

当, *dang,* originated as a picture of "matching rice fields" which are packed closely together. *Dang,* therefore, evokes a sense of fitting perfectly. So we have an image of the channel divergences meshing perfectly with the heart and then entering and scattering throughout it, 当心入散. This is in contrast to *zhong,* 中, which evokes a much more aggressive sense of "hitting the center."[18]

属, *shu,* depicts silkworms trying to stick to mulberry leaves. Hence, when a channel "*shu*" to its related viscus or bowel, it is sticking to it as well as simply homing to it, as when the foot *tai yang* sticks to the urinary bladder 属于膀胱.[16]

散, *san,* evokes an image of the scattering of bamboo, as when the channel divergence of the foot *shao yin* scatters throughout the kidneys 散之肾.[17]

Most modern versions of Chapter 11 of the *Divine Pivot* group the passages pertaining to each confluence together into a single paragraph. Below, we discuss most of the channel divergences' trajectories separately and then address them as confluence pairs. However, we will address the fourth and fifth confluences together. Each passage is presented first in the original Chinese and is then rendered into English as literally and with as little interpretation as possible. Our intent is to first present what the Chinese says as opposed to what it might mean. We will then address the interpretative considerations raised by the passage.

Although we have tried to be as rigorous as possible in our examination of Chapter 11, our goal here is not to attempt to present a single philologically definitive translation. It is our position that the true meaning of the text will be ultimately determined by the manner in which it is most effectively applied and not by sifting through linguistic minutiae. Indeed, the only reality the channel divergences are likely to have is as a tool for guiding therapy. Therefore, our discussion focuses on the potential clinical implications of the various interpretations of the text. In light of this, we present an interpretation of the channel divergences' trajectories based on the assumption that all of the channel divergences separate from the main channels at the confluence (*he*)[20] holes at the knees and elbows. We are aware that such an interpretation puts the greatest number of words in the mouths of the authors of Chapter 11 of the *Divine Pivot* and that we are essentially presuming to rewrite the channel divergences' trajectories. Be that as it may, we believe that this interpretation has a sound basis in the text itself. More importantly, Shima has based his approach to channel divergence therapy on the confluence holes, and it is our opinion that a confluence hole interpretation is abundantly supported by the clinical results it yields.[21] Perhaps more than any other layer of the channel and vessel system as a whole, the channel divergence system is only real insofar as it may be effectively applied in clinical practice.

One of the most important questions to clinicians is where the channel divergences actually begin since this has a direct bearing on how they can be accessed. This, in turn, raises the issue of how the word *zheng* is interpreted. While we readily admit to the possibility of other legitimate interpretations, we are of the opinion that *zheng* refers to the channel divergence as opposed to the main channel.

What follows is a translation of the passages dealing with the channel divergences which originally appeared in Chapter 11 of the *Divine Pivot*. This text also appears in the *Zhen Jiu Jia Yi Jing* (*Systematic Classic of Acupuncture & Moxibustion*) in the chapter titled, "On The 12 Channels, Their Network Vessels, Branches, & Divergences." Because many researchers believe that the *Systematic Classic* is ultimately a more reliable text than the various versions of the *Inner Classic* now extant, we have elected to use *the Systematic Classic* as our source for this translation.

14　The Channel Divergences

From Chapter 11 of the *Ling Shu* (*Divine Pivot*)

Ling Shu Introduction
Source Text

黃帝問於岐伯曰　余聞　人之合於天道也、內有五藏、以應五音、五色、五時、五味、五位也　外有六府、以應六律　六律建陰陽諸經、而合之十二月、十二辰、十二節、十二時、十二經水、十二經脈者　此五藏六府之所以應天道

夫十二經脈者、人之所以生、病之所以成、人之所以治、病之所以起、學之所始、工之所止也　麤之所易、上之所難也　請問　其離合出入奈何

岐伯稽首再拜曰　明乎哉問也　此麤之所過、上之所息也　請卒言之

Huang Di inquired of Qi Bo:

I have heard that humankind is in accord with the way of heaven. Thus they have five viscera internally and these correspond to the five notes, five colors, five flavors, five seasons,[22] and five directions.[23] They also have six bowels externally which correspond with the six pitch-pipes.[24] These are analogous to the yin and yang channels[25] and in accordance with the 12 months, 12 *chen*,[26] 12 solar terms of the year,[27] 12 watches,[28] 12 great waters, and the 12 channels. Thus these five viscera and six bowels correspond to the way of heaven.

The 12 channels are responsible for life in humans and the development of illness. They concern the treatment and the origins of a person's illness. They must be studied by the beginner and yet provide the skilled with limitations [they cannot exceed]. The mediocre practitioner finds them easy while the superior practitioner finds them difficult.

[Huang Di inquired:]

Tell me about that which is independent, that which is united, and about the comings and goings of qi between them.

Qi Bo responded:

These [issues] are neglected by the mediocre, while the superior are familiar with them. Please allow me to inform you about them.

Authors' commentary on the text:

The discussion of the channel divergences in the *Divine Pivot* does not immediately begin with a description of their trajectories. Instead, it begins with a discourse on how the cosmos is reflected in the human organism. We are first instructed that heaven has five of this and six of that and that humanity, as an expression of heaven, is no different. This heavenly correspondence extends to the 12 channels which, despite their apparent simplicity, are actually quite difficult to comprehend. Nowhere is this characterization more accurate than in the case of the channel divergences.

At the end of Huang Di's discourse regarding heaven and humanity as expressed in the subtleties of the channel system, he inquires about *li, he, chu,* and *ru*. As we have already seen, these terms are frequently used when describing the trajectories of the channel divergences. It is, therefore, reasonable to assume that Huang Di's request is limited to information pertaining to the separations and confluences, comings and goings of the channels themselves. Most translators therefore render this sentence as: "Tell me about the separations and confluences between the channels and the comings and goings of qi between them."

This is a perfectly serviceable understanding, as far as it goes. However, such a reading ultimately limits the scope of Huang Di's request and ignores the larger context of the discussion. It is equally plausible that Huang Di also wants to know about the places of connection and separation between the channel system and the cosmos. This latter interpretation more fully accounts for Huang Di's initial explanation of the relationship between heaven and humanity. His concern lies not only with the anatomical vagaries of the channel system, but with the larger issue of how that system interacts with the world at large. Thus, we might legitimately read Huang Di's request in the following manner: "Tell me about where the channels and heaven are independent from one another and the cosmos, and where they are united; about the comings and goings of qi between heaven and earth and humanity."

Interpreted in this spirit, this initial preface suggests that what follows might also speak to the question of how the channel system communicates with the cosmos. Given the text that follows, it may indeed be that the channel divergences are presented here as being among the primary conduits for communication of this nature. While so much is left unsaid that it is impossible to make a definitive statement about this one way or another, a great deal is implied in what is explicitly stated. As we will see, the arcane references to pointing to heaven and pointing to earth in the fifth and fourth confluences respectively are more readily understandable when placed in the context of this cosmological preface. From here, Chapter 11 proceeds to a description of the trajectories of the channel divergences.

THE FIRST CONFLUENCE

The primary of the foot *tai yang* diverges and enters the guo. It ascends to a point five cubits below the coccyx where it enters the anus. From there, it homes to the urinary bladder and disperses in the kidneys. It then travels along the paravertebral sinews to hit the heart and disperse into it. The direct ascends along the paravertebral sinews to the nape where it homes to the (foot) tai yang channel. This constitutes a single channel.

16 The Channel Divergences

AUTHORS' COMMENTARY ON THE TEXT:

This first passage concerns itself with the channel divergence of the urinary bladder and is the most elaborate of all the trajectory descriptions of the channel divergences. Nevertheless, it is still relatively opaque. As with all of the channel divergences, it is referred to exclusively by its three yin-three yang designation, thus emphasizing the resonances conveyed by this conceptual framework. It is generally accepted that the *guo* in question is the popliteal fossa. However, a number of questions arise as to just what happens here behind the knee. How can the channel divergence diverge and enter here? Up until this point, it is ostensibly still part of the stream of the main urinary bladder channel. How does its transit of the popliteal fossa differ from the trajectory of the main channel? The answer to this question lies in an understanding of the word *ru* that conveys the meaning of moving deeply. The channel divergence does not simply separate from the main channel laterally. Rather it plunges beneath the main channel in its trajectory up the posterior aspect of the thigh.

If we interpret the *zheng* as the main channel, we would gloss the first sentence in the following manner: "From the main channel of the foot *tai yang*, a divergence enters the popliteal fossa, connecting with the foot *tai yang* urinary bladder channel." For those convinced that the *zheng* is the main channel, this same grammatical interpretation may be applied, to a greater or lesser extent, to most of the channel divergences.

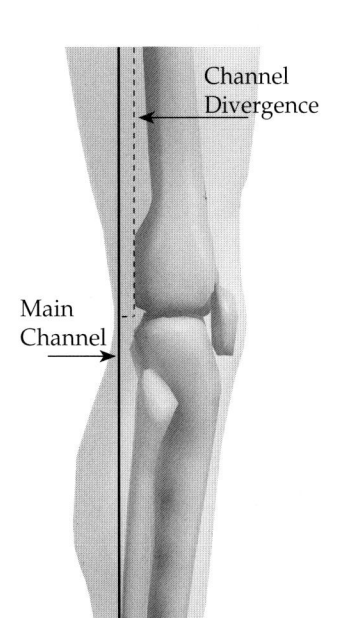

Interpreting *zheng* as the channel divergence, however, we would read the first sentence as: "The primary channel divergence of the foot *tai yang* diverges from the main channel and enters the popliteal fossa, connecting with the foot *tai yang* urinary bladder channel.

FIRST CONFLUENCE
SOURCE TEXT

足太陽之正、別入於膕中 其一道下尻五寸、別入於肛、屬於膀胱、散之腎

循脊當心入散 直者從脊上出於項、復屬於太陽 此為一經也

足少陰之正、至膕中、別走太陽而合、上至腎 當十四椎出屬帶脈 直者繫

舌本、復出於項、合於太陽 此為一合 成以諸陰之別、皆為正也

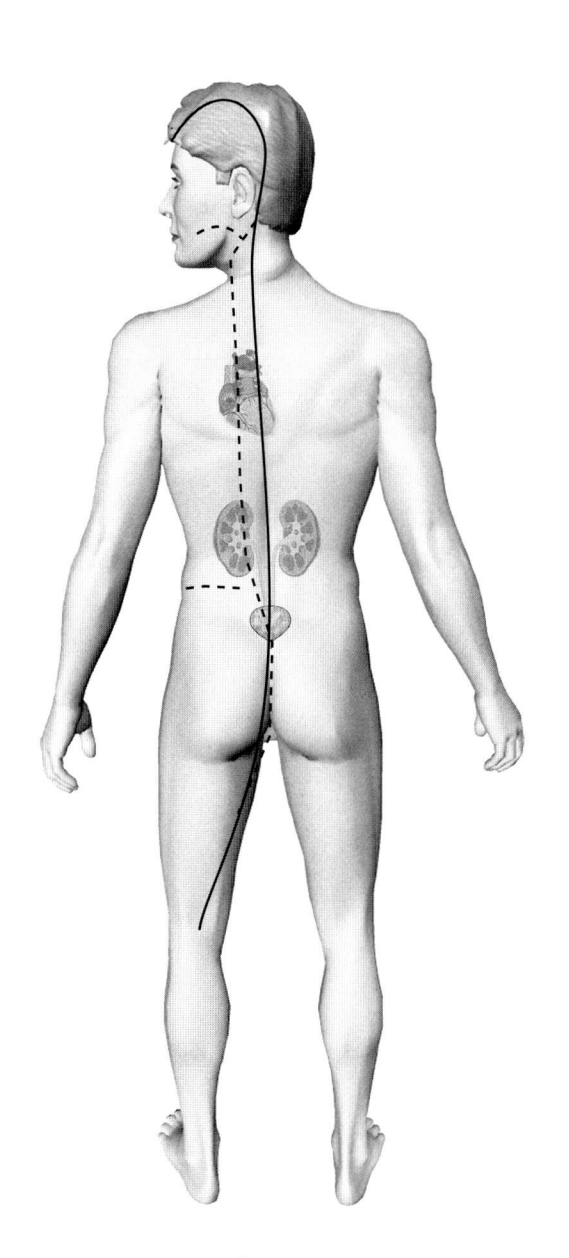

Clearly, all readings of the trajectories for the first confluence support a confluence hole interpretation. This interpretation is predicated, at least in part, on the assumption that the *Divine Pivot* authors explicitly described the trajectories of the first confluence with the intention that its fundamental characteristics be applied to the other confluences whose trajectories are more sketchily described. Tadashi Irie has adopted this same rationale in positing dendritic branches of each channel divergence extending to the paravertebral region in general and the governing vessel in particular.[29]

The *Divine Pivot* authors' use of the word *dang* with respect to the heart, evoking an image of striking, is also of interest. In this context, the trajectory of the channel divergence of the urinary bladder first hits the heart and then dissipates within it. Here is where we first encounter the channel divergence branching with the word *zhi*. The most plausible interpretation is that *zhi* is a direct branch of the channel divergence, and, in this case, it seems fairly clear that the *zhi* is a direct branch that continues along the paravertebrals without venturing into the heart.[30] Finally, we are reassured that the various convolutions of this channel divergence notwithstanding, we are still talking about a single channel.

FIRST CONFLUENCE

The primary of the foot *shao yin* reaches the popliteal fossa where it diverges toward and unites with the *tai yang*. It ascends to the kidneys and, at the 14th vertebra, emerges to home to the *dai* vessel. The direct [branch] links to the root of the tongue and emerges again at the nape of the neck to unite with the foot *tai yang*. This is the first confluence.

18　The Channel Divergences

AUTHORS' COMMENTARY ON THE TEXT:

SECOND CONFLUENCE
SOURCE TEXT

足厥陰之正、別跗上、上至毛際、合於少陽、與別俱行 此爲二合也

足少陽之正、繞髀入毛際、合於厥陰 別者入季脅之間、循胸裏屬膽 散之 上肝 貫心以上挾咽 出頤頷中、散於面、繫系目系 合少陽於外眥也

The first thing we notice about the kidney channel divergence is that once it reaches the popliteal fossa it must travel laterally to unite with the channel divergence of the urinary bladder. Perhaps because the main kidney channel is already travelling relatively deeply, it diverges (*bie*) but does not need to enter (*ru*) to unite with the *tai yang*. While the urinary bladder divergence homes (*shu*) to the urinary bladder viscus, the kidney channel divergence ascends to reach (*zhi*) the kidneys. The kidney channel divergence's emerging (*chu*) to connect with the *dai* vessel suggests that the trajectory of the channel divergence is deep relative to the trajectory of the girdling vessel. Although the two channels communicate at the popliteal fossa, they have separate trajectories. Nevertheless, taken as a pair, these two channels constitute a single confluence. This is in contrast to the various branches of the trajectory of the channel divergence of the urinary bladder alone, which constitutes a single channel.

The kidney channel divergence has a direct branch that does not home to the *dai* vessel, but continues upward from either the kidneys or the 14th vertebrae to link with the root of the tongue.

Finally, the *Systematic Classic* cites the *Jiu Xu* (*Nine Hills*) as saying that the *zheng* refers to any divergence from the yin channels. An interpretation offered by such an early source would seem to carry great weight. Unfortunately, it makes no sense whatsoever, either logically or grammatically.

THE SECOND CONFLUENCE

The primary of the foot *shao yang* curves around the upper thigh and enters the region of the pubic hair where it unites with the *jue yin*. This divergence then enters between the free ribs from where it travels along the inside of the chest and then homes to the gallbladder, dispersing over the liver and penetrating the heart. It ascends passing by the pharynx where it emerges at the jowl and disperses in the face. It links to the eye tie and finally unites with the *shao yang* channel at the outer canthus.

Authors' commentary on the text:

We encounter the first substantial ambiguity regarding where the channel divergence actually begins with the gallbladder channel divergence. The *zheng* of the foot *shao yang* curves around the thigh to enter the pubic region. Since the trajectory of the main gallbladder channel obviously does not follow this course, it is most logical to interpret *zheng* as referring to the channel divergence. Nevertheless, we are still faced with the question of where the channel divergence originated. We do not encounter the word divergence (*bie*) until it enters the ribs, and the channel divergence obviously does not begin here. Thus, the *bie* in question is either a secondary branch or simply clarifying that we are still talking about the channel divergence as opposed to the main channel. Most commentators do not posit a secondary branch at this point. The *bie* is not juxtaposed with a *zhi* or direct branch, and most of the action seems to be occurring along the *bie*. The authors of Chapter 11 tend to mix their use of terms in a rather confusing manner, and, in this case, the *zheng* and the *bie* appear to be one and the same.

Assuming that the *zheng* follows an identical or at least parallel trajectory to that of the main channel, we would read the first sentence as:

The primary channel divergence of the foot *shao yang* follows the pathway of the main channel until it curves around the upper thigh and enters the region of the pubic hair where it unites with the foot *jue yin*.

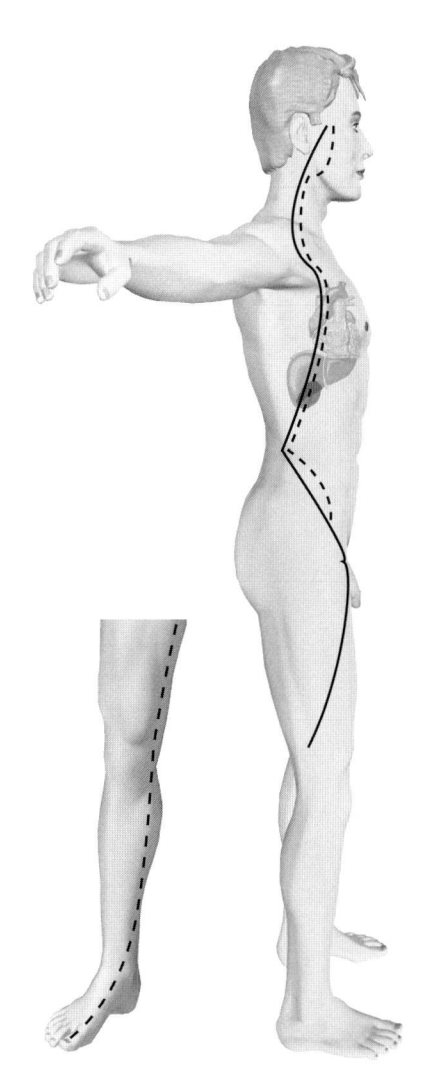

SECOND CONFLUENCE

If the *zheng* is indeed separate from the main channel prior to the thigh then we have to imagine where it might have separated. Our hypothesis, based on the first confluence, is that the separation occurs at the knee. Interpreted in this way, the passage would read as follows

> The primary channel divergence of the foot *shao yang* diverges at the knee and ascends to curve around the upper thigh. From here it enters the region of the pubic hair where it unites with the *jue yin*.

The trajectory of the gallbladder channel divergence does not just contact the heart, it penetrates and transects the heart (*guan xin*). This is a much more potent image than simply striking and dissipating around or communicating with the heart in the case of the urinary bladder. We are left to wonder if the gallbladder's connection with the heart is meant to be more potent than that of the urinary bladder. In light of this, it is interesting to recall that the gallbladder lies opposite the heart in the Chinese clock, thus establishing a potent dynamic between the two.

From the heart, the gallbladder channel divergence ultimately communicates with the eye tie (*mu xi*) and the outer canthus. Wiseman and Ye define the eye tie as something like the optic nerve. They cite the *Divine Pivot* as stating:

> Evils strike the nape of the neck and, encountering vacuity of the body, they enter deeply, following the eye tie to the brain. When they enter the brain, the brain spins. When the brain spins, it causes tension in the eye tie. When the eye tie is tense, the vision of the eye becomes dizzy and spins.[31]

The termination of the second confluence is generally accepted as being *Tong Zi Liao* (GB 1) which is indeed located at the outer canthus.

The primary of the foot *jue yin* diverges from the dorsum of the foot. It ascends to the region of the pubic hair to unite with the *shao yang* and continues its course with the *shao yang*. This is the second confluence.

AUTHORS' COMMENTARY ON THE TEXT:

With the channel divergence of the liver, we see how sketchy the *Divine Pivot*'s descriptions of the trajectories of the yin channel divergences can be. The yin channel divergences are really just tacked on to the trajectories of their yang confluence pairs. In this passage, the *zheng* diverges from either the dorsum of the foot (*fu*) or the knee (*xi*). Most sources assert that it is the dorsum of the foot and that knee is a typographical error. On the other hand, reading it as knee yields a more consistent interpretation overall. This is the only real issue of contention in this passage. Interestingly, Low states that the *zheng* separates from the main channel on the medial aspect of the lower leg, specifically at *Li Gou* (Liv 5), basically splitting the difference.[32] The following interpretation is based on the presumption that the original text is indeed correct and that the channel diverges from the knee.

Confluence hole interpretation:

The primary channel divergence of the foot *jue yin* diverges from the knee. It ascends to the region of the pubic hair to unite with foot *shao yang* and continues its course with the (foot) *shao yang*. This constitutes the second confluence.

The Third Confluence

The primary of the foot *yang ming* ascends to reach the upper thigh, then enters the abdomen. It homes to the stomach, dispersing in the spleen and flowing into the heart above. It proceeds upward, travelling along the pharynx, emerging from the mouth and arriving at the root of the nose and the suborbital region to link with the eye tie and join the *yang ming*.

Authors' commentary on the text:

The stomach channel divergence again presents us with the question of where the channel actually starts. If the *zheng* is indeed the divergence, then it already exists prior to its entry into the abdomen because the passage explicitly states that it ascends to reach the upper thigh. This trajectory ascends to flow into (*tong*) the heart, evoking an image less penetrating than the *guan* of the gallbladder but perhaps more active than the *dang* and *san* occurring in the urinary bladder. Again, the termination of reunion of the divergence with the main channel is assumed to be at its origin at *Cheng Qi* (St 1).

Confluence hole interpretation:

The primary channel divergence of the foot *yang ming* separates from the main channel at the knee and ascends to the upper thigh. It then enters the abdomen and homes to the stomach, dispersing in the spleen and communicating with the

Third Confluence Source Text

足陽明之正、上至髀、入於腹裏、屬胃、散之脾 上通於心、上循咽出於口、上頞頞、還繫目系 合於陽明也

足太陰之正、上至髀、合於陽明、與別俱行、上結於咽、貫舌中 此為三合也

heart above. It proceeds upward, travelling along the pharynx, emerging from the mouth and arriving at the root of the nose and the suborbital region to link with the eye tie and join the main channel of the foot *yang ming*.

THIRD CONFLUENCE YIN CHANNEL

The primary of the foot *tai yin* ascends to reach the upper thigh and unite with the *yang ming*. With its divergence it travels and ascends to bind in the throat and penetrate the root of the tongue. This is the third confluence.

AUTHORS' COMMENTARY ON THE TEXT:

Completing the third confluence, the spleen channel divergence is another channel divergence with only a rudimentary trajectory described by the authors of the *Divine Pivot*. The question of where the channel divergence originates crops up here as well. Another ambiguity is where exactly it reunites with its yang pair. We must assume that the reunion occurs at *Cheng Qi* (St 1).

CONFLUENCE HOLE INTERPRETATION:

The primary channel divergence of the foot *tai yin* diverges from the pathway of the main channel at the knee and ascends to the upper thigh to unite with the (foot) *yang ming*. Travelling together with its paired yang channel it ascends to bind in the throat and penetrates the root of the tongue. This is the third union.

THIRD CONFLUENCE

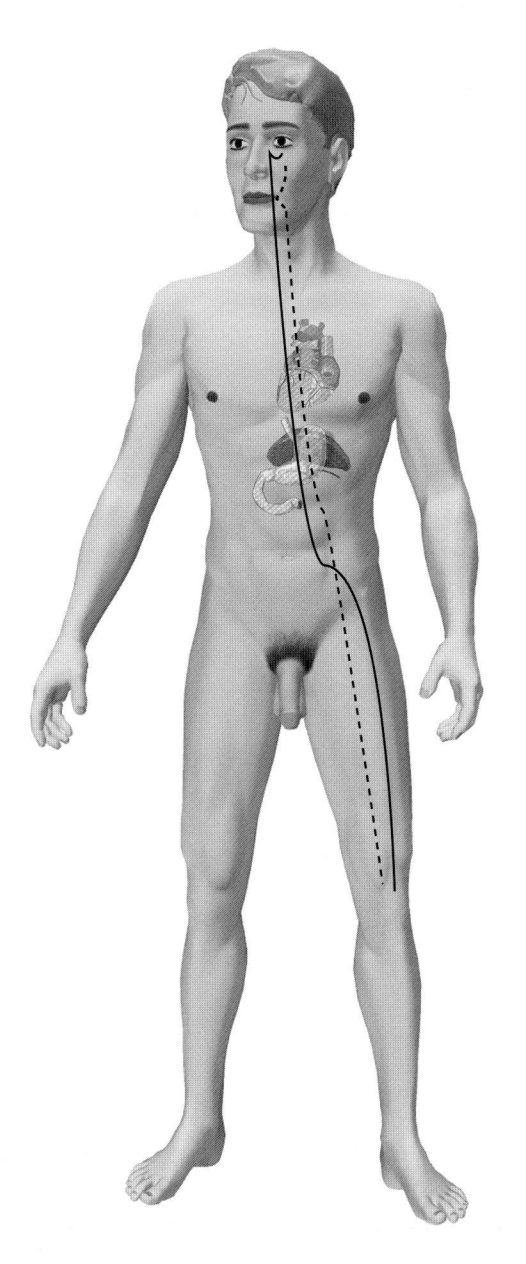

Fourth & Fifth Confluence Source Text

手少陽之正、指天、別於巔、入缺盆、下走三焦、散於胸中也。

手心主之正、別下淵腋三寸、入胸中、別屬三焦、出循喉嚨、出耳後、合少陽完骨之下。此為五合也。

手太陽之正、指地別於肩解、入腋走心、繫小腸也

手少陰之正、別入於淵腋兩筋之間、屬於心 上走喉嚨、出於面、合目內眥

此為四合也

Fourth & Fifth Confluences

The primary of the hand *tai yang* points to the earth. The divergence enters at the shoulder joint. It then enters the axilla and travels to the heart, finally linking with the small intestine.

The primary of the hand *shao yin* diverges to enter the armpit abyss between two sinews. It then homes to the heart and follows the throat upward to emerge at the face and joins the eye at the inner canthus. This constitutes the fourth confluence.

The primary of the hand *shao yang* points to heaven. It diverges at the vertex, entering the supraclavicular fossa, descending through the triple warmer, and dispersing in the chest.

The primary of the hand *jue yin* diverges three *cun* below the axilla. It enters the chest, homing to the triple burner and then coming out to follow the throat. After that, it emerges behind the auricle to join the shao yang below the mastoid bone. This is the fifth confluence.

Authors' commentary on the text:

The fourth and fifth confluences are undoubtedly the most interesting and perplexing of the channel divergences. They are best discussed within the context of one another so we will deal with them together. Given the terse nature of the description of the channel divergences contained in the *Divine Pivot*, it is curious that the words "points to earth (*zhi di*)" and "points to heaven (*zhi tian*)" would appear at the beginning of the discussion of the fourth and fifth confluences respectively. The meaning of these two phrases is unclear, and subsequent commentaries provide only a partial explanation at best. The *Great Treatise* dismisses the reference to earth as a simple directional indicator:

Earth means down. The primary of the hand *tai yang* travels from the hand to the shoulder from where it travels downward to the heart and links with the small intestine such that it points to earth.[33]

The implication here is that the trajectory of this channel divergence points to earth because it runs downward from the shoulder to the heart and small intestine. This explanation is unsatisfying. If the trajectory of the hand *yang ming* channel divergence follows a similar course, then the question remains as to why it is necessary to specifically point out this downward path. What does it mean that the hand *tai yang* descends so precipitously, and what are the clinical implications of such a characteristic?

Zhang Jie-bin provides us with a somewhat expanded explanation to that offered by the *Great Treatise*, the implications of which are profound. Chapter 3 of Volume 7 of the *Lei Jing* (*Categorization of the Classic*), "On the Separations & Unions of the 12 Channels," states:

FOURTH CONFLUENCE

> Points to earth [means that] earth pertains to yin and represents the internal residence of heaven. The hand *tai yang* moves through the vessels internally and diverges at the shoulder separation (*jie*). It enters the axilla and travels to the heart from where it links to the small intestine. Thus, ascending and descending, exteriorization and interiorization occur naturally and, [therefore, this channel] is said to point to earth.[34]

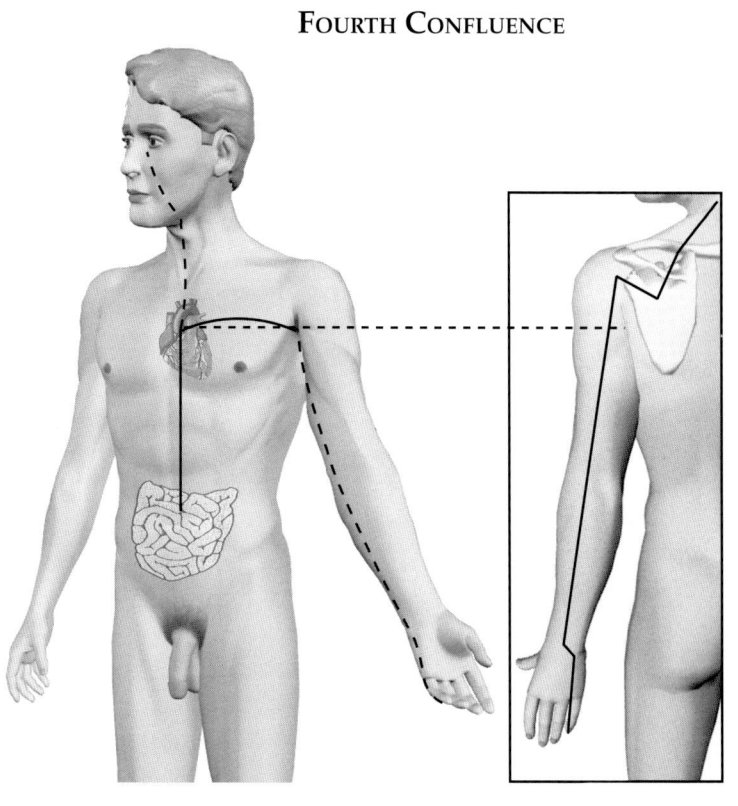

The first thing we are told in the above passage is that earth pertains to yin. Yin, in the context of Zhang's commentary, suggests descent, storage, and internal movement. Zhang's interpretation links the image of downward movement with the internalization of heavenly influence. In addition, it establishes the hand *tai yang* as the central axis for the physiological functions of ascent and descent and the externalization and internalization of qi within the body. Therefore, the channel divergence of the hand *tai yang* may be understood as being involved in the transmission of heavenly qi inward to the heart where it is known to reside. As the yang channel of the confluence pair, it is actively involved in this process, whereas the hand *shao yin* channel of the confluence pair may be understood as representing the receptive aspect of the same basic process.

The concept of pointing to earth cannot be understood outside of the context of its correlated idea that appears in the passage describing the trajectories of the fifth confluence. By contrast, the overall function of the fourth confluence is much more earthly or yin than the heavenly fifth confluence. They are clearly linked in some way, even in the most superficial interpretation of their meaning, and their relationship to one another may shed some light on the larger issue of how the channel divergence system functions as a whole. The *Categorization of the Classic* states:

Points to heaven [means that] heaven pertains to yang and the movement outward to earth. "The primary of the hand *shao yang* ascends to diverge at the vertex. From there it enters the empty basin (*que pen*) and descends to travel to the triple burner and dissipate in the chest. It then outwardly envelops the viscera and bowels and so it is said to point to heaven."[35]

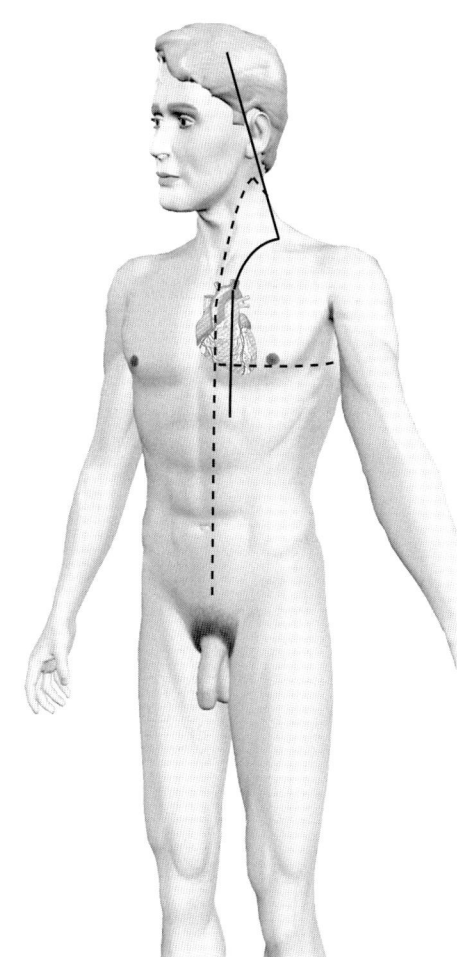

In his initial statement on the matter, Zhang equates the initial ascending trajectory of this channel divergence toward the vertex as pointing to heaven. However, the overall movement of the trajectory of the hand *shao yang* channel divergence is decidedly downward. At this juncture a closer look at the word *zhi* is in order. Most English language translations render the phrases *zhi di* and *zhi tian* as "points to earth" and "points to heaven" respectively. In reading *zhi* as "points toward," we assume that the channels themselves are pointing in the direction of either heaven or earth as the case may be. While such a reading is certainly justifiable, it imposes some limitations on how we may understand this phrase and its meaning within the larger context of the channel divergences.

Most literally, a *zhi* is a finger and, by extension, a pointer, indicator, or referent. It may also be used as a verb meaning to depend on or to count on. Thus, when we say points

FIFTH CONFLUENCE

to heaven or earth, we also mean refers to heaven or earth and, potentially even, depends on heaven or earth. It is not too great a stretch to say that the primary of the hand *shao yang* "evokes" heaven. Understood from this perspective, *zhi tian* is less about the longitudinal relationship between the hand *shao yang* and heaven, than it is about the capacity of the hand *shao yang* triple burner to spread and exteriorize the heavenly influence. This is essentially a yang function. Conversely, *zhi di* refers to the capacity of the hand *tai yang* to guide the heavenly influence inward from the exterior where it may reside in the heart. This capacity for storage and inward movement is a yin function. Earth is evoked as the quiescent and material counterpoint to the more active and diffuse nature of heaven.

The relationships implicit in the above interpretation are further clarified when we remember that each of the yin-yang confluence pairs forms a single functional channel. The primary of the hand *tai yang* small intestine cannot be understood outside of the functions of the hand *shao yin* heart channel. The characteristics of the two channels are interwoven in the channel divergence pairing, and this is why such pairings are referred to as confluences.

Although it is the hand *tai yang* channel divergence that is explicitly said to evoke earth, it does so in its capacity as a yang channel for active engagement. At least according to Zhang, the ultimate locus for the interiorization is the heart sovereign. The same relationship holds true for the hand *shao yang* triple burner channel and the hand *jue yin* pericardium channel. The triple burner is the active expression of the function of the heart master which, in turn, does the actual work of the heart. Thus we have an earthly evocation of the fourth confluence conveying heavenly influence inward to the heart for storage. The fifth confluence represents a more celestial evocation disseminating this heavenly influence in a much more general way into the chest and then outward throughout the body via the triple burner. Regardless of whether we are pointing to heaven or earth, it is a heavenly influence that is being called upon. The question again arises as to how and from where such an influence is being propagated.

The yang channel of the fifth confluence pair is undeniably the oddest of all the channel divergences, beginning as it does from the vertex. It quite literally originates beyond the terminus of the hand *shao yang* channel at *Si Zhu Kong* (TB 23), and, as such, the hand *shao yang* channel divergence is the only channel divergence trajectory that is truly separate from its associated principle channel. The proximity of the terminus of the triple burner channel to *Bai Hui* (GV 20) notwithstanding, no connection between these two holes is recognized in the source literature.

In light of Huang Di's introductory preface, we posit that the most plausible interpretation of the hand *shao yang* triple burner channel is that it establishes a link between external heavenly influences and the triple burner as a whole, including the ancestral (*zong*) qi in the chest. Where the yang channel of the pair communicates first with the triple burner and then dissipates into the chest, the yin channel

CENTRIFUGAL TRANSMISSION OF ORIGINAL YANG VIA THE CHANNEL DIVERGENCES

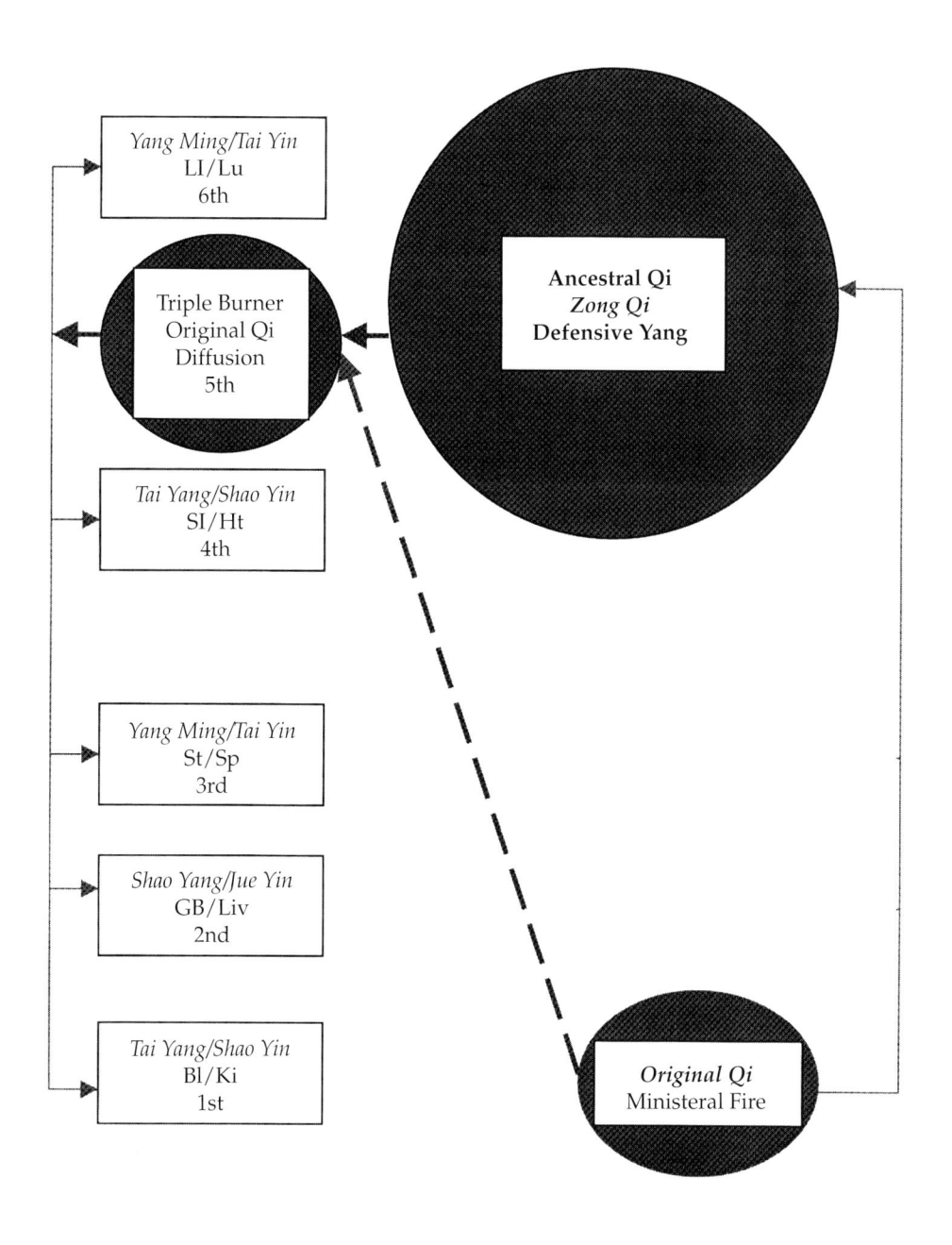

Yang Ming/Tai Yin
LI/Lu
6th

Triple Burner
Original Qi
Diffusion
5th

Ancestral Qi
Zong Qi
Defensive Yang

Tai Yang/Shao Yin
SI/Ht
4th

Yang Ming/Tai Yin
St/Sp
3rd

Shao Yang/Jue Yin
GB/Liv
2nd

Tai Yang/Shao Yin
Bl/Ki
1st

Original Qi
Ministeral Fire

Centripetal Transmission of Heavenly Yang via the Channel Divergences

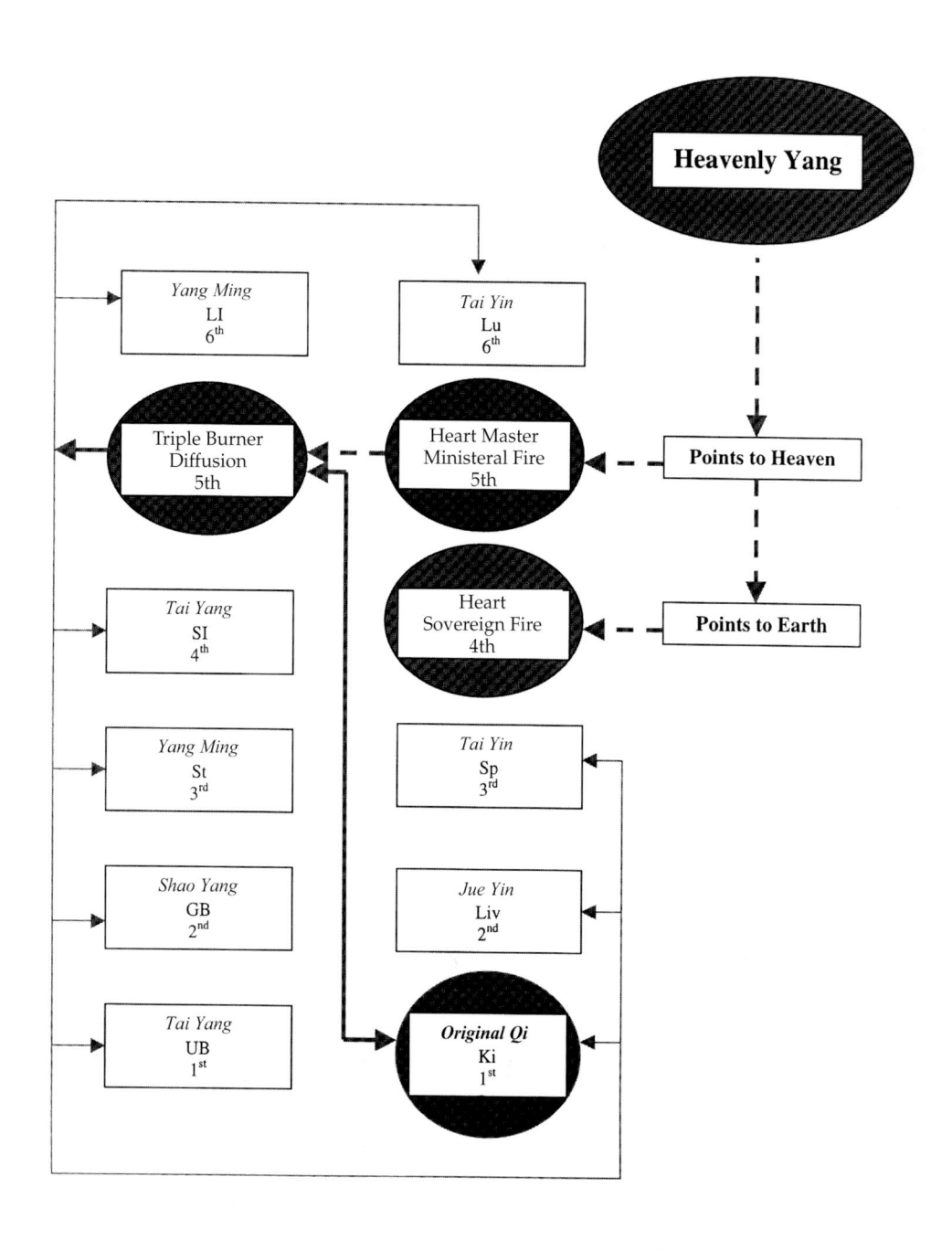

	Yang Ming LI 6th	*Tai Yin* Lu 6th
	Triple Burner Diffusion 5th	Heart Master Ministeral Fire 5th
	Tai Yang SI 4th	Heart Sovereign Fire 4th
	Yang Ming St 3rd	*Tai Yin* Sp 3rd
	Shao Yang GB 2nd	*Jue Yin* Liv 2nd
	Tai Yang UB 1st	*Original Qi* Ki 1st

Heavenly Yang → Points to Heaven → Points to Earth

of the fifth confluence pair enters first directly into the chest and then communicates with the triple burner. This yin-yang confluence pair is clearly central to the communication between the qi of the chest and the functions of the triple burner. Within the context of the overall channel system, the fifth confluence is a central link between the body as a whole and the influence of heaven. Understood in this way, it is no wonder that the fifth confluence originates at the vertex where it can most readily absorb macrocosmic influences and that it is said to "evoke heaven."

Assigning to the channel divergences a role as conduit for heavenly resonance also helps to explain why the channel divergences are conceptualized as "confluences," an issue we will address in the next chapter. In light of this, we may understand the channel divergences as the primary pathways by which a heavenly resonance is transmitted to the viscera, heart, and triple burner in the otherwise closed circulation of the main channels.

Anatomically, Armpit Abyss is generally understood to be *Yuan Ye* (GB 22). The two sinews are the pectoralis muscle anteriorly and the latissimus dorsi posteriorly. Since the heart is the source viscus of this channel divergence, it is not surprising that it homes (*shu*) to the heart. This connection is not simply one of passing through but of returning. It is interesting that this channel divergence does not specifically unite with its paired yang channel but with the eye. This direct connection between the heart and the eye is why the spirit light (*shen ming*) is manifest in the eye.

The termination of the fourth confluence at the inner canthus is most likely *Jing Ming* (Bl 1). However, the end point of the fifth confluence is less clear. Some commentators are content to leave the emergence of the fifth confluence below the mastoid bone vague. Tadashi Irie, however specifies its emergence at the suitably named "completion bone," *Wan Gu* (GB 12), not on the paired hand *shao yang* channel, but on the foot *shao yang* channel. The reasoning for this choice is apparently entirely empirical.

CONFLUENCE HOLE INTERPRETATION:

The primary of the hand *shao yin* diverges from the pathway of the main channel at the elbow to enter Armpit Abyss between two sinews. It then homes to the heart and follows the throat upward to emerge at the face and joins the eye at the inner canthus. This constitutes the fourth confluence.

The primary channel divergence of the hand *shao yang* points to heaven. One branch communicates with the vertex, another divergent branch separates at the elbow and enters the supraclavicular fossa to descend through the triple burner and dissipate in the chest.

The primary channel divergence of the hand heart–governor diverges from the main channel at the elbow and travels to an area three *cun* below the axilla

Sixth Confluence Source Text

手陽明之正、從手循膺乳、別於肩髃、入柱骨、下走大腸、屬於肺、上循喉嚨、出缺盆、合於陽明也

手太陰之正、別入淵腋少陰之前、入走肺、散之大腸、上出缺盆、循喉嚨、復合陽明　此六合也

where it enters the chest. From here it, homes to the triple burner and then emerges to travel to the throat. After that, it emerges again behind the auricle to join the (hand) *shao yang* below the mastoid bone. This is the fifth confluence.

The Sixth Confluence

The primary of the hand *yang ming* travels from the hand to the breast. A divergence at the shoulder joint enters the neck bone. From here it descends to the large intestine, homing to the lungs. It then ascends and travels toward the throat to emerge at the supraclavicular fossa to unite with the *yang ming*.

Authors' commentary on the text:

Its rather convoluted trajectory notwithstanding, the yang facet of the sixth confluence presents us with only a few interpretive problems. The "shoulder joint" is a fairly large area, and the precise location of the "neck bone" is rather obscure. Most interpreters posit that the neck bone is the spine at the nape of the neck. It is worth noting, however, that its only proximity to the heart is via the lung in its trajectory through the chest.

Confluence hole interpretation:

The primary of the hand *yang ming* travels from the hand to the breast, diverging from the main channel at the elbow. The primary parallels the main channel until a secondary divergence at the shoulder joint descends to enter the neck bone. From here it descends to the large intestine, homing to the lungs. It then ascends and travels toward the throat to emerge at the supraclavicular fossa to reunite with the *yang ming*.

Sixth Confluence Yin Channel

The primary of the hand *tai yin* diverges to enter the armpit abyss in front of the *shao yin*, travelling to enter the lungs, and disperses in the large intestine. A branch emerges at the supraclavicular fossa and then follows the throat to reunite with the *yang ming*. This constitutes the sixth confluence.

AUTHORS' COMMENTARY ON THE TEXT:

The lung channel divergence has a straightforward trajectory that sports an unambiguous secondary branch that is central to its confluence with the channel divergence of the large intestine. Although *que pen* is an anatomical region as well as the name of an acupuncture hole, the emergence of the sixth confluence is generally thought to occur specifically at *Que Pen* (St 12).

CONFLUENCE HOLE INTERPRETATION:

The primary (channel divergence) of the hand *tai yin* diverges from the main channel at the elbow and ascends to enter the Armpit Abyss (*i.e.*, the area of *Yuan Ye*, GB 22). It travels in front of the (hand) *shao yin* to enter the lungs and disperses in the large intestine. It emerges at the supraclavicular fossa and then follows the throat to join the (hand) *yang ming*. This is the sixth confluence.

CHANNELS, WHAT CHANNELS?

From the discussions above, it should now be apparent to the reader that the classical Chi-

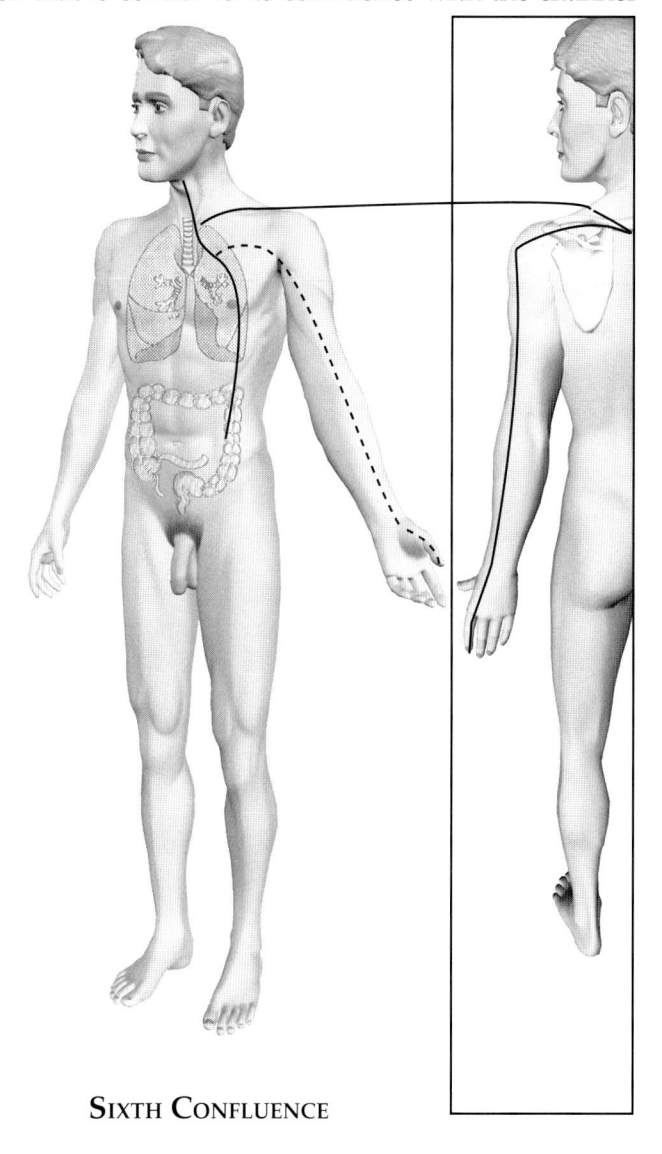

SIXTH CONFLUENCE

nese source materials on the channel divergences offer little in the way of concrete clinically useful information concerning these pathways. It has been our experience that the more we study the source literature on the channel divergences, the less we know with any certainty. In fact, this may be the greatest lesson the channel divergences have to offer modern students of acupuncture. The enigmatic nature of the channel divergences prompts us to question both our conscious and unconscious assumptions concerning the Chinese channel system as a whole. What were the authors of the *Inner Classic* actually trying to convey in their use of

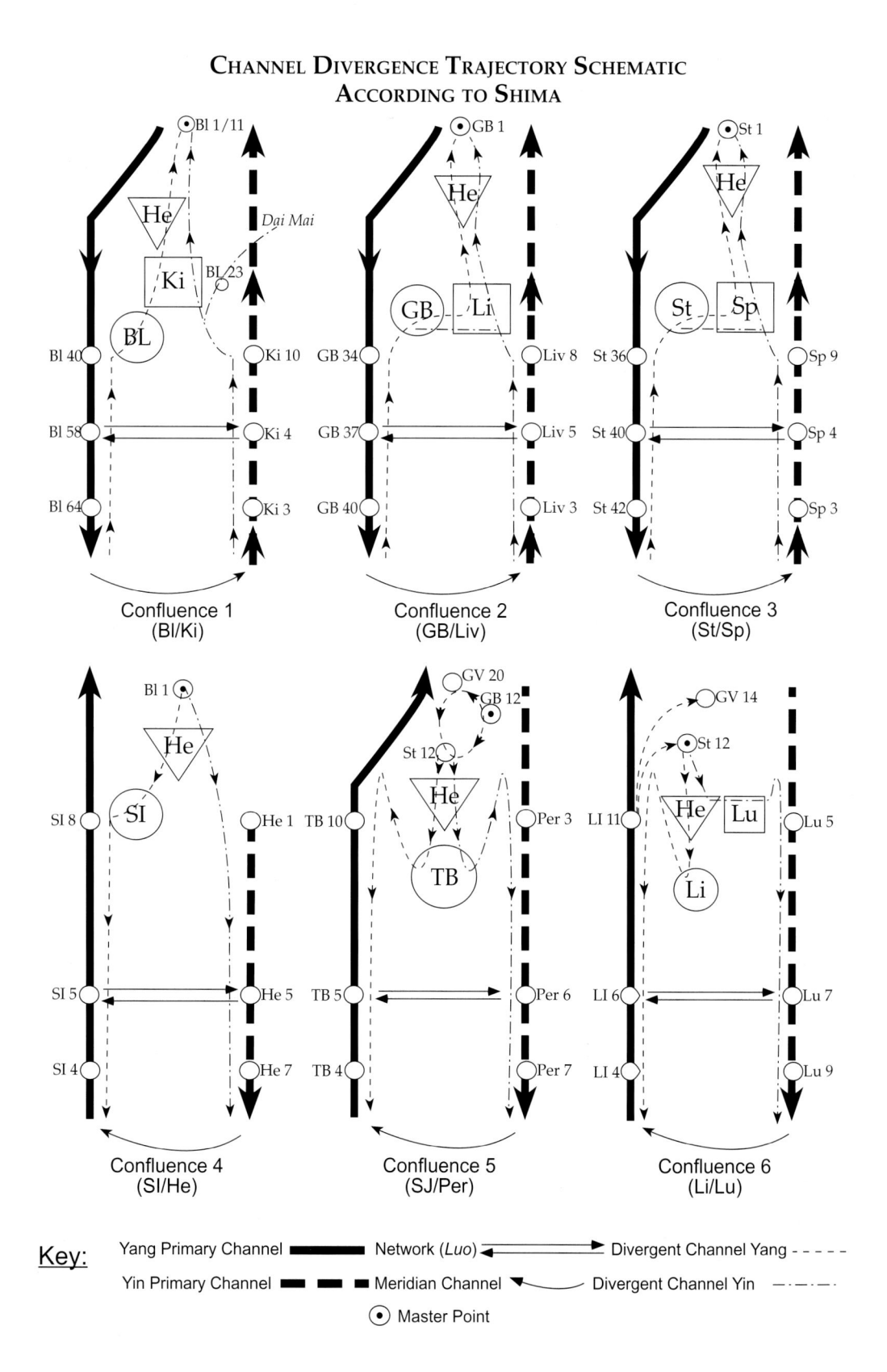

32　The Channel Divergences

CHANNEL DIVERGENCE TRAJECTORY SCHEMATIC ACCORDING TO SHIMA

Confluence 1 (Bl/Ki)

Confluence 2 (GB/Liv)

Confluence 3 (St/Sp)

Confluence 4 (SI/He)

Confluence 5 (SJ/Per)

Confluence 6 (LI/Lu)

Key:
- Yang Primary Channel ▬▬▬
- Network (*Luo*) ◄────►
- Divergent Channel Yang - - - -
- Yin Primary Channel ▬ ▬ ▬
- Meridian Channel
- Divergent Channel Yin —·—·—
- ⊙ Master Point

the word qi and their descriptions of the channels and network vessels? Are the channel divergences essentially a theoretical postscript, and, if so, what does that imply with regard to the rest of the channels?

Even when reading the *Inner Classic* in the original Chinese, most of us inevitably approach the text with a host of preconceptions about this material based on our experience living in the modern world. For instance, a simple convention such as translating the term qi as energy sets us up for a myriad of unconscious assumptions regarding the channel system that its original developers did not hold. This point is central to any understanding of the qi and/or the channel system. In the most practical sense, the channels *are* qi; they are not simply the structures that qi flows through. Despite the most rigorous scientific efforts to identify a physiological referent for the channels, none has been found, and yet acupuncturists manipulate the channels every day. How is this possible? Most acupuncturists would probably answer that they determine the location of a channel or an acupuncture hole on a channel by determining where the qi is or is not. Thus, it is fair to assert that the channels themselves are defined by the presence or absence of qi.[36]

Because there is no satisfactory English translation of the Chinese word qi, we are compelled to talk about it in a variety of ways. We may discuss the fact that it expresses itself in terms of measurable physiological influences in the body.[37] Indeed, most people who experience qi, experience it very concretely. It is the sensation that runs up our arm when we contact an acupuncture hole or runs through our bodies when we do *tai ji quan*. Qi is also snow. Qi is bamboo. These are tangible things. But then too, the rhythm or cadence of a well-crafted poem is also referred to as the qi pulse (*qi yun*). Whatever it is, qi is not just energy. Thus, we are forced to evoke qi in a more abstract manner in an attempt to unite these disparate experiences.

Unschuld's translation of qi as "influence" is much more evocative of the range of meaning Chinese have traditionally associated with the word qi.[8] In their effort to present a comprehensive definition of qi, Birch and Felt talk about it as a dynamic.

> Qi is not in essence a thing, an entity; it is a dynamic. It is associated with movement and process.[39]

While a process-oriented, information-based dynamic such as this does not exclude an energetic or even a materialistic understanding of qi, it compels us to think of qi in much broader terms than as some as yet undefined "stuff" flowing through the body. Nevertheless, we must understand that qi is not just an abstract concept either. All of these descriptions are approximations. The best we can do is to say "qi is like this."

It is extremely difficult to shed our own intellectual baggage in attempting to approach a text such as the *Inner Classic* on its own terms and in the context of the worldview in which it was written. No one really knows how the Chinese mind worked 2,400 years ago, but it is safe to say that the fundamental approach to truth and knowing during the formative stages of the *Inner Classic* in the Han dynasty differed significantly from our modern notions of epistemology. A rudimentary exploration of the Han worldview provides us with a useful basis for interpreting the channel system in as close to its original context as we can hope to achieve today. Before one can begin to extrapolate, it is best to know from what one is extrapolating.

The modern philosopher Zhang Dong-sun has identified three distinguishing characteristics of classical Chinese epistemology:

1. Each relationship within a pair is bidirectional. In other words, each partner in a relationship influences the other. Thus, relationships are intricate and complex, and each member of the relationship is different after the relationship has been established and changes with it.

2. All relationships are mediated by layer after layer of intervening experience rather than being unmediated and direct.

3. Knowledge is always a kind of interpretation rather than a copy or representation.[40]

Clearly, these characteristics suggest that those writing during this period tended to privilege information not on the basis of what something is but on how to interact with it. This is contrasted with the modern approach to knowing which now dominates scientific inquiry. Zhang explains:

> In putting a question about anything, it is characteristic of Western mentality to ask "What is it" and then, later, "How should one react to it?" The Chinese mentality does not emphasize the "what" but rather the "how." Western thought is characterized by the "what priority attitude," Chinese by the "how priority attitude."[41]

Such a "how priority" worldview definitely extends to the literature that provides the core philosophical framework for the *Inner Classic*.

> The *Daodejing* does not purport to provide an adequate and compelling description of what *dao* and *de* might mean as an ontological explanation for the world around us; rather it seeks to engage us and to provide guidance in how we ought to interact with the phenomena, human and otherwise, that give us context in the world. "Knowing," then, in classical China is not a knowing what that provides some understanding of the environing conditions of the natural world, but is rather a knowing how to be adept in relationships, and how, in optimizing the possibilities that these relations provide, to develop trust in their viability.[42]

This perspective is by no means limited to the Daoist cannon. Hall and Ames describe the Confucian approach to knowing (*zhi*) in the following manner:

> *Chi* (*zhi*) is a process of articulating and determining the world rather than a passive cognizance of a predetermined reality. To *chi* (*zhi*) is to influence the process of existence within a range of one's viable possibilities.[43]

This worldview is inevitably embedded in the structure of the Chinese language. Classical Chinese is, by its very nature, rather vague by comparison to modern English. Most Chinese sentences are not propositions at all, and propositions are required for expressing semantic or propositional truth.[44] Indeed, Chad Hansen has argued that the Chinese had no concept of truth as we think of it today. According to Hansen, a pragmatic interpretation of classical Chinese provides a more coherent understanding of textual material than a semantic or truth-based approach to interpretation.[45]

The implications of these philosophical and linguistic characteristics for our understanding of the classical Chinese medical literature are profound. We are left with the realization that, in all likelihood, the authors of the *Inner Classic* were less concerned with imparting knowledge of what the channel system is than with how to interact with it. The information in question cannot be understood from the standpoint of purely passive observation. Zhuang-zi provides us with one of the seminal statements on early Chinese epistemology that speaks directly to this point.

> Zhuang-zi and Hui-zi were strolling across the bridge over the Hao River. Zhuang-zi observed, "The minnows swim out and about as they please. This is the way they enjoy themselves."
>
> Hui-zi replied, "You are not a fish. How do you know what they enjoy?"[46]
>
> Zhuang-zi returned, "You are not a fish. How do you know what they enjoy?"
>
> Hui-zi said, "I am not you. So I certainly don't know what you know. But it follows that, since you are certainly not a fish, you don't know what is enjoyment for the fish either."
>
> Zhuang-zi said, "Let's get back to your basic question. When you asked, 'How do you know what the fish enjoy?' you already knew that I know what the fish enjoy or you wouldn't have asked me. I know it from here on the Hao River."[47]

The modern sinologist Roger Ames interprets this passage in the following manner:

> Knowledge is always proximate as the condition of an experience rather than of an isolated experiencer. Situation has primacy, and agency is an abstraction from it. Knowledge is a tracing out and mapping of the productive patterns (里, *li*) of one's environs in such a manner as to move efficaciously and without obstruction.[48]

It is because Zhuangzi is continuous with his surrounds that "knowledge" of the situation emerges, where the fishes are no less entailed in the realization of the happy experience between Zhuangzi and Huizi. It is the situation rather than some discrete agent that is properly described (and prescribed) as happy. The event is realized in the doing of it. And language both articulates (*ming*) and commands into being (*ming*) the relationships that constitute Zhuangzi in his world.[49]

Zhuang-zi and Hui-zi could just as easily have been talking about the channels and network vessels, for they are no less a part of our experienced reality than the fish in the Hao River. It is likely that, for the authors of the *Divine Pivot*, their understanding of the channels was entirely contingent upon their interaction with them. Because they had little interest in semantic concepts of truth, it would not have occurred to them that the channels are something "out there" that we have to learn to perceive. Everything we know about classical Chinese thought suggests that their minds simply did not work this way. Such a perspective certainly changed over time, but, according to sinologists such as Ames, Hall, and Zhang Dong-sun, this was the worldview when the *Inner Classic* was compiled. We are left with the impression that any existence the channels have is predicated upon our direct interacting with them. Again, it is Zhuang-zi who articulates this so beautifully.

> A path becomes a path by people walking it.
> A thing being called something becomes it.
> Why is it so?
> It is because it is so.
> Why is it not something other than what it is?
> It is because it is not.[50]

Of course, the reason we walk a path such as this is that it might lead us somewhere useful. Similarly, the channel system evolved as a vehicle for meaningful intervention in alleviating suffering. As we have said, the compilers of the *Inner Classic* were primarily concerned with efficacy. If it worked, then it was real.[5]

The descriptions of the channel trajectories in the *Inner Classic* may not propose to map discrete entities that are unobservable by modern science, so much as they simply provide a context for interacting with the body in a meaningful way. Birch and Felt argue that the channel system may be best understood as conceptual tools framed in the context of an information system.

> To understand acupuncture, qi can be thought of as the observable results of the body's information exchange mechanisms. The plural is important. Although a capitalized Qi can be proposed through the idea of a universal stratum, in the human body information exchange occurs by a variety of mechanisms. Thus the idea of a multi-dimensional array of communications paths that are influenced by the physical and energetic universe gives us a very useful tool for thinking about our relationship to the environment.[52]

A perspective such as this is particularly germane to the channel divergences. The channel divergences are well understood as a facet of the body's information exchange mechanism. As we have already said, we are not asserting that either qi or the channel system is just an idea. As clinicians, we experience both qi and the channels as concrete things every day. However, from the standpoint of clinical practice, it may be more productive to focus our understanding on how we can most efficaciously manipulate this experience rather than overly concerning ourselves with what it is in any physical sense. Modern research may or may not ever identify a scientifically reproducible material basis for the channel system, although such a discovery would undoubtedly increase the scope of clinical tools available to acupuncturists and increase its efficacy as a treatment modality. It would be a mistake, however, to entirely abandon the original how-priority understanding of the channels in favor of a purely biophysical model of acupuncture phenomena. Doing so would unnecessarily limit the potential of the channel system as a means of influencing positive change within the body.

The *Inner Classic* is by no means homogenous in its vision of medical practice. It is clear that the various schools of thought represented in the *Inner Classic* each had a specific idea in mind despite the fact that these ideas may, at times, be at odds with one another. It becomes much easier to reconcile these contradictions if we view them from the perspective of this "how priority attitude," the foremost concern of which was the manipulation of the conceptual tools that got the job done.

Despite the fact that the majority of the channel divergence therapies we will discuss in the present work were developed in the past 50 years, they are still the products of a conceptual system predicated upon a how-priority attitude. As we have already mentioned, the approach of the Japanese to the theoretical questions raised by the channel divergences has predominantly been to sidestep them completely and focus on therapy. Nevertheless, the therapies themselves all reflect implicit assumptions about the nature of the channel divergences even if their developers have chosen not to discuss them. It may be that in skirting these philosophical and theoretical matters, the modern channel divergence specialists presented herein have simply embodied one of the essential lessons of the channel divergences.

The fact that the wellspring of Chinese medical wisdom is riddled with contradictions does not absolve us, however, from the responsibility of interpreting what the texts say and mean to the best of our ability. Some interpretations of the texts are most certainly more "right" than others. One is more likely to be successful in developing an efficacious modern treatment style based on a classical text if one has interpreted that text correctly. Still, it must be admitted that treatment styles based on textual misinterpretation can be wrong and still be efficacious. In a sense, one may be right for the wrong reasons. Having said that, it has been our personal experience that those therapies based on clear textual misinterpretation are among the least potent channel divergence protocols that we have seen. As vague as some passages may be, they are, nonetheless, pointing us in a specific direction. However we may choose to embellish the original vision of the *Inner Classic,* we must do our best to identify how its originators conceived it. While it is important, when studying the classical Chinese medical literature to read between the lines, we must not read between the characters.

The authors of this book are first and foremost clinicians and, like our predecessors, our primary interest is also in what works. Why then, have we spilled so much ink wrangling over sinological and theoretical matters that are largely unresolvable? The reason is that all of the therapies described in this book are ultimately based on some initial set of theoretical premises. Although even the originators of these therapies may have little interest in them, we believe that these theoretical premises are a crucial component in understanding the therapies themselves. Perhaps more importantly, we have endeavored to provide the reader with the tools for drawing his or her own conclusions about this most enigmatic facet of the Chinese channel and network vessel system. As we proceed to discussing the variety of ideas regarding the nature of the qi flowing through the channel divergences and the clinical implications of these assumptions, it is useful to bear this in mind.

Readers will observe that the electro-acupuncture treatment methods in this book follow the common convention of assigning positive and negative poles to acupuncture points as a means of designating the direction of electrical current. Those familiar with the physics of electricity, particularly as it functions in AC current, will note that this is not a completely accurate reflection of what is occurring between the two leads of an electro acupuncture device. Since the acupuncturists profiled in the present work are undoubtedly aware of the fundamental laws of physics, it is clear that the assignment of positive and negative leads must be understood as nothing more than functional designations that facilitate optimal clinical outcomes. As we will see again, and again, emphasis is less on theory, than on what yields an effective result.

Endnotes

[1] See Bensky & O'Connor: 492
[2] See Oleson
[3] Kespi: 360
[4] Seki, 1986: 45
[5] Irie, 1987: 49
[6] See Bensky & O'Connor, 1981: 75-81, and Ni, 1996: 5-7
[7] Page 93
[8] *Ling Shu Ji Jiao Shi (Annotated Divine Pivot)*: 284
[9] Shibazaki: 1173-1174
[10] Yang & Chace: 96
[11] Shibazaki: 1173-1174
[12] Personal communication with Irie: 1986

[13] Irie, 1989: 45
[14] Todo: 684
[15] *Ibid*.: 141
[16] *Ibid*.: 386
[17] *Ibid*.: 570
[18] *Ibid*.: 377
[19] *Ibid*.: 889
[20] Wiseman refers to *he* holes as uniting holes.
[21] In Chapter 8 we will present Shima's treatment style in depth, and present two of his case histories which feature his use of a confluence hole-based channel divergence strategy.
[22] Spring, summer, long summer, autumn, and winter
[23] *I.e.*, east, south, west, north, and center
[24] These are 12 bamboo pipes of varied lengths, giving 12 standardized pitches of half tones each having a specific name. From the lowest to the highest, these are *Huang Zhong, Da Lu, Tai Cu, Jia Zhong, Gu Xi, Zhong Lu, Rui Bin, Lin Zhong, Yi Ze, Nan Lu, Wu She,* and *Ying Zhong*. They are evenly divided into two groups. Those which are odd-numbered are yang, while those that are even-numbered are yin.
[25] The channels are grouped in terms of ying and yang in order to match the six pitch pipes. There are actually 12 pipes, but they are divided into yin and yang groups of six pipes each.
[26] These 12 *chen* are the 12 earthly branches. They are commonly used in the premodern Chinese medical literature for listing things in order.
[27] The 12 solar terms are the Beginning of Spring, Waking of Insects, Clear Brightness, Beginning of Summer, Grain in Ear, Slight Heat, Beginning of Autumn, White Dew, Cold Dew, Beginning of Winter, Great Snow, and Slight Cold.
[28] The 12 watches are Midnight (B1), Cockcrow (B2), Calm Dawn (B3), Sunrise (B4), Breakfast (B5), Outlying Region (B6), Midday (B7), Sun Descent (B8), Late Afternoon (B9), Sundown (B10), Dusk (B11), and Serenity (B12). Note that, after the Han dynasty, the 12 watches began to be called after the 12 earthly branches.
[29] Irie: 1989
[30] See Bensky & O'Connor, 1981
[31] Wiseman and Ye: 192
[32] Low: 136
[33] *Huang Di Nei Jing Tai Su (Great Treatise on Huang Di's Inner Classic)*, Vol. 9, "On The Channels, Vessels, Primaries & Divergences"
[34] *Lei Jing (Categorization of the Classic)*: 209
[35] *Ibid*.
[36] Practitioners of many Japanese styles of acupuncture would assert that reactivity of some sort defines the presence of an acupuncture hole or channel. This may include a subjective sense of qi, hardness, or induration, heat or cold. Practitioners of other styles might define this same reactivity not as the presence of qi but as a reflection of its absence. Therefore we believe it is safest not to limit our definition of the channels exclusively to the presence of qi.
[37] Birch & Felt: 157-163
[38] Unschuld, 1990: 8
[39] Birch & Felt: 100
[40] Zhang Dong-sun cited in Ames: 221
[41] *Ibid*.: 221
[42] *Ibid*.: 150
[43] Hall and Ames, 1987: 55
[44] Hansen, 1985: 493
[45] *Ibid*.: 493
[46] According to Graham, 安智 *an zhi* may also be read as "from where do you know what the fish enjoy" or "in what context do you know this?"
[47] *Zhuang-zi*, Chapter 17 "Autumn Waters," translated by Graham, 1981: 123
[48] Ames: 220
[49] *Ibid*.: 221
[50] *Zhuang-zi*, Chapter 2, "The Sorting Which Evens Things Out," trans. by Angus Graham, 1981: 53

[51] A rough corollary of this idea in Western philosophy is instrumentalism. Mauntner, 1996: 277 describes instrumentalism as the view that theories, especially in the sciences, are not strictly speaking, true or false but are to be regarded as tools. Their main use is to assist in predictions, in making the transition from one set of data to another. This is a view of science adopted by pragmatists such as Pierce, Dewey, and James. It essentially rejects truth in favor of usefulness.

[52] Birch & Felt, 1999: 109

2

THE NATURE OF THE
CHANNEL DIVERGENCES

THE SIX CONFLUENCES

One area that needs investigating in our efforts to gain some insight as to what the authors of the *Divine Pivot* may have had in mind with regard to the channel divergences is their use of the term "the six confluences (*liu he*)" to refer to the six channel divergence pairs. The use of terms such as channels (*jing*) and vessels (*mai*) are, at least partially, a reflection of the Chinese preoccupation with irrigation, water control, and its relationship to the land in general.[1] If the terms used to describe other layers of the channel system are also direct reflections of the larger Chinese worldview, it is likely that the choice of the term "six confluences" evokes some larger resonance as well. What then are the six confluences?

According to the *Ci Yuan* (*Sea of Words*), there are at least three meanings of the compound term *liu he* that the authors of the *Inner Classic* may have had in mind when they used this term. First, this term suggests a confluence of the six directions, *i.e.*, heaven, earth, and the four directions, north, south, east, and west. Chapter 2 of *Zhuang-zi*, "On the Equality of All Things," states:

> What is outside the six confluences, the sage lets be present and does not sort. Whatever lies within the province of the six confluences, the sage sorts but does not argue about what is right.[2, 3]

The above passage from *Zhuang-zi* implies that the six confluences may be used to define the boundaries of both space and time. Indeed, it is not uncommon to see *liu he* simply translated as "the universe." The six confluences also define the parameters of one's influence. The sage does not bother him or herself with what they cannot control or influence. They simply acknowledge the presence of what-

42   The Channel Divergences

ever lies outside the boundaries of space and time. In other words, concrete concerns lying within the boundaries of the six confluences must be placed in their proper context, but this sorting should not be a topic of contention. Another interpretation of this passage definitively places the sage outside any limits imposed by space and time.[4] These three interpretations imply that the six confluences are the foundation upon which the phenomenal world is built and that they literally define consensual reality for those of us who have not yet achieved sagehood.

Those readers who have been exposed to the writings of Yoshio Manaka through Steven Birch and Kiiko Matsumoto will be familiar with the polyhedron model of the extraordinary vessels.[5] It is interesting that this same geometric pattern also perfectly defines the boundaries of the six confluences.

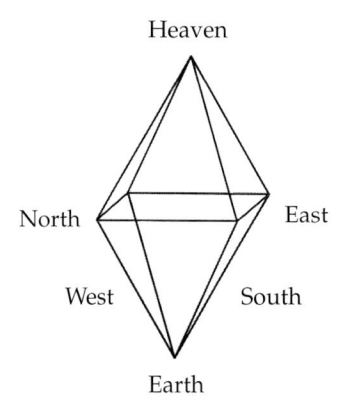

One of the fundamental ways in which human beings structure their experience of the world is through the marking of the seasons. Seasonal resonances are central to ancient Chinese culture as is evidenced by the seasonal assignation to each of the five phases. Similarly, the confluences may be used to mark the junctures between the seasons of the year. For instance, the *Huai Nan Zi*, states:

> Six confluences are early spring with early autumn, mid-spring with mid-autumn, late spring with late autumn, early summer with early winter, mid-summer with mid-winter, [and] late summer with late winter.[5]

The equation of the six confluences with the six directions is echoed much later in the Tang dynasty in the third stanza of Li Po's poem, *Gu Feng* "Ancient Traditions", which says:

> Emperor Qin conquers all six directions.
> How heroic the tiger looks![6]

Ancient Chinese astrology also uses six pairs or confluences (based on the 12 earthly branches) as a means of determining auspicious dates by matching the branches of month and date. For instance *Zi* (Rat) is paired with *Chou* (Cow), *Yin* (Tiger) with *Hai* (Pig), etc. The *Yu Dai Xin Yong* (*New Poems From the Jade dynasty*) contains a poem by Jiao Zhong-qing's wife which states:

Six pairs should correspond properly.
The thirtieth day [of the month] is most auspicious [to get married].[7]

As the reader can see, once again the six confluences are integral components in the Chinese measurement of time. However, in this case, they do not mark the junctures between seasonal transitions. Instead, the six confluences describe the junctures of two distinct but inter-related methods of measuring the passage of time.

Clearly, the six confluences evoke a distinctly heavenly resonance, literally providing structure to space in the six directions and to time in the six seasonal junctures. The relationship of the six confluences to time and timing also evokes a sense of the necessity of administering acupuncture to the right person, at the right time, and in a perfect manner when one has the correct diagnosis. Certainly, the authors of the *Inner Classic* seem to have paid great attention to timing of this sort with their concern for needling the correct acupuncture hole in the correct season and at just the right moment.

Thus, the term "six confluences" has a number of cultural and philosophical connotations, and it is highly unlikely that the authors of the *Inner Classic* selected this term at random without reference to any of these connotations. In the previous chapter, we examined the potential implications of Emperor Huang's preface to Qi Bo's elucidation of the channel divergences. The *Divine Pivot* authors' choice of the term confluences resonates strongly with the heavenly role for the channel divergences described in the previous chapter. We see the six confluences mentioned in the *Elementary Questions* on a number of other occasions in the context of heavenly influences:

> Whatever lies in heaven and earth and within the six confluences, (including) the qi of the seven rivers, the nine orifices, the five storehouses, the 12 articulations, all of these things communicate with the heavenly qi.
> *Elementary Questions,* Chapter 3, "On the Communication of Life's Qi with Heaven"

> In discussing the human form the sages of antiquity discriminated viscera from bowels and identified the extremities of the network vessels and channels and the communication of these with the six confluences.
> *Elementary Questions,* Chapter 5, "On the Correspondences of Yin & Yang"

> As for the communication with the spirit light, the confluence of metal, wood, water, fire, and earth with the four seasons, the eight winds and the six confluences are no different from this.
> *Elementary Questions,* Chapter 11, "The Extra Treatise on the Five Viscera"

The Depth of the Channel Divergences

As we have seen, due to the cryptic nature of Chapter 11 of the *Divine Pivot*, its authors define some of the fundamental characteristics of the channel divergences vaguely at best. This situation extends even to their relative depth and the nature of the qi that flows through them. The British acupuncturist Royston Low asserts that the channel divergences are a mid-depth layer of a stratified channel system.[8] A middle depth positioning of the channel divergences is central to his ideas regarding the nature of the qi flowing in them and his strategy for accessing them, and we will address his perspective more fully in the next section. However, most other sources, both Asian and Occidental, posit a deep trajectory for the channel divergences relative to the other layers of the channel and network vessel system. The French acupuncturists Duron, Laville-Mery, and Borsarello, for instance, describe the layering of channels and network vessels in the following manner:[9]

Channel Layering According to Duron
Skin (*Pi*)
Channel Sinews (*Jing Jin*)
Network (*Luo*)
Main Channel (*Da Jing*)
Channel Divergence (*Jing Bie*)
Viscera & Bowels (*Zang Fu*)

This interpretation makes the greatest sense to the present authors based on our understanding of the extant source material and on our experience in the clinical application of the channel divergences.

In the final analysis, it must be admitted that all of this is, of course, purely theoretical. Given that there is, as yet, no objective means of establishing the location of the channels or even of the existence of qi, it is difficult to say with any certainty whether one layer of the channel system lies beneath another. The purpose of such conjecture is only to provide a context for developing treatment protocols which must then withstand the rigors of clinical testing.

The Nature of the Qi in the Channel Divergences

Directly related to the question of depth is the issue of the nature of the qi that flows in the channel divergences. The *Divine Pivot* is silent on this matter. However, some Western sources state unequivocally that defensive qi and defensive qi alone flows through these channels.[10,11] This assumption is central to several approaches to channel divergences therapy. However, to a large extent, Japanese sources sidestep this issue completely, proceeding directly to treatment without describing the nature of the qi they are manipulating. At least, they have not committed themselves to paper on this issue. Nevertheless, their selection of acupuncture holes for accessing the channel divergences strongly implies the role of original (*yuan*) qi in channel divergence dynamics. Clearly, some of the Japanese channel divergence specialists believe that the channel divergences are, in fact, the deepest of all the channels, deeper even than the extraordinary vessels and, as such, must certainly convey constructive (*ying*) and probably original (*yuan*) qi. The fact that the channel divergences are particularly useful in addressing deep visceral conditions characterized by organic pathologies would seem to the authors to confirm this hypothesis.

While the nature of the qi that flows through the channel divergences is largely a superfluous theoretical concern to many clinicians, it nonetheless bears heavily on how we understand these enigmatic pathways and how we use them. Let us first examine the proposition that the channel divergences are the exclusive provenance of the defensive qi and consider the ramifications of this idea for the clinical use of these channels. Interestingly, Royston Low posits one of the more fanciful but well known interpretations of the channel divergences. He contends that the channel divergences are mid-level channels through which defensive qi alone circulates. While he acknowledges their direct connection to their associated viscera and bowels, he suggests that the channel divergences serve as an intermediary buffer into which "pernicious influences"(*xie qi*) ideally enters prior to attacking the major channel. Therefore, patients suffering from an affliction of the channel divergences have much the same symptoms as if the patients' main channels were afflicted. However, the symptoms will be less severe than those presenting in a main channel. Low cites a passage from Chapter 63 of the *Elementary Questions*, "On Cross Needling," as evidence of this position. Low's rendering is as follows:

> When the vicious energy comes to reside in the human body as a guest, it must come to reside in the skin and the hair first: if the vicious energy persists to stay without leaving, it will enter the body and reside in the Tiny Meridians; if the vicious energy persists to stay without leaving, it will enter further into the body and reside in the Reticular Meridians, internally affecting the five viscera and spreading in the stomach and intestines, causing harm to both the Yin and Yang as well as the five viscera; such are the sequences of attack by the vicious energy, from the skin and hair toward the five viscera, which should be treated by the meridians. If, however, the vicious energy resides in the skin and hair as guest and then enters into the Tiny Meridians to stay there without leaving, blocking up the passages of the Reticular Meridians, unable to flow into the Master Meridians, it will flow in the great links as guest, it often causes disease on the right side with symptoms on the left side. Although the Reticular Meridians are associated with the Master Meridians in the upper or lower, or the left or right regions, their energy spreads in the four extremities with no regular residence not entering into the points on the meridians. This is why the reverse needling should be applied.
>
> The Huang Di asked: Could you tell me about the reverse technique of needling in which the affected left side should be treated by the right side, and the affected right side should be left side? How do you distinguish this type of needling from the opposite technique of needling?

Qi Bo replied: When the vicious energy comes to reside in the meridians as guest, it may cause disease on the right side while the left side is in excess, or it may cause disease on the left side while the right side is in excess; it may cause disease on the right side while the pain on the left has not yet recovered, due to the shifting of Yin from Yang and vice versa; under such circumstances, the patient should be treated by the opposite technique of needling, because the vicious energy attacks the Master Meridians, not the Reticular Meridians. Therefore the disease of the Reticular Meridians as distinguished from the diseases of the Master Meridians should be treated by the reverse technique of needling.[12]

Royston Low goes on to say: "In the latter chapter, apparently, the use of the term Reticular Meridians refers to the Distinct Meridians rather than to the tendino-muscular meridians, with which the word is usually associated."[13] He does not, however, provide any reasons for this assumption.

The *Divine Pivot* describes cross-needling, (Low's reverse needling) as a method that involves pricking the *jing* well holes on the opposite side of the body from the afflicted channel. The text clearly states that cross-needling is a means of draining pathogenic influences from the network vessels (*luo*). For instance, if the hand *yang ming* large intestine network vessel on the left side is affected, then *Shang Yang* (LI 1) should be pricked on the right. According to Low, the network vessels referred to in Chapter 63 of *Elementary Questions* are, in actuality, the channel divergences. Within the Chinese literature, this interpretation can be traced at least as far back as the Qing dynasty when Zhang Yi-nan, commenting on the *Inner Classic*, rather cryptically includes the trajectories of the channel divergences in his notes to the chapter on cross-needling, thereby linking cross-needling with the channel divergences.[14] Unfortunately, Zhang provides no further information on this matter.

According to Low, if one reads luo 络 network as bie 别 divergence, then much of this interpretation falls logically into place. The chapter on cross-needling is obviously concerned with the presence of pathogenic qi on a relatively superficial level and with preventing the penetration of that pathogenic qi into the main channel. Therefore, it makes sense that the channel divergences are mid-depth and that the channel divergences are the exclusive domain of defensive qi, just as we know the network vessels to be. In addition, this substantiates the notion that the symptomology of the channel divergences is an identical but attenuated version of that of the main channels. Nevertheless, it seems that the entire basis for Low's interpretation rests on Zhang's understanding of a single character as it appears in a very few sentences. However, there are a number of problems with reading *luo* as divergence in these sentences, and it is our opinion that this interpretation is founded on shaky theoretical ground.

A Confusion of Divergences

Part of the confusion regarding the words *bie* and *luo* is due to the fact that the trajectories of the network vessels connecting pairs of yin and yang main channels are also referred to as divergences (*bie*) within the classical Chinese literature. Most Chinese commentaries on the channel divergences take care to point out that the divergence (*bie*) of the channel divergences is fundamentally different from the divergence (*bie*) associated with the network vessels. We will encounter a number of similarities between therapies directed toward the network vessels and the channel divergences but theoretically at least, they are distinctly different systems.

The Text Itself

Chapter 63 of the *Divine Pivot* itself is, perhaps, the best argument for interpreting *luo* as network vessel rather than channel divergence. The author of that chapter is careful to distinguish between cross-needling which addresses the *luo* and grand needling (*ju ci*) which specifically addresses the main channels. The relationship between the main channels and the network vessels is well established elsewhere in the *Inner Classic*. Chapter 10 of the *Divine Pivot*, "On the Channels & Vessels," deals with this matter at length. The dynamic between the main channels and the network vessels defines the relationship between the constructive flowing in the main channels and the defensive flowing outside them *in the network vessels*. Because the network vessels contain defensive qi, they defend the main channels from attack by external pathogens. Why is it necessary to posit another layer of the channel system as carrying defensive qi? Clearly, most occurrences of the character *luo* in the *Inner Classic* are best read as "network", "connecting," "reticular," or "spirally wraps," depending on the context and one's terminological predilection. Therefore, what basis is there for reading *luo* as "divergence" in this context? If read as divergence, at what point in the chapter may one resume reading *luo* as network, reticular, or connecting vessel?

An Absence of Discrimination Between Channel Layers

Chapter 34 of the *Divine Pivot*, "On the Five Chaotic Conditions," instructs us to bleed the *luo* using cross-needling to remove blood stasis. Since bleeding appears throughout the *Inner Classic* as one of the primary therapies for draining pathogens from the network vessels, it seems likely that this technique was aimed exclusively at the network vessels. Indeed, the vast majority of commentators throughout history have concurred that cross-needling is a network vessel therapy. The possibility of using cross-needling as a channel divergence therapy raises a number of interesting considerations regarding the relationship between these two channel layers. However, it also brings up some troubling problems as well. If cross-needling may be used to access both the channel divergences and the network vessels, then how can we be sure which layer of pathways we are accessing when we use this technique? Thus, it seems to the authors that the cross-needling argument cannot, at least by itself, be used as evidence for the exclusive flow of defensive qi in the channel divergences.

THE CHANNEL DIVERGENCES & THE MAIN CHANNELS

At this point, it may be useful to review what we know regarding the various species of qi. Chapter 18 of the *Divine Pivot*, "On the Generation & Meeting of the Constructive & Defensive," says that, "The constructive circulates within the vessels and the defensive circulates outside the vessels." The distinction being made here is that constructive qi flows within the main channels, while defensive qi flows around them. As we have already seen, the channel divergences may rightly be perceived as being among the most primary vessels in the entire channel system. As such, it can be argued that they have much more in common with the main channels, which convey constructive qi, than they do with the secondary vessels which convey defensive qi.

THE DIRECTIONALITY OF THE QI-FLOW IN THE CHANNEL DIVERGENCES

Directly related to the question of what species of qi flows in the channel divergences is the question of in what direction it flows. It is universally accepted that the qi in the main channels (*jing*) flows in the direction of its classically described trajectory. For instance, the qi in the main hand *tai yin* lung channel flows distally from the chest. The Western convention of numbering the first hole on the torso, *Zhong Fu* (Lu 1), and the last hole at the corner of the nail on the thumb, *Shao Shang* (Lu 11), reflects this understanding. However, the trajectory of the hand *tai yin* channel sinew (*jing jin*) which carries defensive qi begins at the corner of the nail on the thumb and travels proximally toward the torso. We generally assume that the flow of qi in all the channels travels in the direction of its stated trajectory, but this is most definitely open to debate.

Birch and Felt observe that only the constructive or channel qi is explicitly described as actually flowing in the channels.[15] What happens with the other kinds of qi is admittedly rather vague. However, one of the fundamental qualities of qi is that it moves. Certainly, the defensive qi is conveyed from the exterior during the day to the interior at night, and source qi is disseminated throughout the body via the triple burner. Given this indirect evidence, we believe that it is safe to say that all the qi in the body flows. The question is, then, in what direction does it flow in the channel divergences?

Based on the *Great Treatise*'s discussion of the discrepancies between the flow of qi in the channel divergences and that in the main channels, it is reasonable to infer that the qi in the channel divergences also flows in the same direction as their stated trajectories. Generally speaking, the trajectories of the channel divergences run from distal to proximal and pedal to cephalic.[16] This is consistent with all the superficial secondary vessels—the network vessels, the channel sinews, and the cutaneous regions—which travel proximally toward the torso and head. Further, the classics explicitly state that defensive qi alone inhabits these channels. With this in mind, one may infer that defensive qi flows in a similar manner within the channel divergences. Be that as it may, the trajectories of the channel divergences differ from the other secondary vessels in a number of important ways. First, even given a mid-depth interpretation, they travel much more deeply than do the other so-called secondary vessels. Second, although the trajectories of the other secondary channels are described as beginning at or near the *jing* well or *luo* network holes of their associated channels, the descriptions of the channel divergences begin much more proximally than that.[17]

The trajectories of the channel divergences prior to where they "diverge" from the major channels are, depending on one's interpretation, either obscure or nonexistent. Many investigators, both European and Japanese, seem to assume that the channel divergences have some clinical trajectory parallel to but distinct from the main channels extending distal to the place where they actually diverge from the main channel.[18] In the Shanghai acupuncture textbook we know as *Acupuncture, A Comprehensive Text,* the authors of the text describe the channel divergences' trajectories in the conventional manner. However, their illustrations typically depict the trajectories as originating at the extremities in a manner identical to that of the main channels.[19] This is, to some degree, necessary because on the foot yang and hand yin channels, the trajectories of the channel divergences run contrary to the trajectories of the main channels. Chapter 11 of the *Divine Pivot* makes no mention of any trajectory for any of the channel divergences prior to where they diverge from the main channel. As we have already seen, while the text itself often implies some preexisting channel divergence trajectory, the channel divergence is only discussed from its point of divergence onward.[20]

If we adopt a literal reading of Chapter 11 of the *Divine Pivot* and interpret the channel divergences as actually originating at the *bie*, it becomes difficult to understand how only defensive qi could flow through them. Clearly, the channel divergences are not diverging (*bie*) from the secondary vessels that contain defensive qi, but from the main channels that contain constructive and, to some extent, original qi. By definition, the main channels cannot contain defensive qi, at least not in a condition of health. Even if we accept the premise that defensive and constructive qi always flow together in the same direction, they most definitely flow separately from one another. In addition to positing a contrary flow of defensive qi, Chapter 34 of the *Divine Pivot*, "On the Five Chaotic Conditions," clearly states that the presence of defensive qi in the main channels is the very definition of chaotic qi.

> Emperor Huang asked: What are counterflow and chaos?
>
> Qi Bo answered: The clear qi is yin, while the turbid qi is yang. The constructive qi

flows in the same direction as the vessels, while the defensive qi flows in the opposite direction. When the clear and turbid interfere with one another and are in chaos in the chest, this is called massive disturbance.

Nevertheless, since many approaches to channel divergence therapy access these pathways via acupuncture holes located considerably distal to their points of divergence, we must also explore the possibility that, for all intents and purposes, the channel divergences themselves begin somewhere distal to the actual point of divergence. Perhaps in keeping with the other secondary vessels, channel divergences originate at the *jing* well holes and simply parallel the main channels until they strike out on their own at the point of divergence. This would add weight to the cross-needling strategy for accessing them and further reinforce a hypothetical relationship between the network vessels, the channel divergences, and the defensive qi. Be that as it may, it is clear that, while defensive qi may indeed be conveyed along the channel divergence trajectories, defensive qi is not the only species of qi to take this path.

Royston Low says that the channel divergences provide another vector for the circulation of defensive qi.[21] After all, many of the channel divergences do terminate at the eyes which are the starting point of the daytime circulation of defensive qi. Chapter 62 of the *Divine Pivot*, "On Regulating the Channels," says that defensive qi circulates in the yang channels during the day and in the yin viscera during the night. The circulation of defensive qi through the yang channels begins at the eyes where it is transmitted along the hand and foot *tai yang* bladder and small intestine channels. Although there are a number of interpretations of just how defensive qi arrives at the eyes, Chapter 18 of the *Divine Pivot*, "On the Generation & Meeting of the Constructive & Defensive," states that, "Constructive qi issues from the middle burner, while defensive qi issues from the upper burner." Whether or not this is a textual error is the subject of some disagreement. However, the relationship between defense qi and the qi of the chest is well established. The ancestral qi (*zong qi*), the qi of the chest, and the upper sea of qi (*shang qi hai*) are at least partially understood as "the constructive and defensive qi derived from food and drink and combined with the respiration to accumulate in the chest."[22]

All of these considerations begin to coalesce when we remember that the few explicit statements regarding the channel divergences concern their trajectories through the heart and chest. The most accurate statement we can make on this matter is that the channel divergences all link with or pass through the qi of the chest, the ancestral qi. What does it mean that the channel divergences pass through the chest?

An Alternative Model

To truly understand ancestral qi, we must understand its relationship to original qi. The ancestral qi is the active expression of the original qi. Original qi is stored in the lower burner in the lower sea of qi, while ancestral qi is stored in the upper burner in the upper sea of qi. Ancestral qi is composed of latter heaven qi,[23] and original qi is composed of both latter heaven and former heaven qi. While the original qi is focused in the life gate (*ming men*) between the two kidneys, the ancestral qi is accumulated in the chest center (*dan zhong*) between the two breasts. The integration of these two types of qi is known as true qi (*zhen qi*). Chapter 75 of the *Divine Pivot*, "Needling Norms of True & Evil [Qi]," talking about the measured needling of true pathogens, asserts, "The true qi is the merging of qi received from heaven and grain qi made manifest in the body." In this way, we can see that the ancestral qi and the original qi are intimately related and that original qi manifests itself on a day-to-day basis through the ancestral qi. This dynamic occurs throughout the body, but it occurs most specifically in the sea of qi in the chest.

Zhang Jie-bin comments in his *Lei Jing* (*Categorization of the Classic*) that, "The chest center is the sea of qi," and, "The chest center is located in the middle of the chest between the two breasts."[24] Furthermore:

> The heart commands because it is the sovereign. There must be a sending out of orders, messages and decrees, and the chest center governs and commands qi to spread out and to distribute yin as well as yang.[25]

Here we see that this chest center is the active envoy of the heart and is responsible for the communication between the heart and all the rest of the qi. Although the channel divergences of the lung and triple burner do not pass directly through the heart, they are, nonetheless, in indirect communication with it via their passage through the upper sea of qi.

Clearly, the authors of Chapter 11 of the *Divine Pivot* were not interested in providing us with explicit guidance with respect to the channel divergences. They were content to simply point us in a general direction. As we have already noted, one of the few things we really know about these channels is that they pass through the chest, some specifically through the heart and the rest through the chest cavity in general. We believe that the implication here is that, in traversing the chest, all of the channel divergences connect the viscera and bowel qi with the true qi, *i.e.*, the integration of ancestral and original qi. This hypothesis fits all the basic information we have regarding the channel divergences. Furthermore, it explains why the channel divergences have proven so clinically useful in treating not only deep visceral pathologies but also in addressing disharmonies more commonly associated with the defensive qi.

This hypothesis is consistent with our image of the channel divergences as a fundamental axis between the interior and exterior of the body. The channel divergences may provide an essential pathway for the internalization of the predominantly *external* defensive qi back into the core and for the externalization of the fundamentally *internal* original qi to the periphery. Thus, it becomes apparent how original yang (*yuan yang*) not only contacts but also potentizes defensive yang (*wei yang*).

Our purpose here in questioning the predominant model of channel divergences therapy in the West is not simply academic posturing. The cross-needling interpretation of the channel divergences is instructive in a number of important ways. Using this model, we end up with the channel divergences system performing much the same function as the network vessels in preventing pathogens from entering the main channels. When all is said and done, pricking *jing* well holes can be an effective treatment strategy toward this end regardless of whether one believes one is accessing the channel divergences or the network vessels. On the other hand, a cross-needling interpretation of the channel divergences clearly creates a number of assumptions of its own (one major assumption being that the defensive qi alone flows in the channel divergences) and these assumptions feed back into one's overall picture of this layer of pathways. In our opinion, these assumptions ultimately limit the potential clinical application of the channel divergences as a therapeutic concept. We believe that the alternative model of visceral qi and ancestral qi circulation through the channel divergences we have presented is consistent with the available source material *and* allows for a much wider range of clinical application. Conversely, it is our experience that such a conceptual framework most accurately reflects the effects of the channel divergence system we have observed clinically.

ENDNOTES

[1] Unschuld, 1985: 83
[2] Li shi-zhen's *Qi Jing Ba Mai Kao* (*A Personal Critique of the Eight Vessels of the Extraordinary Channels*) equates the *dai* vessel with the six conflunces. "The *dai* vessel horizontally binds all the vessels so it is referred to as the six confluences." The *yang wei* governs the exterior, the influence of which is analogous to heaven. The *yin wei* governs the interior, the influence of which is analogous to earth. The *yin* and *yang qiao* vessels govern the yin and yang channels on the sides of the body and taken together, this influence is analogous to east and west. The *chong*, *ren* and *du* govern the vertical axis of the body, the influence of which is analogous to north and south. The *dai* vessel links the entire body together such that its influence is analogous to the six confluences. Just as the six confluences provide a unifying concept for spatial relations, the *dai* vessel organizes all of the extraordinary channels into a unified whole. Just as the six confluences are a concept that unifies spatial relations, the *dai* vessel unifies the extraordinary vessels. This is not to infer, however, that the extraordinary vessels are synonymous with the channel divergences.
[3] This interpretation of this passage is from Kuang-ming Wu: 146. For the sake of clarity in the present discussion, we have changed his "six cosmic correlates" to the six confluences.
[4] Personal communication with the Sinologist Huang Ying-jun
[5] *Huai Nan Zi*: 141
[6] *Ci Yuan (Word Source)*: 164
[7] *Ibid*. 164
[8] Low: 131
[9] Duron, et al.: 66
[10] Kespi: 359
[11] Low: 131
[12] Low: 129-130
[13] *Ibid*.

[14] Zhang Yi-nan: Vol. 7: 43
[15] Birch and Felt, 1999: 149
[16] The trajectory of the hand *shao yang* triple burner channel divergence is an exception to this rule. Its trajectory runs downward from the vertex.
[17] There are two distinct but related types of network vessels. The most commonly recognized type of network or connecting vessels in the West are the pathways which connect yin-yang pairs of channels via the *luo* holes. While the trajectories of these pathways are explicitly described in the *Ling Shu*, they are clearly conceptualized as being a component of a much larger and more diffuse network vessel system. As such, they are referred to as network branches (*luo zhi*). Network vessels as a larger and more general concept are described in Chapter 10 of the *Ling Shu* as: "The vessels that can be seen are the network vessels. They travel along pathways which are inaccessible [to the main channels], coming and going, and spreading throughout the skin. The trajectories of these network vessels roughly parallel the major channels. There are two basic methods for needling this larger network vessel system. The first involves bleeding the binding (*jie*) places where blood vessels are apparent. The second involves needling the *jing* well holes using the cross-needling technique." This latter technique suggests that the trajectories of the network vessels, as an overall system, begin at the *jing* well holes.
[18] Seki, Irie, Kespi, Low
[19] Bensky & O'Connor: 76-80
[20] Admittedly, many styles of channel divergence treatment rely on hole selections that lie distal to the actual *bie*, or hole of divergence, some of which are, in our opinion, more clinically useful than others. While the final proof may well be in the empirical pudding, we must for the time being restrict ourselves to the textual material itself, lest we lose ourselves in circular logic. For that matter, mainstream extraordinary vessel therapies demonstrate that it is not necessary to have a direct connection between a hole and the channel it purports to access for it to have an influence. There is no direct connection between Lu 7 and the *ren mai*, and yet this hole is considered the key hole for accessing that vessel.
[21] Low: 127
[22] *Nei Jing Jiang Yang (An Exposition on The Inner Classic)*: 48
[23] Ancestral qi is source qi. Wiseman and Ye define source qi as "the basic form of qi in the body which is made up of a combination of three other forms: the essential qi of the kidney; qi of grain and water, derived through the transformative function of the spleen; and air (great qi) drawn in through the lung. Source qi springs from the kidney (or life gate) and is stored in the cinnabar field. It is the basis of all physiological activity.: 548
[24] *Lei Jing (The Categorization of the Classic)*, Shi Er Guan "The Twelve Officials": 30
[25] *Ibid.*

3

CHANNEL DIVERGENCE DIAGNOSTICS

Although they may potentially be used for virtually any complaint, the channel divergences are particularly effective for deep viscera and bowel disorders and for some pain syndromes. Having decided to use this particular layer of the channel and network vessel system for treatment, we must now decide which of the channel divergences is most appropriate for the problem at hand. The major Japanese-based channel divergences treatment systems all rely to a greater or lesser extent on the following criteria:

> Viscera & Bowel Symptom Presentation
> Pulse Diagnosis
> Abdominal Diagnosis
> Akabane Diagnosis

These diagnostic methods tend to be mixed, matched, and cross-referenced to ensure an optimum channel divergence selection. Because the channel divergences exert a profound influence on the channel system as a whole, many of the methods used to diagnose them are quite simple. Any method of evaluation that tells us about the state of the main channels and viscera in a general way can supply us with the information we need to decide which of the channel divergences to treat. Be that as it may, many of the same Japanese acupuncturists who were involved in developing the channel divergences as a viable therapeutic system were also involved in developing a remarkable array of elaborate and sophisticated diagnostic methods. Although a fecund cross-fertilization of ideas within the Topological Acupuncture Society persisted until Manaka's death in the late 1980s, each investigator was, nevertheless, striving to develop their own unique and distinctive style. Arcane diagnostic methodologies involving magnets and tuning forks go a long way toward defining a personal approach. When all is said and done, however, it is our opinion that many of these sophisticated diagnostic criteria may be of greater use as research tools than as day-to-day methods of clinical diagnosis for the busy acupuncturist.

The plethora of diagnostic methods that have been applied to the channel system raises a number of interesting questions regarding the superiority of one diagnostic method over another or, for that matter, what exactly is being diagnosed. Whatever the methodology, the diagnostic process is undeniably among the most subjective facets of acupuncture practice. In the interest of presenting the most acceptable and familiar face to the biomedical community, it might be preferable to foster the impression that acupuncture diagnosis is an entirely quantifiable process and, as such, it should be possible to determine the primacy of one diagnostic criteria over another. However, anyone who has spent any time in clinical practice must admit that there is much that is unquantifiable in the diagnostic process. Given this reality, we are of the opinion that the diagnostic method or methods that allow an individual practitioner to most effectively "tune in" to a patient in the most complete manner possible will be the preferred diagnostic criteria for that practitioner. Thus, one practitioner may find pulse diagnosis the most useful tool for them, while another may prefer Omura's bi-digital O-ring testing.[1] It should be noted that the distinction between diagnosis and treatment is more than a little vague in many Japanese acupuncture systems. There is a well-known axiom that, "Diagnosis is treatment and treatment is diagnosis" (診斷即治潦療, *shin dan soku chi ryo*). This is especially true with abdominal diagnosis and channel palpation. As we will see, the ongoing and overall process of integrating diagnosis and treatment is, perhaps, the most definitive method for selecting an effective channel divergence for treatment.

Viscera & Bowel Symptom Presentation

Among the above-mentioned diagnostic methods, viscera and bowel symptomology is undoubtedly the most straightforward. One simply selects the second confluence pair, the liver and gallbladder, to treat a typical liver disorder, such as hepatitis, or a gallbladder disease, such as cholecystitis. Similarly, one selects the sixth confluence pair, the lungs and large intestine, to treat constipation and/or asthma. While the simplicity of this approach has much to recommend it, it provides little guidance when one is faced with complex patients presenting with multiple visceral imbalances and many symptomatic complaints. In such instances, we must prioritize our treatment strategy to address the core channel divergences involved and treat them accordingly. This means that, in many situations, we must proceed to an examination of the pulse.

Pulse Examination

Diagnosis of the channel divergences via the pulse may be approached in a number of ways. One of the simplest is also among the most popular. That is, one selects the appropriate channel divergence by determining the most imbalanced pulse. Naturally, the notion of "most imbalanced" can mean a variety of things. In some patients, the most imbalanced pulse is the weakest and most sunken pulse. In other patients, it is the strongest and most wiry pulse.[2] Given that pulses can and do change from moment to moment, the pulse is best taken on a number of occasions to establish which pulses are, indeed, the most consistently imbalanced. Shima typically recommends that a practitioner take the pulse weekly for a month before deciding on an appropriate channel divergence. This is particularly important for individuals who are just beginning to use the channel divergences. Because this layer of the channel and network system provides a direct link to the deepest aspects of visceral function, its potential for causing disruption is as great as its capacity for alleviating suffering. Therefore, channel divergences' treatments should be well thought out prior to administration.

Those practitioners who rely on immediate feedback from the pulse to ascertain the effectiveness of the treatment will probably find channel divergence treatments to their liking. It is our experience that acupuncture's effects on the level of the channel divergences is strongly reflected in the pulse. For instance, properly applied channel divergences protocols will typically cause weak pulses to become stronger, and more rooted, while wiry pulses tend to become more supple.

Abdominal Diagnosis

Abdominal diagnosis occupies a central position in many styles of acupuncture originating in Japan. Indeed, abdominal diagnosis is one of the distinguishing features of what we in the West refer to as "Japanese acupuncture." It is only natural then that the developers of channel divergences therapies would turn to the abdomen for diagnostic insight in accessing the channel divergence. Because abdominal conformations are somewhat less changeable than the pulse or Akabane testing, they are less fickle indicators of which channel divergence or divergences are the primary areas of imbalance within the body.

A fundamental principle of channel divergence therapy is that, if one can diagnose a viscus or bowel pathology, then one has essentially already selected a potential channel divergence. Thus, simple abdominal indicators work quite well in helping us determine which channel divergences to treat. The most basic system of abdominal diagnosis is a five-phase system derived from a number of vague statements regarding the abdomen in the 16th and 67th difficult issues of the *Classic of Difficult Issues*. The most specific information on abdominal palpation is contained in the 16th difficult issue which discusses diagnosis based on observation of palpitation of the aorta above, below, and lateral to the umbilicus. This appears to have been the starting point of all the various styles of Japanese abdominal diagnosis. In general, abdominal palpation for the purposes of acupuncture therapy requires substantially more pressure than the touch required for herbal prescribing, although some acupuncture-based styles of palpation, such as those of the so-called meridian schools, are quite superficial. There are, in fact, many different Japanese maps of the *hara* which can yield conflicting information. Therefore, most practitioners of abdominal diagnosis tend to limit themselves to one or two of these models to avoid confusion. Nevertheless, if one intends to evaluate the abdomen in terms of both acupuncture and herbal therapies, the more superficial herbal palpation is generally performed first.

Virtually any system of abdominal palpation may conceivably be used to determine which channel divergences to treat. Some channel divergence practitioners simply palpate the alarm (*mu*) holes on the abdomen, while others prefer more elaborate diagnostic criteria. Prior to his development of a vessel diagnosis specific to the channel divergences, Tadashi Irie relied heavily on the reactivity of the alarm holes on the abdomen as a means of determining which confluence to needle. For example, reactivity at *Zhong Wan* (CV 12) and *Zhang Men* (Liv 13) in the absence of more pronounced reactivity elsewhere would strongly indicate that the third channel divergence confluence, the spleen and stomach pair, was the confluence to needle.

In the final analysis, however, it is difficult to say that one method of abdominal diagnosis yields a more reliable result than another. In light of this, we will first discuss one of the simplest forms of abdominal palpation as a method for determining an appropriate channel divergence confluence pair. Perhaps the most popular style of abdominal diagnosis in Japan today is known as Kinoshita style, and it is taught as the standard abdominal pattern at acupuncture schools in Japan today. It focuses largely on the yin viscera (*zang*) and represents a fairly accurate reflection of the original discussions in the *Classic of Difficult Issues*. In this system, the subcardiac area corresponds to the heart. The area surrounding the umbilicus corresponds to the spleen. The region below the umbilicus corresponds to the kidneys, the area

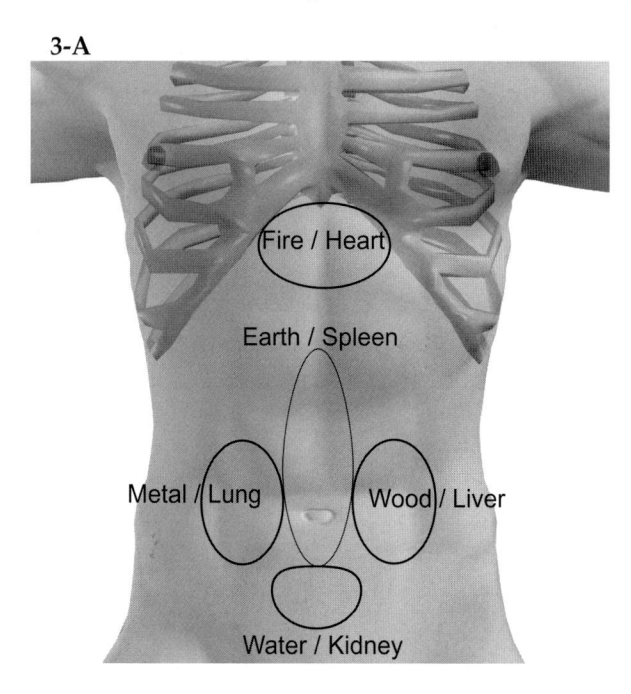

3-A

to the left of the umbilicus corresponds to the liver, and the region to the right of the umbilicus corresponds to the lungs. (See chart 3-A.) The region of maximum abdominal reactivity established by manual palpation determines the appropriate channel divergence pair.

The question of what constitutes reactivity in abdominal diagnosis is a large one. Pressure pain upon palpation is undoubtedly the clearest form of reactivity. In general, the sorest spot is the most reactive. However, many areas may not be sore at all. Instead, the clinician may experience localized tension or a knotted feeling under his or her hand. Conversely, they may feel a depression or sense of emptiness, heat, or cold. Under the right circumstances, these sensations may override the patient's experience of pain upon palpation in determining the most reactive region or hole.

A few channel divergence practitioners are on record as favoring the more obscure Oda-Mubunryu abdominal diagnosis method developed in the 16th century by Isai Misonou and popularized by Yoshio Manaka. This style provides a more elaborate map of visceral and bowel correspondences on the abdominal terrain. For more information on abdominal palpation in general, the reader is referred to Matsumoto and Birch's *Hara Diagnosis: Reflections on the Sea*.

AKABANE DIAGNOSIS

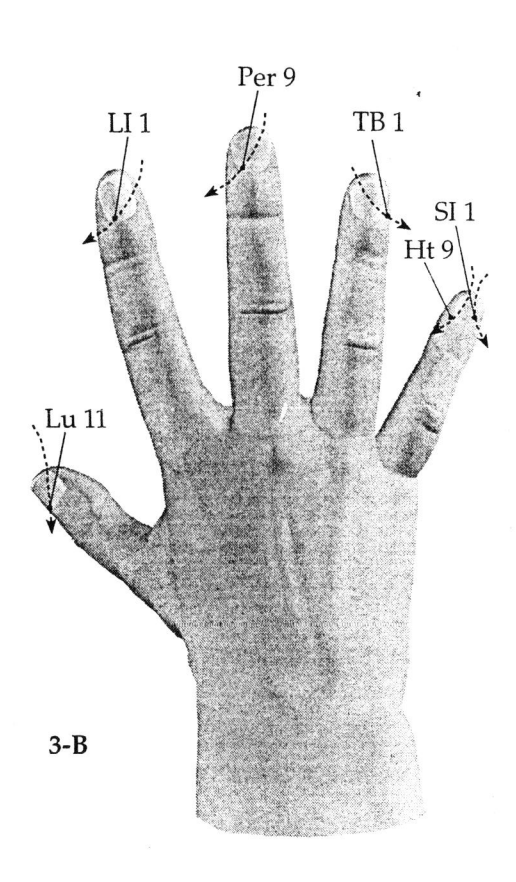

Developed 50 years ago, Akabane diagnosis and therapy is a very modern innovation by acupuncture standards. Nonetheless, it has found a place in many styles of acupuncture practice throughout the world. For instance, Akabane diagnosis affected such seminal influences on Western acupuncture as James Tin-yao So and J. R. Worsley. Kobei Akabane's central interest was in right/left imbalances in the major channel system, and it was his belief that, once these imbalances were resolved, the rest of the channel system would balance itself. Toward this end, he developed a method of determining these right/left imbalances by evaluating the sensitivity of the *jing* well holes on each of the extremities.

Akabane's initial insight came when he applied direct moxibustion to a *jing* well hole on the toe of a diabetic patient. The patient made a dramatic recovery despite the fact that he had inadvertently produced a substantial burn. This piqued Akabane's interest in the role of *jing* well holes in both reflecting and regulating channel activity. Over the course of his investigations, it became clear to Akabane that the heat-sensing nerve receptors were the most sensitive, and thermal stimulation of these receptors was an ideal means of evaluating the channels. He experimented further with non-scarring moxa cones on the *jing* well holes and eventually refined his methodology with the use of an incense stick drawn across the hole.

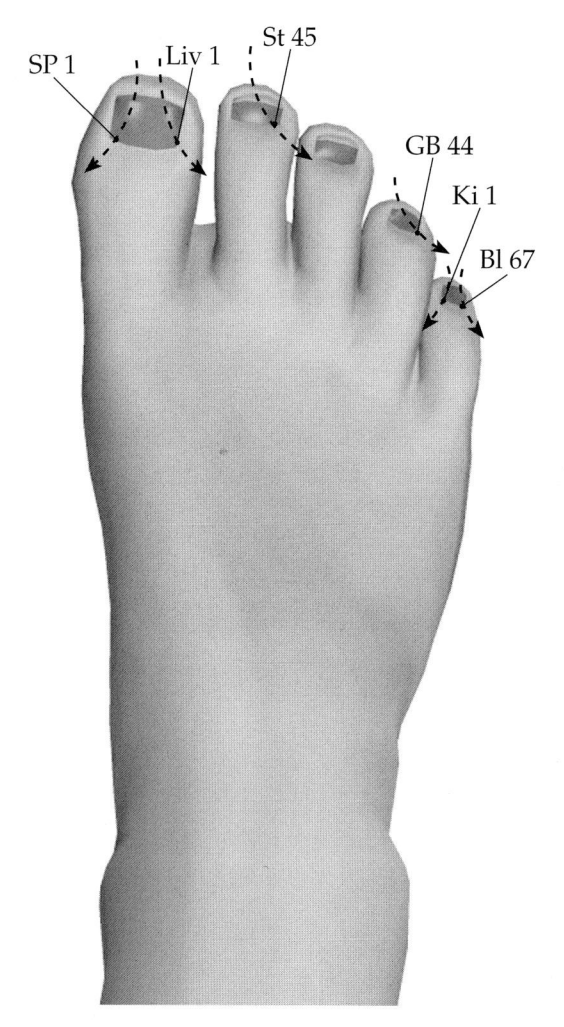

The basic method developed by Akabane is as follows: A thick stick of incense is drawn lightly and rapidly across a *jing* well hole on a diagonal axis from distal to proximal. The number of strokes required to elicit a heat response from the patient is then tabulated. Somewhere between five and 10 strokes is considered normal. Anything less than five strokes is considered an indicator of repletion in that channel, while anything over 10 strokes reflects a vacuity condition. For instance, if the spleen *jing* well hole on the right requires three strokes and the spleen *jing* well hole on the left requires 25 stokes, this reflects an obvious left/right imbalance. The spleen channel on the right is replete, while the spleen channel on the left is vacuous. The numerical difference between the values on the left and the values on the right is considered the "deviation." Whichever channels reflect the widest discrepancy or deviation between left and right are considered to be the most imbalanced. Although another channel, for instance, the kidney channel, may appear to be in a much greater state of vacuity based on a higher number of strokes required to elicit a heat response, the deviation may still be lower than that of the spleen channel in our example. In this case, the spleen channel is still considered to be the most imbalanced.

Channel	Left	Right	Deviation
Sp	25	3	22
Ki	45	55	10

Akabane's own approach to treatment was very simple. He treated the back transport holes (*bei shu xue*) corresponding to the most imbalanced channels, applying moxa to the vacuous side and needling the replete side. Because it was Akabane's contention that these right/left imbalances were the central issue in all diseases, having rectified them, all other pathologies would take care of themselves. Therefore, he limited his practice to the treatment of the back transport holes and the local use of interdermal needles (*hinaishin*). He apparently had little interest in any layer of the channel and network vessel system beyond the main channels.[3]

Kazuko Itaya and Yoshio Manaka found Akabane's treatment style very interesting and studied it in some depth, devising more mechanical means of evaluating the heat-pain threshold response.[4] Their work was instrumental in popularizing Akabane testing among other members of the Topological Acupuncture Society.

In the early 1980s, Miki Shima expanded the Akabane method further and developed a method for evaluating both the extraordinary vessels and the channel divergences. This Akabane-based method continues to provide the foundation for his diagnosis and subsequent treatment of the channel divergences. We will discuss Miki Shima's application of this method in Chapter 8. For the present, let us focus our attention on the method itself. Shima's idea was to look at the basic data gleaned from testing the *jing* well holes in new ways. He added together the numerical values of both left and right channels to yield a total value for the entire channel and then compared this with the total left/right values for other channels. In this system, subtracting the smaller total from the larger equaled the deviation. In this way, Shima advanced and refined Akabane's original method to encompass the extraordinary vessels and the channel divergences. This modified Akabane method is Shima's primary diagnostic tool for evaluating the channel divergences.

Take, for instance, the first confluence pair. The Akabane values for the left and right kidney channels are added together, as are the values for the left and right urinary bladder channel. The smaller of these two numbers is then subtracted from the larger to yield a "deviation" reflecting the overall degree of imbalance between the bladder and kidney channels. The same procedure is done for the other five confluence pairs. The pairs with the greatest deviation reflecting the greatest degree of imbalance between pairs are the channel divergences that are then treated.

Tadashi Irie has since asserted that the Akabane method most accurately reflects the condition of the channel sinews as opposed to any of the deeper layers of the channel and network vessel system.[5] This assertion makes a certain amount of sense given that the trajectories of both the channel sinews and the network vessels begin on or near the *jing* well holes. In addition, it is not uncommon that patients who have obvious and profound visceral vacuities often have Akabane readings that reflect a replete condition. The musculature of such individuals is often hypertonic. In these instances, it is the superficial channel sinew layer that is replete, while the underlying channels and viscera are vacuous and depleted.

A full discussion of the channel sinews is beyond the scope of the current work. Nevertheless, the proposition that Akabane testing is primarily a means of evaluating the immediate condition of the channel sinews raises a number of questions for those of us endeavoring to use this method as a means of determining channel divergences strategies. First and foremost among these issues is that, if Akabane testing reflects the channel sinews, how then can it tell us anything at all about the deeper layers of the channels and network vessels? This conundrum is resolved through repeated Akabane testing. While a single Akabane test is only likely to accurately reflect the present condition of the channel sinews, the consistent patterns that emerge from repeated testing should uncover the underlying strata of the main channels. From this information, one may then determine the state of the extraordinary vessels and the channel divergences. Therefore, for the purposes of evaluating the channel divergences, it is generally considered necessary to administer Akabane testing twice weekly for a month. In this manner, a more definitive picture emerges regarding which channel divergences to treat. This is the same reasoning that guides the use of pulse diagnosis in determining the appropriate channel divergences for treatment.

Akabane testing is a relatively simple procedure requiring no more technology than a stick of incense, and patients can easily be taught to test themselves. This testing procedure is considered a therapeutic modality in itself and can comprise an important part of a patient's home treatment plan in addition to providing the clinician with useful information. The gentle influence exerted by stroking the *jing* well holes with a stick of incense acts to supplement depleted channels. The ultimate goal of this procedure is to elicit readings in the 5-10 stroke range. The form on the following page provides an excellent means of organizing and tabulating Akabane findings and may be copied for use by the reader.

Akabane Test Form

TABLE 1: LATERAL POLARIZATIONS

FOOT Channel	R	L	Tot.	Dev.
Spleen				
Liver				
Stomach				
Gallbladder				
Kidney				
Bladder				

HAND Channel	R	L	Tot.	Dev.
Lung				
L. Intestine				
Pericardium				
Triple Burner				
Heart				
S. Intestine				

TABLE 2: CHANNEL DIVERGENCE POLARIZATIONS

	Tot.	Dev.		Tot.	Dev.		Tot.	Dev.
Bl			GB			Ht		
Ki			Liv			SI		
St			PC			Lu		
Sp			TB			LI		

TABLE 3: EXTRA CHANNEL POLARIZATIONS

	Tot.	Dev.		Tot.	Dev.		Tot.	Dev.
SI 3			Lu 7			Lu 7		
Bl 62			Ki 6			Sp 4		
GB 41			PC 6			Ht 5		
TB 5			Sp 4			Ki 6		
LI 5			PC 6					
St 40			Liv 4					

ENDNOTES

[1] See Appendix 10 for a further discussion addressing the question of the validity of Omura's bi-digital O-ring test.
[2] Wiseman's term for *xian mai* is stringlike. The authors prefer wiry.
[3] Akabane, 1950
[4] Manaka, Itaya & Birch: 329
[5] Irie lecture notes, 1988

4

CHANNEL DIVERGENCE THERAPEUTICS

Once we have determined which channel divergence confluence pair we need to stimulate, our next task is to figure out how to actually access it. Toward this end, we have a wide range of options at our disposal. As we have seen, Chapter 11 of the *Divine Pivot* says nothing regarding the channel divergences beyond providing us with their trajectories, leaving subsequent generations to fend for themselves with regard to their clinical application. Modern investigators have taken a number of approaches to the problem of treating the channel divergences as distinct from the main channels.

Regional descriptions of channel trajectories and even acupuncture hole locations are common phenomena that appear throughout the classical literature. In the discussion of the roots and nodes (*gen jie*) that appears in Chapter 5 of the *Divine Pivot*, "On the Roots & Nodes," the node of the *jue yin* is described as being located in the center of the chest. Rather than simply assigning the most prominent acupuncture hole in a stated region to the trajectory in question, many investigators take the literature at face value. This interpretation assumes that when a region is referred to, the acupuncture hole or channel trajectory may appear anywhere within that region, and it is up to the practitioner to determine its precise location. This assessment is based on palpation of the region in question where the practitioner looks for tenderness, knots of tension or areas of flaccidity, and sensations of heat or cold which may even be evaluated with the hand held a few inches above the surface of the skin. Using this approach, the most "reactive" hole, *i.e.*, the hole that exhibits the greatest degree of tenderness, tension, flaccidity, heat, or cold, is then the appropriate hole to needle. As we will see in the next few chapters, various iterations of this strategy were adopted by some of the early Japanese channel divergences investigators. Such an approach, of course, requires a great deal more attention on the part of the practitioner than if they were to adhere to a predetermined set of hole locations.

A more concrete solution to the problem of deciding which holes to needle as a means of accessing the channel divergences is to simply needle the holes cited in the *Divine Pivot* as the origination and end holes of a given channel divergence. For instance, if we intend to access the channel divergence of the urinary bladder, one would needle *Wei Zhong* (Bl 40) and *Tian Zhu* (Bl 10). As we have seen in Chapter 1, however, the issue of where each of the channel divergences actually begins and terminates is very much open to question. As a general rule, the trajectories of the channel divergences are described as passing through areas or regions of the body as opposed to specific acupuncture holes. Investigators have taken two basic approaches to this problem, the simplest of which is to decide what are the best acupuncture hole candidates within a stated region and to simply designate them the "master" or "access" holes as the case may be. Again taking the channel divergence of the urinary bladder as our example, the channel divergence is said to separate from the main channel at the popliteal fossa. While most practitioners assume this to be the acupuncture hole Bl 40, this is clearly an interpolation. Similarly, Chapter 11 of the *Divine Pivot* states that the trajectory of the channel divergence of the bladder "ascends along the paravertebral sinews to the nape where it homes to the [foot] *tai yang* channel." Such a description leaves a great deal of room for interpretation. As we have already seen, the trajectories for the first confluence described in the *Divine Pivot* are among the most definitive of all the channel divergence trajectories, and certain aspects of their topology have been extrapolated to the other five confluences. Things only become less definitive from here. Given the inherent vagueness of the channel divergences trajectories, it is not surprising that a variety of hole combinations pertaining to these channels have developed.

All of the treatment strategies in this chapter reflect certain commonalities in their understanding of the channel divergence system. This is particularly true with regard to acupuncture hole selection for the channel divergences. The designation of the "master return" holes that constitute the termination of the channel divergences is pretty much the same for all the systems in this chapter except the OICS protocol (now called the OIRS), which sidesteps the issue entirely. Nevertheless, the OIRS strategy clearly occupies much of the same conceptual ground with the other French medical treatment strategy we will discuss.

Yi–tian Ni's Tradition

TCM acupuncture as a formalized style does relatively little with the channel divergences in terms of treatment. The lip service that orthodox TCM pays to this layer of the channel system extends primarily to the theoretical framework it provides for explaining the symptom indications of acupuncture holes appearing on channels whose primary trajectories do not specifically traverse the affected area. That is not to say, however, that some acupuncturists trained in the People's Republic of China do not use the channel divergences clinically. Yi-tian Ni was one of these. Her excellent book on the channels and network vessels, *Navigating the Channels of Traditional Chinese Medicine,* discusses the channel divergences in some depth, summarizing the material available in most Chinese language texts on the channels. More importantly, however, her case histories demonstrate that she actually used this information in her clinical practice. Her approach was an integrative one. Rather than using a channel divergence treatment *per se*, Ni's understanding of the channel divergences was blended into her overall treatment strategy, which might also incorporate an appropriate combination of the main channels, the network vessels, the channel sinews, and the extraordinary vessels. Her schema for the channel divergences trajectories is as follows:[1]

CHANNEL	SEPARATING	ENTERING	EMERGING	CONVERGING
Bl	Popliteal Fossa Bl 40	Sacrum 5 *cun* above the Anus	Nape Bl 10	Nape Bl 10
Ki	Popliteal Fossa Ki 10	Same as above	Nape Bl 10	Nape Bl 10
GB	Hip GB 30	External Genitalia	Mandible	GB 1
Liv	Dorsum Foot Liv 3	External Genitalia	Mandible	GB 1
St	Front of Thigh	St 30 area	Mouth	Bl 1
Sp	Front of Thigh	St 30 area Sp 12	Throat	Mouth
SI	Shoulder Joint SI 10	Axillary Fossa	None	None
Ht	Axillary Fossa Ht 1	Axillary Fossa	Face	Bl 1
TB	Vertex GV 20	Supraclavicular Fossa	None	None
Per	Below Axillary Fossa GB 22	Chest	Retroarticular area	Mastoid Process
LI	Hand	Supraclavicular Fossa	Supraclavicular Fossa	LI 18
Lu	Anterior to Axillary Fossa Lu 1	Chest	Supraclavicular Fossa	LI 18

French Medical Treatment Strategies

One of the most clinically useful discussions on the channel divergences currently extant in the English language appears in Joseph Helms' *Acupuncture Energetics*. Presented within the context of the Medical Acupuncture style, Helms outlines a cogent approach to what he calls the "distinct meridians" in the treatment of both internal and musculoskeletal disorders. Helms draws his material from the French sources of Soulie de Morant and Chamfrault. However, his discussion pares away much of the dense theoretical overlay characteristic of many French writings on acupuncture. The methodology he presents is both practical and relatively straightforward.

While Helms has his own terminology for the various acupuncture hole pairings necessary to activate a channel divergence, his choice of terms reflects some of his assumptions regarding the nature of the channel divergences and, therefore, warrants some examination. In the following discussion, we will use Helms' terminology followed by our own in the interest of promoting clarity and consistency. Like the present authors, Helms adopts the term "access" to denote the holes on the extremities that pertain to the channel divergences. However, he refers to the cephalic channel divergence holes as "return" holes (our master holes). This choice of words reflects the assumption that it is at these acupuncture holes that the qi flowing through a given channel divergence "returns" or is reunited with the qi flowing in the main channel. Helms presents the opinion that defensive qi flows through the channel divergences, and so, with this in mind, we may also infer that these return holes provide a pathway for defensive qi to return to the interior of the body. This is the position adopted by Royston Low.[2]

In the system presented by Helms, the access and return/master holes are combined with "focusing" holes. As their name suggests, these holes focus the influence of the treatment on the region or viscus one wishes to address. Focusing holes are most often the alarm or back transport holes of the viscera associated with a given channel divergence. The return hole and access hole pairings for the channel divergences cited by Helms are listed below.

Channel Divergence Couplings According to Helms		
Confluence Pair	Return Hole/Master Hole	Access Hole
Kidneys/Urinary Bladder	Bl 10	Ki 10 /Bl 40
Spleen/Stomach	Bl 1 (St 1)	Sp 12/ St 30
Liver/Gallbladder	GB 1	Liv 12/ GB 30
Heart/Small Intestine	Bl 1	Ht 1/ SI 10
Pericardium/Triple Burner	GV 20	Per 1/ TB 16
Lungs/Large Intestine	LI 18	Lu 1/ LI 15

Helms goes on to prescribe a specific methodology for activating the channel divergences which is as follows:

1. First, needle the access holes bilaterally on both the yin and yang confluence pair.

2. Next, needle the return/master hole bilaterally on the yang channel of the confluence pair.

3. Finally, focus the site of the treatment by appropriate use of the back transport or front alarm holes or local holes for the anatomical region.

Helms specifically states that the access and focusing holes should be needled using "tonification" or neutral technique depending on the nature of the problem being treated.

> An acute hepatitis (yang in nature) would demand inserting the needles with a neutral technique, achieving *De Qi*, and leaving them untouched to disperse. A case of chronic bronchitis (yin in nature) would require tonification of the needles.[3]

Therefore, the superior return/master hole would be needled with a neutral technique unless it is also a focusing hole. Finally, Helms frequently administers electrical stimulation to the channel divergences, recommending 2-8Hz per second for what he terms "energy tonification" in the case of chronic problems and 70Hz per second for "energy movement" in case of acute problems requiring a more draining technique.

Helms is careful to echo the sentiments of many channel divergence specialists that treatment on this level is a strong intervention and that patients should be discouraged from over-exertion subsequent to therapy. Furthermore, he also instructs that channel divergences treatments should be short, lasting not more than 10-15 minutes. Along these lines, it is the authors' experience that electrical stimulation is often counterproductive in the case of patients who are in advanced states of depletion. Unfortunately, these are the very patients for whom channel divergences therapy can be so effective. Conversely, it is our experience that electrical stimulation on the level of the channel divergences can be quite effective in addressing pain patterns presenting in relatively healthy or strong individuals.

Finally, almost as a postscript, Joseph Helms mentions that:

> It is the practice of some disciplines of acupuncture to piqure in tonification the tendinomuscular extremity hole associated with the meridian and organ being addressed with the distinct meridian output. This is done on the side contralateral to the organs' anatomical location, or bilaterally for paired or centrally located organs. Stimulating this hole activates the defensive energy for the disturbed organ. This technique reinforces the effect of the distinct meridian treatment and may be added to the above protocol if the clinical results are not promptly satisfactory.[4]

It is unfortunate that Helms does not say from which acupuncture style this notion originates, because this is a fascinating idea. Here we see the use of cross-needling technique within the context of channel divergences therapy. However, it is now being associated not only with the channel divergences but with the channel sinews as well. According to Helms, this technique further focuses the defensive qi on the disturbed organ.

In his introductory remarks on the channel divergences, Helms mentions that, "Traditional sources state that *wei qi* is the exclusive form of energy circulating in the distinct meridian."[5] As we have seen, this convention equating the defensive qi with the channel divergences, although possibly Chinese in origin, was most fully developed in Europe. It is interesting as well that Helms uses the words "activates the defensive energy for the disturbed organ" rather than, for instance, "the disturbed meridian." This suggests that needling the *jing* well hole in conjunction with a channel divergences treatment potentiates the clinical effect by somehow shunting defensive qi from the channel sinews inward to the affected viscus.

The material Helms presents is largely practical as opposed to theoretical, and his text is clearly focused on the business of training physicians to do acupuncture. Therefore, the mechanism for this influence is not explained. As a means of draining pathogens from the network vessels, the *jing* well holes effectively function as spigots, bleeding off excess qi and blood from the superficial channel layers. In this case, the qi is drawn distally. Nevertheless, the defensive qi circulating in the network vessels and channel sinews is understood by many clinicians to flow proximally or centripetally. Thus, administering supplementation at the *jing* well hole could conceivably further promote the flow of defensive qi along the superficial layers. This could enable the defensive qi to merge more meaningfully with the qi that has been drawn from the core by accessing the channel divergences. The practical concern of actually administering an effective supplementation needle technique to a *jing* well hole is its own thorny issue which we will not tackle at this time.

The above-mentioned potentizing technique reveals once again the vestiges of the connection that has been made in the West between the channel divergences, the network vessels or sinew channels, and the defensive qi. While it is intriguing to consider adding a cross-needling strategy into one's channel divergences repertoire, the current authors have found it to be considerably less useful than the other channel divergences techniques described in the present work. It is our experience that what use cross-needling does have is limited primarily to musculoskeletal as opposed to more viscerally based internal complaints, thus suggesting to us that its essential sphere of influence lies within the network vessels.

The following patient example is reprinted with permission from *Acupuncture Energetics*. Helms makes it clear that this is not truly a case *per se* in that Father Grabowski does not actually exist. He is a composite representation of a wide variety of experiences with a number of patients assembled together for teaching purposes.[6] Nevertheless, this hypothetical clinical sketch serves to illustrate how the channel divergences are conceptualized and applied within the context of the French medical tradition Helms so aptly describes.

FATHER GRABOWSKI INFARCTS HIS BOWEL[7]

Father Anthony Grabowski, who is preoccupied with his bowel noises and sensations even on the most relaxed of days, has undergone emergency surgery to remove a segment of infarcted bowel. Given his preoccupation with his intestines, you are not surprised when he develops a postoperative atonic illness. When you visit him in the surgery department, he is pallid, and gray, with a tone of heavy depression to his voice. You try to cheer him up with reassurance that the operation was without complications, and that you can help him through the next step. Despite your reassurances, he expects the worst.

You know that the spleen-stomach distinct meridian couplet is useful for any abdominal disturbance, with special effectiveness for problems of postoperative atony. His abdomen is taped, but there is no problem inserting the inguinal *access* points of Sp 12 and St 30, or in taking the *master/return* points at St 1 on the cheek. You decide to use St 25, the *mu* point of the large intestine for the focusing point on the abdomen. It lies just outside the edge of the adhesive tape, at the level of the umbilicus. For good measure you palpate along the *ren mo*, which sends a network of capillary vessels into the abdomen. You do not need to wait very long to hear the results of your treatment program. As you write your chart notes the report from Father Grabowski confirms the accuracy of your input decision, and the effect engenders a feeble smile from the reticent cleric.

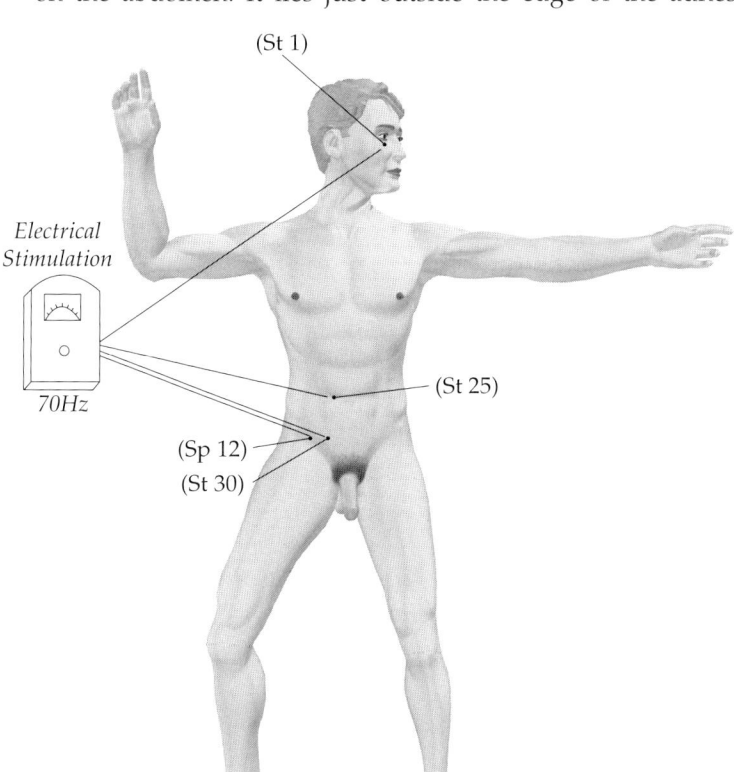

The OICS Channel Divergence Treatment Strategy for Pain [8]

During the late 1970s and early 1980s, the Occidental Institute of Chinese Studies (OICS) was a seminal force in bringing acupuncture materials to the United States. Their sources were largely French-Vietnamese in origin and reflected much of the mystical and theoretical bent of French acupuncture thinking coupled with a certain vagueness regarding the clinical application of those ideas. The OICS advanced course material on the use of the channel divergences to treat pain syndromes was quite possibly the first information in English on this topic to reach the U.S. It consists of a rather elaborate treatment protocol synthesizing a number of notions concerning the channel divergences.

Channel divergence or "distinct meridian" problems are understood in this system as disorders that are unilateral in nature unless they are chronic. They are intermittent and anarchic in that there is no periodicity or discernable cycle to their occurrence. In addition, there will be visceral symptoms presenting in the associated organs. Finally, these symptoms are believed to be less severe than when a pathogen penetrates to the viscus and bowel via the main channel. The OICS protocol indicated for channel divergence pain presentations is as follows:

1. First, treat local areas to disperse the pathogen from the channel divergence.

2. Next, treat the *jing* well hole on the corresponding channel opposite the affected side. This rallies healthy energy from the healthy side to the afflicted side and prevents the pathogen from afflicting the healthy side.

3. Next, supplement the corresponding main channel since it must be in a state of weakness.

4. Next, needle the transport hole on the affected channel to further expel the pathogen.[9]

5. Next, needle the union holes for the channel divergence pertaining to the afflicted side.

6. Finally, needle *Bai Hui* (GV 20) to harmonize everything.

It is immediately apparent from the description of the nature of channel divergence imbalances in this system that this protocol is strongly influenced by Royston Low's interpretation of channel divergence pathodynamics (see Chapter 2). However, the OICS protocol may also be interpreted as a systematic inward progression of therapeutic influence in which the channel divergences are really only the final step.

The first step involves needling local painful holes, the rationale for which is the dissipation of pathogenic qi from the channel divergence. How this is different from the local treatment of the channel sinews is unclear. It is, in fact, much more likely that it is the channel sinew layer that is being stimulated in this step.[10] Needling the *jing* well hole on the opposite side in step two may be understood as a part of the channel divergences treatment to marshal qi from the unaffected side to the diseased side. This is consistent with the assumption that Chapter 62 of the *Elementary Questions,* "On cross-needling," is a discussion of the channel divergences. Although we believe that this interpretation is erroneous and that cross-needling is specifically appropriate for the network vessels, treating the network vessels in this stage of the therapy is a logical step in this progression. Thus, steps one and two effectively function together to clear the most superficial layers of the body.

The supplementation of the corresponding main channel on the affected side is predicated on the assumption that, because there is a pathogen in the network vessel (or channel divergence) which is, therefore, in a state of repletion, the main channel must be in a state of weakness. This relationship is alluded to in Chapter 58 of the *Elementary Questions,* "On the Qi Holes."

Having marshaled the correct qi to the main channel, the transport hole on the affected side is needled to expel pathogenic qi from the body. The rationale for expelling pathogenic qi from the body via the transport holes is unclear. According to the above, the pathogen is, by definition, located in the channel divergence and not in the main channel. While it makes sense to supplement the main channel to prevent the pathogen from entering it, no mechanism has been posited for how the transport holes function to evict a pathogen from the channel divergence. Chapter 44 of the *Divine Pivot,* "[Action in] Accordance With the Qi of the Day & the Divisions of the Four Seasons," recommends transport holes for "diseases that come and go," although such disorders are by no means always channel divergence problems. Chapter 1 of the same text prescribes the transport holes for diseases of the viscera, and channel divergence problems will have a visceral component. Nevertheless, it is stretching acupuncture theory to assert that transport holes specifically access the channel divergences layer. It could be argued that, within the context of the present protocol, the channel divergence layer has already been accessed in steps one and two. However, we have already demonstrated that these procedures are much more likely stimulating the channel sinew and network vessel layers. In light of this, it is more in keeping with orthodox acupuncture theory to interpret steps three and four as focusing on the main channel, as opposed to the channel divergence *per se*.

It is not until step four that we see a definitive channel divergence influence when we are instructed to needle the access and master holes associated with the corresponding channel divergence. The OICS source material does not distinguish between the holes on the upper body and those on the head, preferring the term "union points" to denote the acupuncture holes specifically associated with the channel divergences. However, it is clear that they are to be needled together. Naturally, the protocol reflects its own interpretation regarding precisely what these holes may be. Their interpretation is as follows:

CHANNEL DIVERGENCE COUPLINGS ACCORDING TO OICS		
Kidneys/Urinary Bladder	Bl 40	Bl 10, Ki 10
Liver/Gallbladder	CV 2	GB 1, Liv 5, GB 30, GB 1
Spleen/Stomach	St 30	Bl 1, Ki 11
Heart/Small Intestine	GB 22	Bl 1, Ht 1, SI 10
Pericardium/Triple Burner	Chest Thorax	Per 1, TB 16, GV 20
Lungs/Large Intestine	Chest Thorax	LI 18, Lu 1, LI 15, LI 18

In this step, we return to more consensual ground regarding what a channel divergence treatment should look like. It is interesting that this step appears where it does so late in the protocol. Even assuming that each of the above steps exerted some influence on the channel divergence system, those procedures must be seen as preparation for the main event. Step five is the heart of this channel divergence treatment protocol.

Needling GV 20 in the final step is said to provide for a general rebalancing. In subsequent chapters, we will see that the use of this acupuncture hole within the context of channel divergences therapies may be rationalized from a number of different perspectives.

TREATMENT SCHEME FOR THE OICS CHANNEL DIVERGENCE PROTOCOL

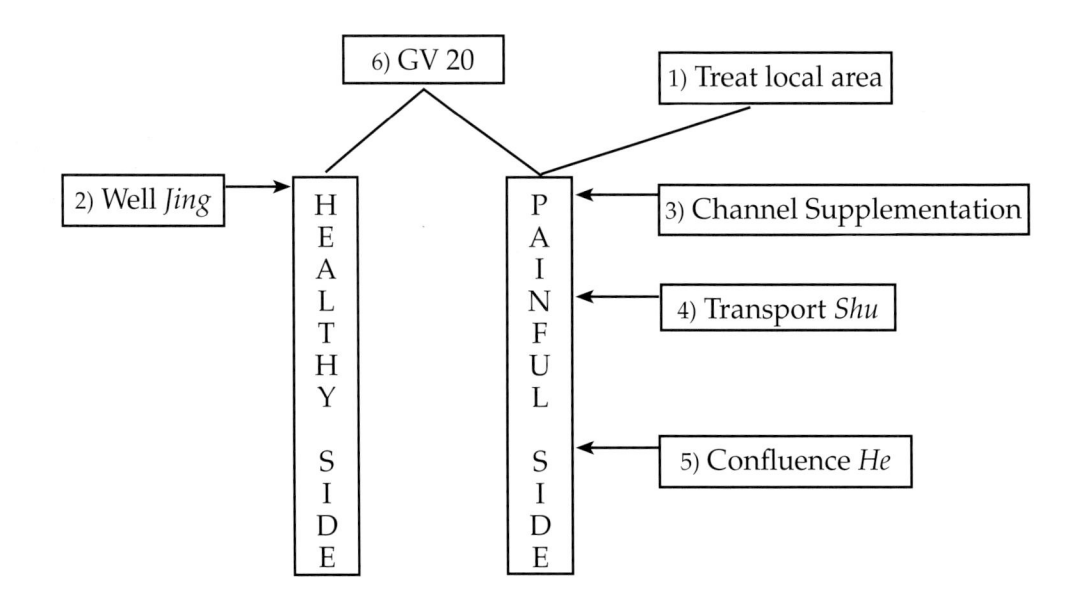

```
                    6) GV 20              1) Treat local area
                       /\
  2) Well Jing  →   H     P      ←  3) Channel Supplementation
                    E     A
                    A     I
                    L     N      ←  4) Transport Shu
                    T     F
                    H     U
                    Y     L
                          
                    S     S      ←  5) Confluence He
                    I     I
                    D     D
                    E     E
```

When viewed critically through the lens of orthodox acupuncture theory, the OICS protocol outlined above makes much more sense as a methodology that sequentially addresses a broad spectrum of the channel and network vessel layers rather than a treatment strategy pertaining exclusively to the channel divergences. Regardless of the theory behind it, the OICS methodology is yet another example of how acupuncture investigators have sought to exploit the intimate connection between the defensive qi circulating in the exterior and the visceral qi residing in the core of the body. Such a concept is implicit in nearly every channel divergence treatment strategy of which we are aware. While we cannot claim to have any personal clinical experience with the OICS channel divergence protocol, we must admit that it is comprehensive in its scope, in fact, almost to the point of vagueness. It evokes an elegant image of gradually working inward in an effort to sweep away a pain producing pathogen even as we recruit visceral qi to actively evict that pathogen outward.

We will now proceed to an examination of the channel divergence methodologies originating in Japan.

Endnotes

[1] Ni: 5-7
[2] Low: 126-132
[3] Helms: 194
[4] *Ibid.*: 195
[5] *Ibid.*: 189
[6] "The patients are imaginary agglomerates…and teaching vehicles." Helms: xix
[7] Reprinted with permission from Helms: 213
[8] Seminar notes from the Occidental Institute of Chinese Studies, 1980
[9] The transport hole referred to here is the transport *shu* hole, the third in the series of transport holes on the extremities.
[10] The same material from which this channel divergence protocol is derived also contains protocols for addressing the tendinomuscular meridians (channel sinews) and for the local treatment of pain. Step one in both of these procedures is the "dispersal of acupuncture points closest to the center of the pain." Regardless of whether one believes one is stimulating the channel sinews or the channel divergences, within the context of the overall system, the technique appears to be the same.

5

Tadashi Irie's Channel Divergence Treatment Style

Tadashi Irie is perhaps the best known and most influential of the channel divergence specialists in Japan. Born in 1927, Irie was first trained as a statistical mathematician. He inherited his father's herbal apothecary with no knowledge of herbs, although he subsequently married a pharmacist and went on to become a master acupuncturist. Irie's frustration with the lack of systematic learning in acupuncture training led him to Yoshio Manaka with whom he studied extensively. Like many of the acupuncturists in Manaka's circle, Irie was keenly interested in the secondary channels, and, as he came into his own as an acupuncturist, he became widely recognized as an authority on channel divergence therapy. Even though he developed treatment methods that ultimately did not rely on them, Irie's set of channel divergence master holes on the head has become the standard for many channel divergence practitioners in Japan regardless of the style they practice.

In contrast to the progressive refinement and simplification evident in the evolution of Kodo Seki's style, Irie's approach to channel divergence therapy is characterized by a high degree of complexity and diagnostic sophistication. He almost always treats more than one channel divergence at a time, and his approach reflects a deep concern for the pathogenesis of disease. Irie's style is, therefore, very much concerned with establishing a hierarchy of importance for the channel divergences involved in any illness, and each layer of this hierarchy requires a different treatment strategy. Irie's treatment style is nothing if not systematic and continually evolving.

Irie's primary focus is on addressing the channel divergence system in as comprehensive manner as possible. Toward this end, he not only determines the most unbalanced side of the primary channel divergence involved, he has also developed different treatment protocols for each of the various channel divergence pairings. For instance, a hand and foot channel divergence pairing requires a slightly different treatment strategy than a hand and hand channel divergence pairing. Finally, he is unique in that he combines his acupuncture treatments with the administration of *kanpo* herbal medicine,[1] and the methodology he uses for determining which formulas to prescribe is a direct outgrowth of his acupuncture diagnostic process. Irie has categorized each of the major *kanpo yaku* formulas as pertaining to one of the six confluences. Some of these categorizations are by no means obvious to the present authors, at least in terms of how these formulas are used in Chinese medicine in China. However, they are based on Irie's own friction-testing method. A listing of Irie's *kanpo yaku* formulas arranged according to the six confluences, appears in Appendix 6. Irie's treatment style is included in the present work specifically because it represents one of the most comprehensive approaches to the channel divergences and because it has been so influential in the development of Miki Shima's own channel divergence style.

Both Tadashi Irie and Kodo Seki have published extensively, and, with each publication we see a step in a process of ongoing development. Their insights have never been presented as *faits accomplis* but as something that was continually evolving. Therefore, it would be a gross misrepresentation of Irie's system (or Seki's system) if we were to present a single stage in its development. It is our opinion that the final methodologies of either acupuncturist is essentially no more useful to other acupuncturists than their works in progress. Each step in their development reveals another facet of the channel divergence system for the reader to consider.

Irie's strongest influence on channel divergence therapy in Japan occurred during the first two stages in his development. During the early 1980s, Irie developed a method of diagnosis combining magnets and either Omura's bi-digital O-ring test or his own friction test. Irie's friction test is extremely simple yet subtle. One places the index finger of one hand on the hole or area to be tested while the index finger of the other hand is rubbed over the top of the adjoining thumb. Irie performs this motion with an elegant waving of the wrist. An experience of sticky resistance between the thumb and index finger is a reflection that the area being tested is weak.

Irie's overall methodology involved the placement of magnets on a series of points positioned on a line traversing the wrist just above the level of the acupuncture hole *Nei Guan* (Per 6) and at a second line positioned three fingerwidths proximal to the first. One of the two above-mentioned tests was then performed with the magnets in place, and the weakest finding determined the appropriate channel divergence to treat.

The Basic Irie Protocol

Master Holes

Tadashi Irie's original work on the channel divergences was published in 1979. In this work, Irie codified the master holes on the head that would become recognized as the standard holes for nearly all other Japanese channel divergence styles. These are as follows:

Channel Divergence Master Holes According to Irie	
First Confluence-Urinary Bladder/Kidneys	*Jing Ming* (Bl 1) or *Da Zhu* (Bl 11)
Second Confluence-Gallbladder/Liver	*Tong Zi Liao* (GB 1)
Third Confluence –Stomach/Spleen	*Cheng Qi* (St 1)
Fourth Confluence –Small Intestine/Heart	*Jing Ming* (Bl 1)
Fifth Confluence-Triple Burner/Pericardium	*Wan Gu* (GB 12)
Sixth Confluence-Large Intestine/Lungs	*Que Pen* (St 12)

Coupling these master holes on the head with distal holes on the extremities is one of the distinguishing characteristics of Japanese channel divergence therapies as a whole. Without a coupling of the holes on the head with holes on their related yin-yang channel pairs, it becomes difficult to say with any degree of confidence that one is activating the channel divergences as opposed to some other layer of the channel and network vessel system. In codifying these holes, Irie quite literally defined channel divergence therapy during that time. It is curious, then, that Irie himself dispensed with the use of the master holes during a later phase in his development.

Directionality

In addition to standardizing the channel divergence master holes on the head, Tadashi Irie also established precedents for the directionality of bias-induction that would be adopted by many other Japanese channel divergence practitioners.[2] The most fundamental issue for the directionality of bias with regard to the channel divergences involves the flow of qi in the channel divergences themselves. If we assume that the description of their trajectories also describes the direction of the flow of qi within the channel, as is the case for the other channels and networks in the body, then we have a problem. Irie's system stipulates that the charge or bias should be induced from the access holes on the legs to the master holes on the head for the first three confluences. This is completely in accord with the assumed flow of qi in the first three confluences. For the fourth, fifth, and sixth confluences, however, the bias is induced from the master holes on the head to the access holes on the upper extremities, ostensibly moving against the assumed flow of qi.

As is so typical of Japanese teachers, Irie has never explained why he adopted this methodology. He has simply claimed that it worked best and has left it to his students to develop a rationale for his decision. One possible explanation is that, with the arms raised, the upper extremities can be conceptualized as superior to the head. Understood in this manner, conducting the qi to the upper extremities is actually in accord with the overall flow of the channel divergences. Another practical explanation is that the upper extremity confluences are especially vulnerable to counterflow. Conducting the qi away from the head in the three upper body confluences helps to prevent side effects such as headache and dizziness.

The Basic Protocol

The core of Irie's basic channel divergence methodology consists of coupling a master hole with a confluence, source, or network hole on an associated yin or yang channel. The method of determining the appropriate channel divergence itself is quite simple and is based on the symptom presentation and pressure pain reactivity at the associated alarm holes on the abdomen. The optimal hole on the appropriate channel divergence is selected based on pressure pain reactivity.

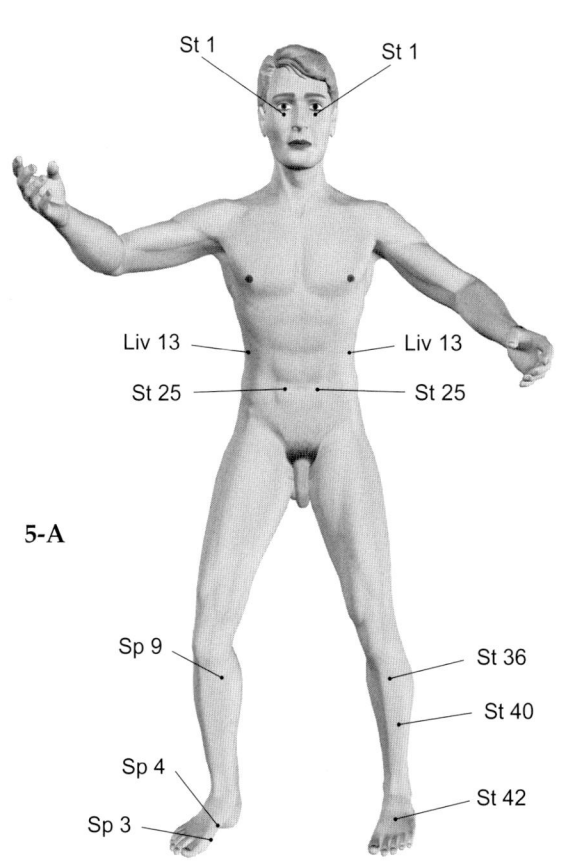

For instance, a patient presenting with diarrhea and abdominal pain who exhibits pressure pain at *Tian Shu* (St 25) and *Zhang Men* (Liv 13) would be treated with the third confluence. *Yin Ling Quan* (Sp 9), *Tai Bai* (Sp 3), and *Gong Sun* (Sp 4) would then be palpated for pressure pain reactivity, and the sorest hole selected. *Zu San Li* (St 36), *Feng Long* (St 40), and *Chong Yang* (St 42) would also be palpated for pressure pain reactivity, and the sorest hole selected. The sorest hole on each channel would then be needled along with the master hole of the second confluence, *i.e.*, *Cheng Qi* (St 1).

When using this basic protocol, Irie stimulated the confluences he was treating with electricity. He specified electrical stimulation of 1-2Hz at one miliampere of current, although he did not specify a waveform. In other writings, Irie did specify that the optimal waveform requires an initial sharp rise and fall followed by a relatively slow repolarization phase. However, he also believed that sawtooth waveforms were acceptable.

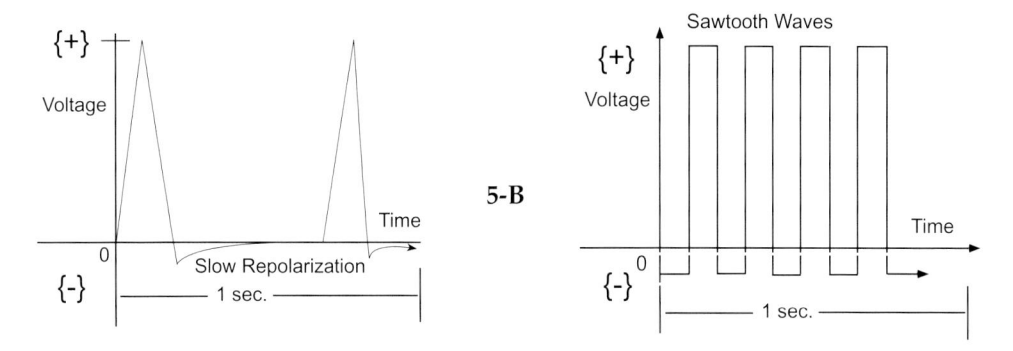

5-B

Be that as it may, subsequent oscilloscope testing of the electro-acupuncture devices he actually used revealed great variability in the actual waveform output.

Needles are inserted to a depth of 5-10mm along the flow of the channel divergence. It is important to remember that the yang channel divergences on the leg and the yin channel divergences on the arms flow in opposite directions from their associated main channels.

Irie's basic protocol is actually quite elegant in its simplicity and is easily administered by any practitioner with a basic sense of Chinese medical pathophysiology and even rudimentary palpatory skills. As such, it is a good place for acupuncturists completely unfamiliar with the channel divergences to begin working.

The Advanced Irie Protocol

Irie's 1990 publication represents a more mature and considerably more complex expression of his approach. Here he incorporates the bi-digital O-ring and friction test diagnosis so characteristic of his later mode of practice. In addition, he developed an elaborate means of diagnosing the channel divergences using magnets applied to the forearm.

Channel Divergence Vessel Diagnosis

The foundation of Irie's diagnostic methodology involves his use of two lines of points proximal to the wrist that he has identified as specifically reflecting the state of the channel divergences. Once these points have been identified, a magnet is placed on each point in succession while the practitioner performs a muscle test as a means of evaluating the relative strength or weakness of the corresponding channel divergence.

Irie has fairly precise specifications for the magnets used in this diagnostic process. At least two 1.5 x 3cm cylinder magnets are required for this initial stage of diagnosis. In addition, two bar magnets are required to determine the subordinate channel divergences involved. A further discussion regarding the specifications of Irie's cylinder and bar magnets and how to assemble them yourself appears in Appendix 8.

We have described the methodology using the O-ring test because readers are more likely to be familiar with it and it is quite a bit easier for most people to use than Irie's friction test.[3] What follows is a description of Irie's diagnostic method.

ESTABLISHING THE DIAGNOSTIC
TERRITORY OF THE CHANNEL
DIVERGENCES ON THE FOREARM:

1. Identify the six pulse positions.
2. Identify *Nei Guan* (Per 6) and describe a line transversely across the wrist one fingerwidth proximal to the level of this acupuncture hole. This is the channel divergence line (CDL). (See 5-C)
3. Mark six points (three points bilaterally) along the CDL, identified as A-F: (See 5-D)
- **Point A** is located on the lung channel of the right hand at the level of the CDL and corresponds to the sixth confluence lung/large intestine.
- **Point B** is located on the pericardium channel of the right hand at the level of the CDL and corresponds to the third confluence spleen/stomach.
- **Point C** is located on the heart channel of the right hand at the level of the CDL and corresponds to the fourth confluence, the pericardium/triple burner.
- **Point D** is located on the lung channel of the left hand at the level of the CDL and corresponds to the fifth confluence, the heart and small intestine.
- **Point E** is located on the pericardium channel of the left hand at the level of the CDL and corresponds to the second confluence, the liver/gallbladder.

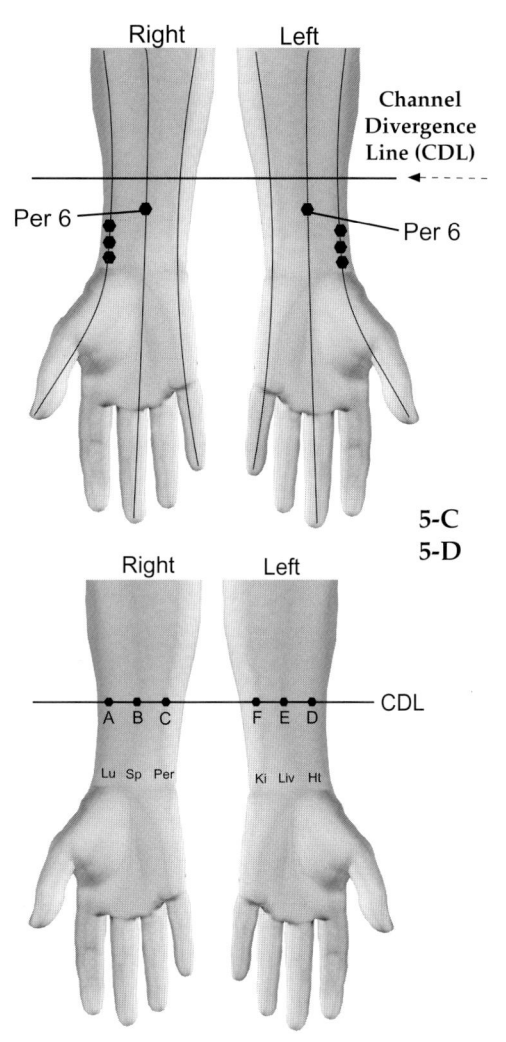

A. Lu LI (The Sixth Confluence)
B. Sp St (The Third Confluence)
C. Per TB (The Fourth Confluence)
D. Ht SI (The Fifth Confluence)
E. Liv GB (The Second Confluence)
F. Ki BL (The First Confluence)

- **Point F** is located on the heart channel of the left hand at the level of the CDL and corresponds to the first confluence, the kidney and urinary bladder.

4. Describe another transverse line located three fingerwidths proximal to the CDL. These points are identified in the same manner as explained above and marked A-F. This line is used in diagnosing the subordinate channel divegence. (See 5-E)

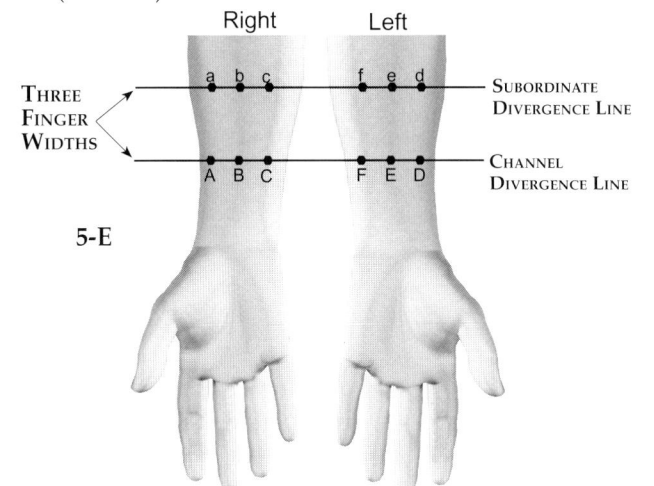

5-E

DETERMINING THE PRIMARY CHANNEL DIVERGENCE:

The first step in the testing process is the determination of the primary channel divergence. As the name implies, this is the main channel divergence requiring treatment. The state of the primary channel divergence determines the overall pattern of treatment.

1. Place a cylinder magnet on the CDL with its north pole oriented toward the ulna. This magnet is taped in place. (See 5-F)
2. Using the cylinder magnet, touch each point on the CDL in succession and bilaterally while performing the O-ring test.
3. The weakest and next weakest O-ring responses are recorded.
4. The primary channel divergence is the channel corresponding to the point that elicits the weakest O-ring response because the weakest O-ring response is understood to reflect the greatest disturbance in the channel system.
5. If the results of this test are inconclusive, then retest the points along the CDL with the north pole of the magnet oriented distally toward the hand (see graphic on next page). In this case, the strongest O-ring

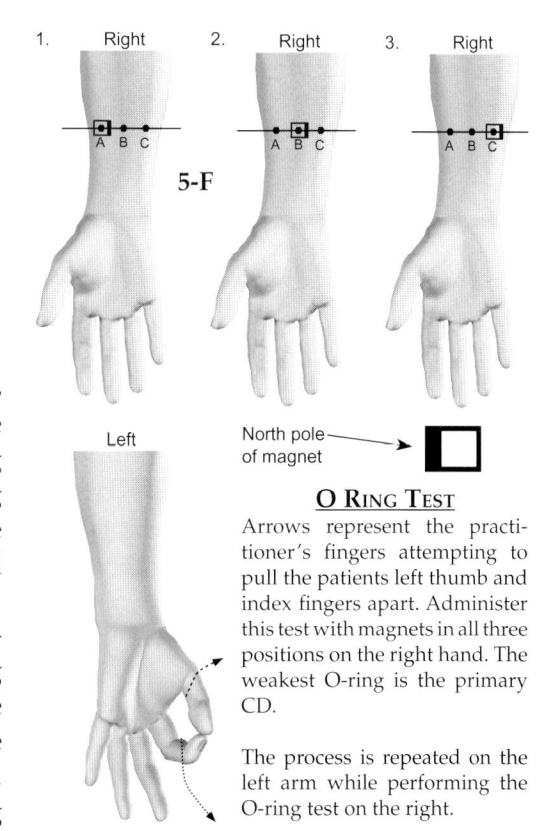

5-F

O RING TEST

Arrows represent the practitioner's fingers attempting to pull the patients left thumb and index fingers apart. Administer this test with magnets in all three positions on the right hand. The weakest O-ring is the primary CD.

The process is repeated on the left arm while performing the O-ring test on the right.

84 The Channel Divergences

response, *i.e.*, the point tested with the most difficult-to-open response of the thumb and forefinger, is the primary channel divergence.

DETERMINING THE VISCERA-BOWEL POLARITY OF THE PRIMARY CHANNEL DIVERGENCE:

Once the primary channel divergence has been established, the practitioner must then determine whether it is necessary to treat the yin channel or the yang channel of the confluence pair, corresponding to the viscera or bowel respectively.

1. Place a cylinder magnet on the primary channel divergence point on the CDL with its north pole oriented distally toward the hand.
2. Perform the O-ring test. A weak test indicates an abnormality of the bowel (*fu*).
3. If the ring is still difficult to open, then reorient the magnet with the north pole oriented proximally toward the elbow. The ring should be easier to open, indicating a visceral (*zang*) imbalance. Here again, the magnet is being used to amplify the weaknesses in the channel system to achieve the optimal combination of channel divergences, and the optimal stimulation of left or right yin and yang channels.

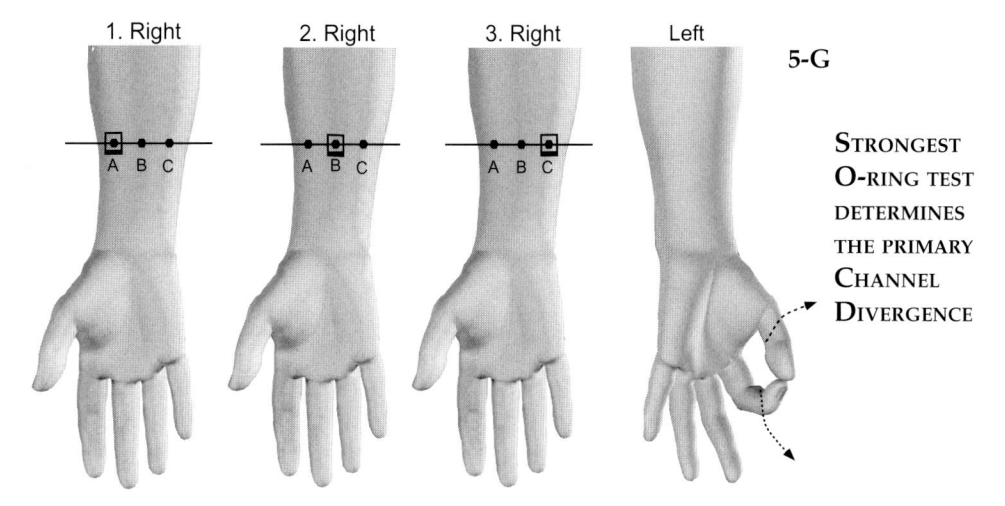

5-G

STRONGEST O-RING TEST DETERMINES THE PRIMARY CHANNEL DIVERGENCE

CONFIRMING THE PRIMARY CHANNEL DIVERGENCE:

The designation of the primary channel divergence is then reconfirmed using other diagnostic methods. This step also establishes which side of the primary channel divergence is most imbalanced.

1. The O-ring test is next applied to the Oda facial points and the Oda abdominal diagnostic points. Both sets of points are arrayed bilaterally, and the test should be administered to both sides of the body. See Appendix 3.
2. Ideally, the associated Oda facial and abdominal points are palpated with the index finger while the O-ring test is administered to the patient. However the palpatory influence tends to last long enough that it is generally sufficient to press vigorously on the points and then administer the O-ring test.

3. A weak O-ring test is indicative of abnormality, and abnormality on a given side establishes which side should be treated first.[4]

Irie almost never uses a single channel divergence or confluence pair alone. The secondary channel divergence is the next most acutely imbalanced channel divergence.

Determining the secondary channel divergence:

1. A cylinder magnet is left on the primary channel divergence point on the CDL with its north pole oriented in whatever direction that produced a weak O-ring test and is then taped in place. A second cylinder magnet is placed on the remaining five points on the CDL in turn which are then tested with the O-ring or friction test in the usual manner. Remember that the second magnet is oriented towards the ulna. The weakest of these tests determines the secondary channel divergence. (See 5-H, A, B, & C)
2. The viscera-bowel polarity is determined by the same method described above for the primary channel divergence. (See 5-H, D & E)
3. Confirmation of the secondary channel divergence is established by the same method described above for the primary channel divergence.
4. The left-right polarity of the primary channel divergence establishes the pattern for treatment so it is not necessary to determine which side of the secondary channel divergence is most imbalanced.

Determining channel divergence pairs:

At this stage in the diagnostic process, we have two channels. Two channel divergence confluence pairs have been identified, and the most imbalanced yin or yang channel within each pair has been designated. The most imbalanced of these two channels has been designated as the primary, and the next most imbalanced has been designated as the secondary.

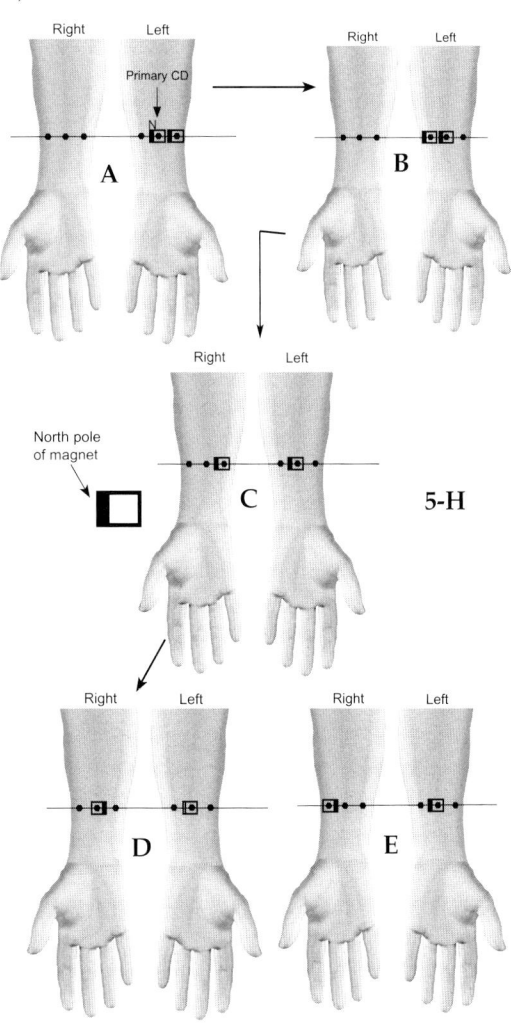

5-H

Determination of secondary CD

In addition, the most imbalanced left or right primary channel has been identified. The relationship between the primary and secondary determines the overall pattern of treatment. Combinations of primary and secondary channel divergences are divided into two categories: 1) those that are paired and 2) those that are unpaired.

Channel divergence combinations are considered paired if they possess similar six-channel nomenclature. Paired channel divergence combinations are further subdivided into pairs according to the location of the primary channel. Each of these subdivisions requires a different selection of acupuncture holes. Thus, we have:

1. The primary is on the foot, and a secondary is on the hand. For instance, the urinary bladder and small intestine channels are paired by virtue of the fact that they are both *tai yang* channels.
2. The primary is on the hand, and the secondary is on the foot. For instance, the heart and kidney channels are paired by virtue of the fact that they are both *shao yin* channels.

Obviously, most of the possible channel combinations are unpaired and fall within four basic categories:

1. The primary is on the hand, and the secondary is on the foot. For instance, the lung and kidney channels are unpaired.
2. The primary is on the foot, and the secondary is on the hand. For instance, the liver and heart channels are unpaired.
3. The primary is on the foot, and the secondary is on the foot. For instance, the gallbladder and urinary bladder channels are unpaired.
4. The primary is on the hand, and the secondary is on the hand. For instance, the heart and lung channels are unpaired.

With the exception of the latter two pairings which are treated identically, each of the above combinations are treated with a different selection of acupuncture holes.

TREATMENT PHASE ONE

TREATMENT OF PRIMARY AND SECONDARY CHANNEL DIVERGENCES:

Once we have established the primary and secondary channel divergence and have determined the relationship of this pair, we have all the information we need to proceed to the initial phase of treatment. At this time, we may also elect to first determine the subordinate channel divergences prior to beginning treatment. However, for the time being, we will discuss this diagnosis as a separate step.

As a general rule, the abnormal or imbalanced side is treated first when administering the first phase of treatment. Bi-metal needles or ion pumping cords are unnecessary at this time. Electro-acupuncture stimulation may be used. However, this modality should be administered at the fairly low intensity of one volt, 2Hz at 1-3 milliamperes for a maximum of four minutes. Needles may be retained for 5-10 minutes during this phase of treatment.

NEEDLING THE ABNORMAL SIDE

Tadashi Irie's treatment protocols for each of the channel divergence combinations first involves the use of just two acupuncture holes focused on the abnormal or imbalanced side. Remember, the abnormal side of the channel divergence is determined in the confirmatory step of the diagnostic process by weak O-ring tests on the face or abdomen.

With the exception of those cases where the primary and secondary are located on the same extremity, the primary is always needled at its network hole. For instance, if the primary is the kidney channel divergence then the acupuncture hole *Da Zhong* (Ki 4) is needled.

Primary hand and secondary foot combinations are treated by administering the second needle to the unaffected side. In the case of paired channels, the second needle is the source hole, while, in the case of unpaired channels, the second needle is the network hole on the unaffected side.

Primary foot and secondary hand combinations are treated uniformly on the abnormal side. In the case of paired channels, the second needle is again the source hole, while, in the case of unpaired channels, the second needle is the cleft (*xi*) acupuncture hole on the unaffected side.

Channel divergence combinations involving two channels on the same extremity are treated with the source hole on the primary channel and the network hole on the secondary channel.

The treatment specifications discussed above are summarized in the following tables for easy reference.

Type	Location		Holes for Treatment on the Abnormal Side of the Primary Channel Divergence		Holes for Treatment on the Normal Side Of the Primary Channel Divergence	
	Primary	Secondary	Primary	Secondary	Int. Ext. Primary	Int. Ext. Secondary
Paired	Hand	Foot	Network	Source-opposite	Source	Network-opposite
	Foot	Hand	Network	Source	Source	Network
Unpaired	Hand	Foot	Network	Network-opposite	Source	Source-opposite
	Foot	Hand	Network	Cleft	Network	Cleft
	Foot	Foot	Source	Network	Source	Network
	Hand	Hand	Source	Network	Source	Network

HOLE DESIGNATIONS FOR PAIRED CHANNEL DIVERGENCES

Hand Primary	Abnormal Side		Normal Side	
	Primary Foot Network *Luo*	Secondary Hand Source *Yuan*	Primary Foot Source *Luo*	Secondary Foot Network *Yuan*
	SI 7	Bl 64	SI 4	Bl 58
	TB 5	GB 40	TB 4	GB 37
	LI 6	St 42	LI 4	St 40
	Lu 7	Sp 3	Lu 9	Sp 4
	Per 6	Liv 3	Per 7	Liv 5
	Ht 5	Ki 3	Ht 7	Ki 4

Foot Primary	Abnormal Side		Normal Side	
	Primary Hand Network *Luo*	Secondary Foot Source *Yuan* Opposite Side	Primary Hand Source *Yuan*	Secondary Foot Network *Luo* Opposite Side
	Bl 58	SI 4	Bl 64	SI 7
	GB 37	TB 4	GB 40	TB 5
	St 40	LI 4	St 42	LI 6
	Sp 4	Lu 9	Sp 3	Lu 7
	Liv 5	Per 7	Liv 3	Per 6
	Ki 4	Ht 7	Ki 3	Ht 5

Tadashi Irie's Style

HOLE DESIGNATIONS FOR UNPAIRED CHANNEL DIVERGENCES

Hand Primary / Foot Secondary	Primary Hand Network *Luo*	Secondary Foot Network *Luo*	Primary Hand Source *Yuan*	Secondary Foot Source *Yuan* Opposite Side
	SI 7	GB 37	SI 4	GB 40
		St 40		St 42
		Sp 4		Sp 3
		Liv 5		Liv 3
		Ki 4		Ki 3
	TB 5	Bl 58	TB 4	Bl 64
		St 40		St 42
		Sp 4		Sp 3
		Liv 5		Liv 3
		Ki 4		Ki 3
	LI 6	Bl 58	LI 4	Bl 64
		GB 37		GB 40
		Sp 4		Sp 3
		Liv 5		Liv 3
		Ki 4		Ki 3
	Lu 7	Bl 58	Lu 9	Bl 64
		GB 37		GB 40
		St 40		St 42
		Liv 5		Liv 3
		Ki 4		Ki 3
	Per 6	Bl 58	Per 7	Bl 64
		GB 37		GB 40
		St 40		St 42
		Sp 4		Sp 3
		Ki 4		Ki 3
	Ht 5	Bl 58	Ht 7	Bl 64
		GB 37		GB 40
		St 40		St 42
		Sp 4		Sp 3
		Liv 5		Liv 3

The Channel Divergences

Hand Primary / Foot Secondary	Abnormal Side		Normal Side	
	Primary Foot Network *Luo*	Secondary Hand Cleft *Xi*	Primary Foot Network *Luo*	Secondary Hand Cleft *Xi*
	Bl 58	TB 7	Bl 58	TB 7
		LI 7		LI 7
		Lu 6		Lu 6
		Per 4		Per 4
		Ht 6		Ht 6
	GB 37	SI 6	GB 37	SI 6
		LI 7		LI 7
		Lu 6		Lu 6
		Per 4		Per 4
		Ht 6		Ht 6
	St 40	SI 6	St 40	SI 6
		Per 7		Per 7
		Lu 6		Lu 6
		Per 4		Per 4
		Ht 6		Ht 6
	Sp 4	SI 6	Sp 4	SI 6
		TB 7		TB 7
		LI 7		LI 7
		Per 4		Per 4
		Ht 6		Ht 6
	Liv 5	SI 6	Liv 5	SI 6
		TB 7		TB 7
		LI 7		LI 7
		Lu 6		Lu 6
		Ht 6		Ht 6
	Ki 4	SI 6	Ki 4	SI 6
		TB 7		TB 7
		LI 7		LI 7
		Lu 6		Lu 6
		Per 6		Per 6

Tadashi Irie's Style

Hand Primary Foot Secondary	Abnormal Side		Normal Side	
	Primary Foot Source *Yuan*	Secondary Foot Network *Luo*	Primary Foot Source *Yuan*	Secondary Foot Network *Luo*
	UB 64	GB 37	Bl 64	GB 37
		St 40		St 40
		Sp 4		Sp 4
		Liv 5		Liv 5
		Ki 4		Ki 4
	GB 40	Bl 58	GB 40	Bl 58
		St 40		St 40
		Sp 4		Sp 4
		Liv 5		Liv 5
		Ki 4		Ki 4
	St 42	Bl 58	St 42	Bl 58
		GB 37		GB 37
		Sp 4		Sp 4
		Liv 5		Liv 5
		Ki 4		Ki 4
	Sp 3	Bl 58	Sp 3	Bl 58
		GB 37		GB 37
		St 40		St 40
		Liv 5		Liv 5
		Ki 4		Ki 4
	Liv 3	Bl 58	Liv 3	Bl 58
		GB 37		GB 37
		St 40		St 40
		Sp 4		Sp 4
		Ki 4		Ki 4
	Ki 3	Bl 58	Ki 3	Bl 58
		GB 37		GB 37
		St 40		St 40
		Sp 4		Sp 4
		Liv 5		Liv 5

The Channel Divergences

Hand Primary Foot Secondary	Abnormal Side		Normal Side	
	Primary Hand Source *Yuan*	Secondary Hand Network *Luo*	Primary Hand Source *Yuan*	Secondary Hand Network *Luo*
	SI 4	TB 5	SI 4	TB 5
		LI 6		LI 6
		Lu 7		Lu 7
		Per 6		Per 6
		Ht 5		Ht 5
	TB 4	SI 7	TB 4	SI 7
		LI 6		LI 6
		Lu 7		Lu 7
		Per 6		Per 6
		Ht 5		Ht 5
	LI 4	SI 7	LI 4	SI 7
		TB 5		TB 5
		Lu 7		Lu 7
		Per 6		Per 6
		Ht 5		Ht 5
	Lu 9	SI 7	Lu 9	SI 7
		TB 5		TB 5
		LI 6		LI 6
		Per 6		Per 6
		Ht 5		Ht 5
	Per 7	SI 7	Per 7	SI 7
		TB 5		TB 5
		LI 6		LI 6
		Lu 7		Lu 7
		Ht 5		Ht 5
	Ht 7	SI 7	Ht 7	SI 7
		TB 5		TB 5
		LI 6		LI 6
		Lu 7		Lu 7
		Per 6		Per 6

DETERMINING THE SUBORDINATE CHANNEL DIVERGENCES:

The subordinate channel divergences are subordinate only in the sense that it is most important to treat the primary and secondary channel divergences prior to addressing the subordinates. Nevertheless, the imbalance at the level of the subordinate channel divergence may in fact reflect the root of the patient's disorder that underlies the primary and secondary channel divergences. Diagnosis of the subordinate channel divergences takes place on the second CDL, the transverse line located three fingerwidths above the main CDL. Points along the subordinate CDL are marked in the same manner as the main CDL. With a few exceptions, the basic testing procedure for the subordinate channel divergences is identical to that for the primary and secondary channel divergences. However, it is also necessary to establish the nature of the relationship of the subordinate channel divergences to one another in order to determine the key channel to treat. While the examiner may discover a number of subordinate channel divergences, the goal is to determine which of these is the pivotal one affecting all the others. Ultimately, only one channel divergence is treated in this stage. The procedure is as follows:

1. The bi-digital O-ring test is used on the subordinate CDL to determine the three or four most imbalanced subordinate channel divergences.
2. When using the bi-digital O-ring test for diagnosis of the subordinate channel divergence the north pole of the cylinder magnet must be first oriented distally toward the hand rather than horizontally. With the cylinder magnet placed in this manner, the task is to determine the weakest O-ring responses.
3. The clinician must randomly choose one of the imbalanced organs identified by the weak O-ring test and place a bar magnet bilaterally on the source hole of that channel with the north pole oriented distally.
4. With the bar magnets in place on the source hole of the affected channel, the clinician retests the remaining weak points on the subordinate CDL with the north pole of the cylinder magnet oriented toward the hand and then notes the weakest responses.
5. Retain the bar magnet on the source hole of the affected channel and place the cylinder magnet on the corresponding point on the second CDL. For instance, if the bar magnet is placed on the kidney channel, then the cylinder magnet would be placed at f. (See figure 5-I, pg. 94.)
6. Test the other weak points along the subordinate CDL that have an engendering (*sheng*) or control (*ke*) cycle relationship to the affected channel. In this example, those would be the lungs at A and the heart at D.
7. Tape another cylinder magnet to these same points (a and d) and perform the O-ring test again. If the O-ring test is stronger with the magnet in place on these points, then the first point is the true source of the weakness in the second point.
8. If this last O-ring test is weaker, then the first point is not the source of the problem. In this case try other points related by cycles and/or reverse the order of placement. If no others become stronger, the one point that helps all the others

94 The Channel Divergences

is the sole source of the problem, and the imbalance is an isolated channel problem.

If the pivotal subordinate channel divergence does not affect any channels other than itself this is an isolated channel problem.

EXAMPLE:

1. If, for instance, the kidney, liver, and spleen are found to be abnormal as evidenced by a weak O-ring test on the second channel divergence line at f, e, and b respectively, then one might randomly select f, the corresponding kidney point. Place a bar magnet on *Tai Xi* (Ki 3), the source hole of the kidney channel with its north pole oriented proximally. The distal orientation of the north pole runs the influence of the magnet against the flow of the channel and is, therefore, draining. (See 5-I)
2. Place another magnet on the Subordinate Channel Divergence Line (SDL) at (e) with the north pole oriented distally and administer the O-ring test. If the liver (e) tests stronger than the kidney (f), then this means that the liver is relatively unaffected by the kidney channel.
3. Remove the bar magnet from Ki 3 on the kidney channel and place it on *Tai Bai* (Sp 3) bilaterally with the north pole oriented proximally, again draining the spleen channel, and perform the O-ring test.
3. Do abdominal diagnosis using the O-ring test, targeting the two or three most imbalanced subordinate channel divergences that have been determined in phase one. Place a "therapeutic" magnet on the abdominal points (e.g., on the kidney point that was the weakest of the paired kidney abdominal points or areas) and test the abdominal points and areas again.
4. If the spleen and liver are corrected, then the kidney is primary and the relationship between the other imbalanced channels is a *sheng* cycle relationship (Ki-Liv).
5. If, on the contrary, the liver corrects the spleen, then the *ke* cycle is in effect.
6. If the spleen alone is corrected, then the problem is an isolated channel divergence problem.

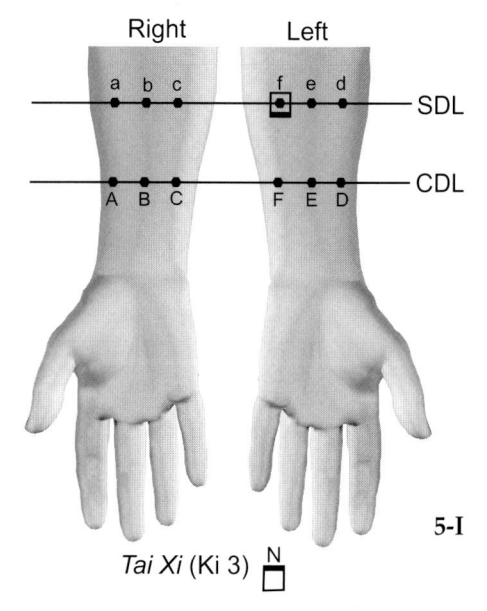

5-I

TREATMENT OF THE SUBORDINATE CHANNEL DIVERGENCE:

Tadashi Irie's treatment strategy for the subordinate channel divergence utilizes Kodo Seki's basic treatment protocols. Only the most imbalanced subordinate channel divergence is treated, and it is stimulated unilaterally. One determines which side to treat by evaluating which of the associated abdominal reflex holes elicits the greatest pressure pain. For instance, if the subordinate channel divergence is the stomach channel, then one would palpate its associated reflex hole, *Tian Shu* (St 25). If left St 25 was more reactive, then one would treat the left side. This is essentially the same methodology used in determining laterality for the primary channel divergence.

Just as with the primary and secondary channel divergences, the subordinate channel divergence are stimulated electrically. However, in this phase, the stimulation is incrementally stronger at 7Hz and 3 volts and 1-5 milliamps for 10-15 minutes. The following treatment protocol will be discussed in depth in the next chapter. It is presented here for easy reference.

Channel & Network Vessel Confluence	Negative Pole	Positive Pole	Primary Treatment
Pericardium & Triple Burner Channels	GB 12	Per 7 TB 4	Yin Channel of Confluence Pair is Primary

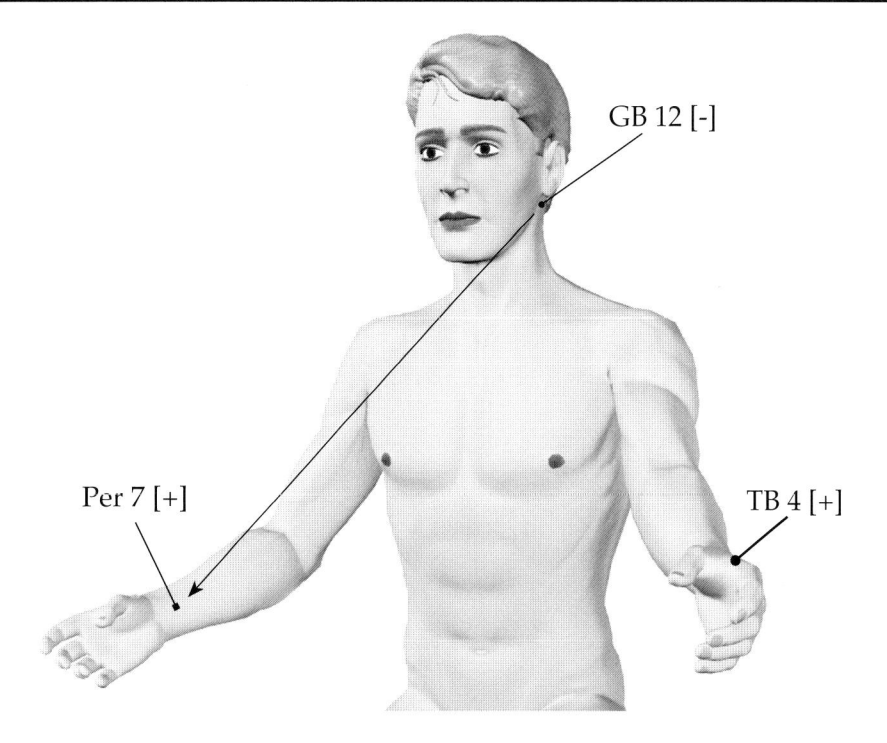

GB 12 [-]

Per 7 [+]

TB 4 [+]

ELECTRO-ACUPUNCTURE PROTOCOL FOR THE SUBORDINATE CHANNEL DIVERGENCE (from Seki)

Interior-Exterior Channels and Network Vessels Point Combination ESA	7Hz 3 volts and 1-5 milliamps		Primary Treatment	Channel Divergence
Channel & Network Vessel Confluence	Negative Pole	Positive Pole		
Kidney & Urinary Bladder Channels	Bl 64 / Ki 3	Bl 11 (Bl 23)[5]	Yin Primary	First Confluence
	Bl 11	Bl 64 / Ki 3	Yang Primary	
Liver & Gallbladder Channels	GB 40 / Liv 3	GB 1	Yin Primary	Second Confluence
	GB 1	GB 40 / Liv 3	Yang Primary	
Spleen & Stomach Channels	St 42 / Sp 3	St 1	Yin Primary	Third Confluence
	St 1	St 42 / Sp 3	Yang Primary	
Heart & Small Intestine Channels	Bl 1	Ht 7 / SI 4	Yin Primary	Fourth Confluence
	Ht 7 / SI 4	Bl 1	Yang Primary	
Pericardium & Triple Burner Channels	GB 12	Per 7 / TB 4	Yin Primary	Fifth Confluence
	Per 7 / TB 4	GB 12	Yang Primary	
Lung & Large Intestine Channels	St 12	Lu 9 / LI 4	Yin Primary	Sixth Confluence
	Lu 9 / LI 4	St 12	Yang Primary	

Irie's advanced channel divergence method is undeniably unwieldy. However, for all its complexity, this protocol is an attempt to systematically address as many facets of the channel divergence system as possible. Irie's methodology allows for the determination of primary, secondary, and symptomatic levels of treatment and provides a means of determining which side to treat. It is sensitive to five phase relationships and even allows for the incorporation of herbal therapies. Few clinicians have adopted Irie's advanced protocol in its entirety. However its overall influence has been profound. The comprehensive nature of Irie's thinking has influenced nearly all of the other Japanese channel divergence specialists, particularly Miki Shima. Irie's attention to questions of treatment laterality provided a seminal influence on Shima's interest in this area, and his adoption of the Akabane technique to channel divergence therapy is a reflection of this. While Irie focused his attention almost exclusively on the channel divergences, both Shima and Naomoto integrated channel divergence and extraordinary vessels therapies and auriculotherapy in an effort to provide the comprehensive influence envisioned by Irie. It is possible that the value of Tadashi Irie's advanced protocol lies more in the directions toward which it points than in the specific means of getting there.

CASE HISTORIES

The authors were unable to find any case histories illustrating Irie's advanced treatment protocols. To our knowledge, he did not publish any. The following cases reflect Tadashi Irie's earlier methodology which is much more accessible in any case. Presenting symptoms and abdominal diagnosis are relatively rudimentary, yet his basic channel divergence treatment protocols achieved excellent results. The cases are presented in the terse manner so characteristic of Japanese acupuncturists and the commentaries following each case are by the present authors.

CASE ONE[6]

A 40 year-old male presented with vomiting from excessive consumption of alcohol the previous evening. The patient was firmly built and still smelled strongly of alcohol. His face was flushed, and he complained of stomach pain. There was pain on palpation at right *Qi Men* (Liv 14) and *Zhong Wan* (CV 12). For this, Irie administered a channel divergence treatment in the following manner.

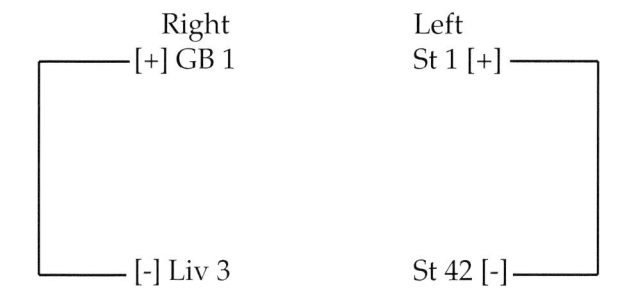

```
        Right            Left
      ┌─[+] GB 1      St 1 [+]─┐
      │                        │
      │                        │
      │                        │
      │                        │
      └─[-] Liv 3     St 42 [-]┘
```

Electrical stimulation was applied to the above acupuncture holes at 1 volt and 4Hz for four minutes, and the patient was cured.

AUTHORS' COMMENT:

This case reflects a relatively straightforward application of the channel divergences. A source hole was selected as an access hole, and this was combined with a master hole on the head. The patient's acute symptoms suggested liver and stomach involvement, and this was confirmed by palpation. We surmise that Irie chose to treat the liver on the right because of the pressure pain on right Liv 14.

Case Two[7]

A 56 year-old male presented with such severe hemorrhoidal pain that he could hardly walk. His condition had worsened three days previously after drinking heavily at a party. Examination revealed severe tenderness at *Kong Zui* (Lu 6) on the right side, and severe tenderness on the right large intestine Hirata Zone.[8] No abdominal examination was performed. For this condition, Irie administered the following channel divergence treatment.

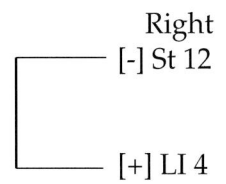

```
            Right
       ┌─── [-] St 12
       │
       │
       └─── [+] LI 4
```

Electrical stimulation was applied to the above acupuncture holes at 1.5 volts and 2Hz, and, within three minutes, the patient could sit down on a sofa, and five minutes later, the pain had disappeared completely. Three months later, the man reported that he had remained free from his hemorrhoidal pain from that time forward from that one treatment.

Authors' Comment:

Case two also involves a very simple application of the channel divergences. Note that, although the problem was clearly limited to the large intestine channel, Irie thought to check the cleft hole on its yin channel pair, the lung. From the perspective of the channel divergences, the large intestine and lung channels are a single functional entity, and, so, reactivity may present on either channel. In this case, we may assume that there was no reactivity on the large intestine channel.

Case Three[9]

A 30 year-old male presented with severe bronchial asthma. He had suffered from asthma for the past six years and been hospitalized several times for this condition. The patient had tried many types of therapy, but he still suffered from severe attacks. His facial color was dark and blue. He reported that his bowel movements resembled rabbit stools and that he was very thirsty. His tongue was narrow, red, and dry, and his pulse was rapid. Examination revealed severe pressure pain at right *Huang Shu* (Ki 16) and *Yin Jiao* (CV 7). Soreness was also elicited at *Dan Zhong* (CV 17) and *Zhong Fu* (Lu 1). However, they were less tender than right Ki 16 and CV 7.

A channel divergence treatment using six minutes of electrical stimulation was administered to the yin channel of the first confluence pair and the yang channel of the sixth confluence pair.

```
        Right              Left
      ┌─ [+] Bl 1        Bl 1 [+] ─┐
      │ ┌─ [-] St 12    St 12 [-] ─┐ │
      │ │                           │ │
      │ └─ [+] LI 11    LI 11 [+] ─┘ │
      │                               │
      │                               │
      └── [-] Ki 3        Ki 3 [-] ──┘
```

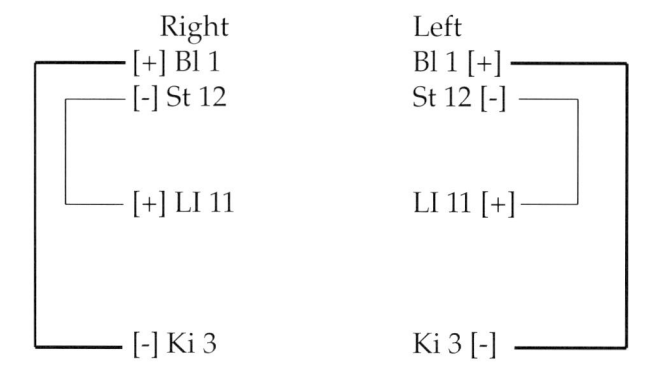

This eased the acute attack of the asthma greatly. Next, electrical stimulation using 1 volt for 50 seconds was administered to the fifth confluence.

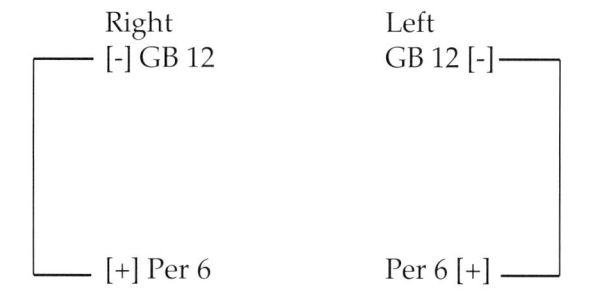

```
        Right              Left
      ┌─ [-] GB 12      GB 12 [-] ─┐
      │                             │
      │                             │
      │                             │
      └─ [+] Per 6       Per 6 [+] ─┘
```

This resolved the pressure pain at CV 17 and the asthma was completely arrested. The patient was then given *Liu Wei Di Huang Wan Jia Wei* (Six Flavors Rehmannia Pills with Added Flavors) for 10 days.[10] He was still being treated regularly and continued to improve at the time this case was originally written. Irie noted that asthma is not easy to cure.

Authors' Comment:

Irie's third case is much more representative of how the present authors use the channel divergences in the context of viscera and bowel disorders. The presenting symptoms and palpatory findings suggested lung-kidney pattern asthma. Irie's choice of access holes is interesting. Irie selected a source hole on the yin channel of the first confluence pair to address the kidney but used the uniting hole on the large intestine channel to address the sixth confluence. This is a very elegant treatment. We see yin channels on the lower extremities paired with yang channels on the upper extremities. Despite the palpatory findings which strongly indicated that the lungs be addressed directly, Irie elected to treat the large intestine. One rationale for this choice may be a biorythmic one. The kidney and large intestine lie opposite each other on the Chinese clock, and there is a potent dynamic between these two channels, particularly in cases of respiratory involvement.

Irie specifically mentions severe pressure pain on CV 17 and Lu 1. However, they were less tender than right Ki 16 and CV 7. This suggested that the kidneys were at the root of the disorder and that the lungs were really just a site where the symptoms manifested. Hence, Irie selected a source hole for the access hole on the yin kidney channels and used a more symptomatic cleft hole on the yang channel of the secondary confluence pair. Since this case was clearly a severe one, he administered the treatment bilaterally.

Although the asthma attack diminished substantially in his first phase of treatment, the pressure pain at CV 17 remained, suggesting some secondary imbalance. Clearly, Irie felt it necessary to address the matter in a more comprehensive manner. CV 17 is the reflex hole of the pericardium and the fifth confluence is, therefore, an obvious choice. His use of the yin channel on the fifth confluence also reflects an understanding that there is often cardiac involvement in long-standing respiratory conditions, and it may be necessary to address the heart and lungs as a functional whole in the context of the gathering or ancestral qi.

As we have already seen, Irie's overall treatment approach is distinctive in that he combines acupuncture and *kanpo yaku* herbal formulas. In addition, he has identified various *kanpo yaku* formulas as influencing specific confluences. Some of these designations are obvious, and some are idiosyncratic. For instance, Irie consolidates his treatment effect in case three using a relatively simple herbal preparation focused on addressing what he clearly identified as the core imbalance.

ENDNOTES

[1] *Kanpo* has two schools; Han dynasty medicine and jin-yuan medicine. These style of Chinese herbal medicine make primary use of the formulas of Zhang Zhong-jing from the *Shang Han Lun (Treatise on Damage [Due to] Cold)* and the *Jin Gui Yao Lue (Essentials from the Golden Cabinet)* as well as the medical literature of the Jin Yuan period.

[2] As we will see, virtually all of the Japanese channel divergences specialists we will discuss employ some sort of strategy to make the qi move between the access and master holes of the confluence pairs. Typically, electricity is used but ion pumping cords, or gold and silver needles are also common means of inducing such a charge or bias.

[3] See Appendix 10 for a description of the bi-digital O-ring testing procedure.

[4] Cancer patients tend to be slow responders to the bi-digital O-ring test. Therefore, the test must be administered very strongly and the tester should allow at least five seconds between each test.

[5] Acupuncture holes in parentheses indicate an optional hole for treatment.

[6] Irie, 1979: 69

[7] *Ibid.*

[8] See Appendix 3 for a discussion of the Hirata Zones.

[9] Irie, 1987: 87

[10] Irie is fond of using a specific modification of Six Flavors Rehmannia Pills. He typically adds Flos Carthamis Tinctori (*Hong Hua*) to the standard prescription containing: *Shu Di Huang* (Radix Rehmanniae Glutinosae Conquitae), *Shan Yu Zhu* (Fructus Corni Officianalis), *Shan Yao* (Radix Dioscoreae Oppositae), *Fu Ling* (Sclerotium Poria Cocos), *Ze Xie* (Rhizoma Alismatis Orientalis), and *Mu Dan Pi* (Cortex Moutan Radicis).

6

Kodo Seki's Channel Divergence Strategies

Kodo Seki was another member of the Japanese Topological Acupuncture Society whose ideas exerted a profound influence on the development of channel divergence therapies in Japan. Seki was originally trained as a thoracic surgeon and maintained a medical practice even as his interest in acupuncture grew. He is a great conceptual synthesizer in addition to being an innovative thinker in his own right. While Seki adopted much of Irie's early diagnostic methodology, Irie himself integrated a number of Seki's treatment protocols into his own treatment strategy. Seki's *Modern Electro-acupuncture Therapeutics* contains a chapter in which he outlines his approach to channel divergence therapy. The bulk of the material he published on the channel divergences appears as a series of charts that summarize his treatment strategies. We will present four of Seki's treatment protocols here. These are representative of his overall approach and the general evolution of his thought.

Diagnostic Parameters

Kodo Seki's diagnostic approach to the channel divergences roughly approximates Irie's. Seki performs pulse diagnosis at the radial artery, palpates for pressure pain along related channels, on the abdominal alarm holes, and along the Hirata Zones on the medial aspect of the leg.[1] In addition, Seki performs more conventional abdominal diagnosis. He cross-references the findings from all of these diagnostic parameters against a patient's symptom presentation to determine the optimal channel divergence to treat.

SEKI'S BASIC ELECTRO-ACUPUNCTURE PROTOCOL

The first characteristic of Seki's basic protocol for the channel divergences is his selection of acupuncture holes for treatment. Seki uses Irie's standard set of master holes on the head and neck pertaining to their respective channel divergence confluence pairs. These are combined with distal holes located on the main channels associated with a given channel divergence. The access holes he chooses are, without exception, source holes. Regardless of whether his strategy is based on theoretical or purely empirical grounds, this hole selection strongly implies that source qi plays a central role in his channel divergence therapy.[2]

Another salient feature of Seki's treatment strategy is his use of relatively strong electrical stimulation, and the manner in which this stimulation is applied has a direct influence on how the channel divergences themselves are used. The direction of flow of the electrical current determines whether it is the yin channel or the yang channel of a given confluence pair that is being stimulated. Seki emphasizes the yin channel of a confluence pair for paresthesias, numbness, atony, or what may be generally understood as vacuity conditions, and the yang channel of a confluence pair for pain syndromes or what may be understood as repletion conditions. The same holes are needled to treat a given channel divergence regardless of whether one is trying to stimulate the yin or the yang channel of that pair. The polarity of the electrical stimulation determines which channel of the pair is of primary influence.

For instance, using Seki's strategy in the case of numbness along the posterior aspect of the lower extremities, we might select the first confluence, the urinary bladder-kidney channel pair, emphasizing the yin channel because the condition is one of numbness or vacuity. Toward this end, we would needle *Jing Gu* (Bl 64) and *Tai Xi* (Ki 3), attaching the negative poles to these points, and then needle *Da Zhu* (Bl 11) and potentially *Shen Shu* (Bl 23), attaching the positive pole to these points. This combination of holes would be electrically stimulated with 7Hz at 3 volts for 5-10 minutes. For lumbar pain, we might also select the first confluence. However, because we are dealing with a pain pattern, we would emphasize the yang channel of the confluence pair. In this case, we would needle the same points, although Bl 64 and Ki 3 would be positive, while Bl 11 would be negative.

In many ways, Seki's methodology seems to contradict our assumptions regarding the flow of qi in the channel divergences.[3] Like most Japanese developers of the channel divergence therapies, he had little interest in theoretical concerns and wrote nothing to explain his reasoning. So we are left to our own devices to figure out his rationale. The explanation that makes the most sense to the current authors approaches the problem from the perspective of the assumed flow of qi. If we think of the positive pole as the place where the qi is going along both the main channel and the channel divergence, and the negative pole as the place where the qi is coming from, then Seki's polarity pairings make sense. In our example of the first confluence emphasizing the yin confluence pair (the kidney channel), we basically have qi running from both Bl 64 and Ki 3 toward Bl 11. We must keep in mind that, for the purposes of the channel divergences, Bl 11 lies on the urinary bladder and kidney channels simultaneously. In this case, the qi of the yin confluence pair is moving in the direction of the flow in its main channel, while the qi of the yang confluence pair is running against it. We suggest that Seki assumes that qi moving through the channel divergences in the same direction as the flow of the main channels exerts a stronger influence than qi moving against it. Hence, in this example the yin channel of the confluence pair is primary.

Channel & Network Vessel Confluence	Negative Pole	Positive Pole	Primary Treatment
Urinary Bladder & Kidney Channels	Bl 11	Bl 64	Yang Channel of Confluence Pair is Primary

URINARY BLADDER & KIDNEY CHANNELS

In making the yang channel of the first confluence pair primary, we are directing the flow of qi from Bl 11 to Bl 64 and Ki 3. This runs against the flow of qi within the main kidney channel but with the flow of qi within the main urinary bladder channel, thus creating a stronger influence on the yang confluence pair. The reader will notice that, for the first, second and third confluences, the positive pole is attached to the master holes on the head to activate the yin confluence pair. This pattern is reversed in the fourth, fifth, and sixth confluences such that attaching the positive pole to the master holes on the head activates the yang channel of a given confluence pair. The above-mentioned rationale makes sense of this apparent contradiction. (See 6-A)

For the sixth confluence, we are instructed to attach the negative pole to *Que Pen* (St 12) and the positive pole to *Tai Yuan* (Lu 9) and *He Gu* (LI 4) to activate the yin channel

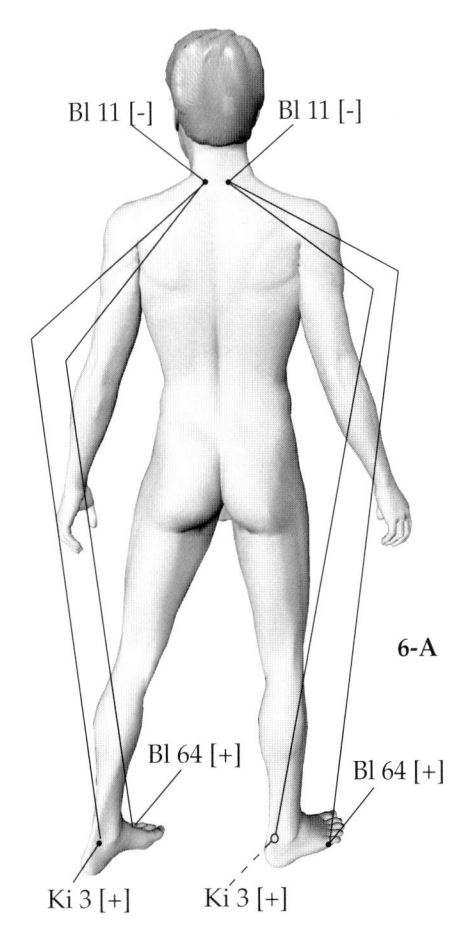

6-A

of the sixth confluence pair. Despite the fact that the recommended linkage is reversed as compared to the first three confluences, the rationale based on the flow of qi remains consistent. In activating the yin channel of the confluence pair, the qi flows most strongly from the negative pole at St 12 to the positive pole at Lu 9 in the direction of the flow of qi in the main lung channel. The connection between St 12 and LI 4 moving against the flow of the main channel of the large intestine takes a secondary role. In activating the yang confluence pair, the qi flows most strongly from the negative pole at LI 4 to the positive pole at St 12 in the direction of the flow of the main channel of the large intestine. The flow of current from Lu 9 to St 12 runs against the flow of qi in the main channel of the lungs and so takes a secondary role.

Channel & Network Vessel Confluence	Negative Pole	Positive Pole	Primary Treatment
Lung & Large Intestine Channels	St 12	Lu 9 LI 4	Yin Channel of Confluence Pair is Primary

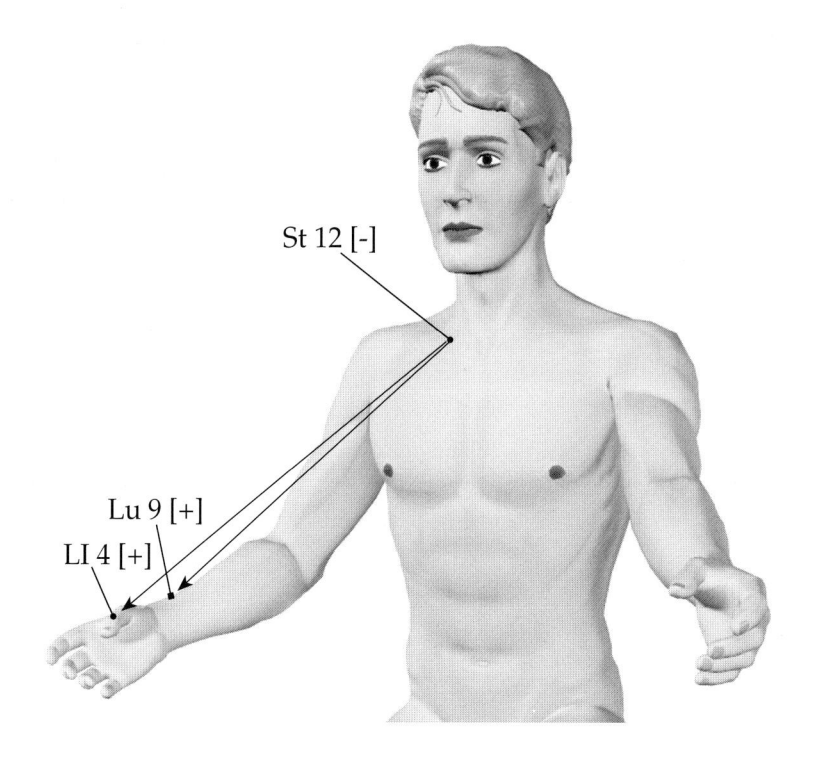

6-B

Seki's treatment strategy is summarized in the following table:

Interior-Exterior Channels and Network Vessels	Point Combination ESA 7Hz 3 volts		Primary Treatment	Channel Divergence
Channel & Network Vessel Confluence	Negative Pole	Positive Pole		
Kidney & Urinary Bladder Channels	Bl 64 Ki 3	Bl 11 Bl 23	Yin Primary	First Confluence
	Bl 11	Bl 64 Ki 3	Yang Primary	
Liver & Gallbladder Channels	GB 40 Liv 3	GB 1	Yin Primary	Second Confluence
	GB 1	GB 40 Liv 3	Yang Primary	
Spleen & Stomach Channels	St 42 Sp 3	St 1	Yin Primary	Third Confluence
	St 1	St 42 Sp 3	Yang Primary	
Heart & Small Intestine Channels	Bl 1	Ht 7 SI 4	Yin Primary	Fourth Confluence
	Ht 7 SI 4	Bl 1	Yang Primary	
Pericardium & Triple Burner Channels	GB 12	Per 7 TB 4	Yin Primary	Fifth Confluence
	Per 7 TB 4	GB 12	Yang Primary	
Lung & Large Intestine Channels	St 12	Lu 9 LI 4	Yin Primary	Sixth Confluence
	Lu 9 LI 4	St 12	Yang Primary	

Seki's Channel and Network Vessel Treatment Strategy

Seki's channel and network vessel treatment strategy is perhaps the most idiosyncratic of his treatment protocols. Nevertheless, it provides a conceptual foundation for his overall approach to the channel divergences. The emphasis here is on the main channel. However, we see that the channel divergence master holes facilitate communication between a variety of functional channel pairs. In addition to allowing for communication between channels that are not directly related, this strategy provides an innovative technique for activating the extraordinary vessels.

Before we can examine the specifics of Seki's channel and network vessel treatment strategy, we must first understand his use of *Bai Hui* (GV 20) and *Tian Tu* (CV 22) which figure prominently in many of his acupuncture protocols. The rationale for needling these holes is based on the understanding that GV 20 is the meeting hole of all the yang channels in the head and neck. In the process of studying the various intersection points of the channel system as a whole, many investigators have questioned whether there might also be an intersection hole for all the yin channels. As we will see in the discussions that follow, CV 22 has been found to function empirically as an intersection hole for the yin channels. Since all of the channel divergences terminate in the head, CV 22 and GV 20 theoretically provide a direct vector for communication between any channel in the body. Seki referred to the pairing of these two holes as his "bypass treatment." We will investigate the ramifications of this concept further in the next section. For the present, it is sufficient to grasp the idea that CV 22 is an intersection hole for all of the yin channels.

The first hole we are instructed to stimulate to initiate the circuit appears to be based on empirical experience as opposed to some fixed theoretical rule. This access hole may be either a source, network, or extraordinary vessel meeting hole. Which of these hole categories one actually uses depends on the channel pair one is activating.

Having stimulated one of the above-mentioned holes on the first channel of the functional pair, one then connects this to one of the Seki bypass holes (GV 20 or CV 22) and, perhaps, a relevant channel divergence master hole. Here we see that the channel divergence master hole is often considered optional and is so designated by its appearance in parentheses in the table on page 109. The implication is that, by stimulating either CV 22 or GV 20, we are essentially bypassing the necessity for activating the channel divergence master hole. We may choose to bypass the channel divergence master hole entirely by needling one of the bypass holes, or we may reinforce the internal connection between the channel divergence master holes and the bypass holes by needling them both.

Once we have directed the qi to the bypass holes (GV 20 or CV 22), it is then a simple matter to direct the qi to the second channel of the pair. This final acupuncture hole in the circuit is most often a network hole. However, it may also be a source or extraordinary vessel meeting hole. Seki focuses the actual direction of influence from one acupuncture hole to another with electrical stimulation just as he does in the first treatment protocol described above. Like the first protocol, Seki administers an electrical stimulus of 7Hz at 3 volts. The access hole on the source channel of the pair is always connected to a negative pole, while the final hole on the circuit is always positive. This leaves us with the question of how to connect the bypass holes and or the channel divergence master holes which are the key to the entire circuit.

We must remember that, in this system, GV 20 is indicated when activating yang channels and CV 22 is indicated when working with yin channels. Seki shows a clear preference for connecting GV 20 to a negative pole and CV 22 to a positive pole. Such a rationale may be understood if we consider that GV 20 has a very yang and upbearing nature that is best addressed with a complementary yin-negative influence lest we draw too much qi into the upper part of the body. In the grossest terms, it is most likely safest to drain GV 20.[4] Conversely, CV 22 has a downbearing yin nature that will likely respond best to a yang or positive stimulus.

Let us now examine the first example from the summary table so we can see how these principles are applied to various channel pairs. Here we have a pairing of the *yang ming* channels of the large intestine and the stomach. *He Gu* (LI 4) is needled and connected with a negative pole. The positive lead is connected to *Cheng Qi* (St 1). This draws the qi from the large intestine channel into the head. Because there is an internal connection between St 1 and GV 20, simply needling this hole draws the qi here of its own accord. We have selected GV 20 as opposed to CV 22 because we are primarily activating the yang channels. A negative pole is attached to GV 20 and a positive lead is attached to *Xian Gu* (St 43) to complete the circuit.

	Negative	Positive
Large Intestine Stomach *Yang ming* functional pair	GV 20 ⟶ St 43 ⬑ LI 4 ⟶ St 1	

When activating channel pairs that pertain to the extraordinary vessels, Seki adds a further refinement to the protocol we have just described. The table below illustrates a pairing of the spleen and pericardium channels which are the two channels involved in activating the *chong* vessel and the *yin wei* vessel. In Seki's system, the standard extraordinary vessel meeting holes are always used whenever one is stimulating a channel pair relating to the extraordinary vessels. We must, therefore, needle *Gong Sun* (Sp 4), the meeting hole of the *chong* vessel, and to this we attach a negative lead. CV 22 is connected to the corresponding positive lead because we are needling yin channels. We then needle *Qi She* (St 11). Because of the internal connection of all the yin channels to CV 22, the qi flows from CV 22 to St 11 to which we attach a negative lead. We complete the circuit by attaching a positive lead to *Nei Guan* (Per 6). Finally, when treating the extraordinary vessels, Seki combines electrical stimulation therapy with a much more subtle bioelectric influence by attaching ion pumping cords to the extraordinary vessel meeting holes in the circuit. In this case, the black or negative clip is attached to Per 6, while the red or positive clip is attached to Sp 4. Seki notes that, when the entire circuit is connected in this way, the *chong* vessel is the primary vessel that is influenced, and the *yin wei* vessel is influenced only adjunctively. Seki's ion pumping connections are consistent for all four extraordinary vessel pairs.

Extraordinary Vessel Pair	Electrostimulation	IP Connection
Spleen Pericardium *Chong Mai* *(Yin Wei Mai)*	St 11 ⇌ Per 6 Sp 4 → CV 22	Per 6 [-] Sp 4 [+] IP \

Once again, the rationale for these connections requires some theoretical gymnastics on our part. The standard ion pumping cord protocol for the extraordinary vessels requires that the black or negative clip be attached to the main hole of the extraordinary vessel, while the red chord is attached to the access hole. If we accept this methodology as valid, then we may interpret the ion pumping cord extraordinary vessel connections as secondary feedback mechanisms. In our current example, we have a charge or influence originating from Sp 4 and terminating at Per 6.[5] This is the predominant direction of influence and determines the primary extraordinary vessel that is to be activated. The addition of the ion pumping cords running a charge from Per 6 to Sp 4 provides a complementary and balancing stimuli to the primary connection.

Aside from the variability Seki exercises in his selection of origination holes for the patterns outlined here, he is also rather inconsistent with his allocation of channel divergence master holes. These inconsistencies may simply be the result of clinical empiricism. Regardless of the demands of theory, Seki clearly believes that the following patterns yield the best results. Seki himself must have been aware of both the complexity and the somewhat *ad hoc* nature of this system because he both refined and simplified his methodology in subsequent writings. We will explore his revised system next. However, before we do so, we need to say a few more things regarding the current methodology because it is clearly an important milestone in Seki's thinking about the channel divergences.

Seki developed his channel and network vessel strategy primarily as a symptomatic treatment for musculoskeletal problems. Although it is not even a channel divergence treatment *per se*, it nevertheless makes skillful use of the channel divergence master holes and the internal connections they facilitate. Taken as a whole, this strategy is unique for a number of reasons. First and foremost, it is a sophisticated methodology for promoting communication between channels that do not influence one another directly. This is especially meaningful when we consider that traditional theories provide us with relatively few options for achieving this end. Of course, we have the network vessel connections between yin-yang pairs. But this pathway is limited in its scope to those specific yin-yang channel pairs. If we wish to promote communication between channels that are not directly linked by the circulation of qi in the main channels, we must refer to a lengthy list of intersection holes and to try and make some coherent use of these connections.

Seki's system of utilizing the channel divergence master holes and his notion of bypass holes provides us with a methodology for promoting direct communication between any two channels in the body using a relatively small number of needles. We need only remember eight acupuncture holes on the head, but these allow us to move about the channel system freely. This is a freedom of both breadth and depth because such an approach not only promotes communication on the level of the main channels, but, in accessing the channel divergences, it brings very deep layers of qi into direct contact with the exterior of the body. As we will see, Seki's approach provides a template for some very innovative applications of the channel divergence system and its integration with the main channels and extraordinary vessels.

CHANNEL & NETWORK VESSEL TREATMENT PROTOCOL

Main Channel	Electro-stim. 7Hz 3V Neg. Pos.	Extraordinary Vessel	General Category	IP Connection
Large Intestine Stomach	GV 20 → St 43 ↖ LI 4 → St 1	Enters the 9th & 10th Vessel	Yang Ming	
Small Intestine Urinary bladder	GV 20 → Bl 62 ↖ SI 4 → St 1	Du (Yang Qiao)	Tai Yang	BL 62 B SI 3 R
Triple Warmer Gallbladder	GV 20 → GB 41 ↖ TB 5 → GB 21	Yang Wei (Dai)	Shao Yang	GB 41 B TB 5 R
Spleen Heart	Bl 1 → Ht 5 ↖ Sp 1 → CV 22			
Kidney Pericardium	GB 12 → TB 5 ↖ Ki 4 → CV 22			
Liver Lung	GB 1 → Lu 7 ↖ Liv 3 → CV 22			

Channel & Network Vessel Treatment Protocol

Main Channel	Electro-stim. 7Hz 3V Neg. Pos.	Extraordinary Vessel	General Category	IP Connection
Spleen Lung	St 12 → Lu 7 ↖ ↘ Sp 1 → CV 22		*Tai Yin*	
Kidney Heart	Bl 1 → Ht 5 ↖ ↘ Ki 4 → CV 22		*Shao Yin*	
Liver Heart	GB 12 → Per 7 ↖ ↘ Liv 3 → CV 22		*Jue Yin*	
Spleen Pericardium	St 11 → Per 6 ↖ ↘ Sp 4 → CV 22	*Chong* (Yin Wei)		Per 6 B Sp 4 R
Kidney Lung	Bl 2 → Lu 7 ↖ ↘ Ki 6 → CV 22	*Yin Qiao* (Ren)		Lu 7 B Ki 6 R
Liver Heart	GB 1 → Ht 5 ↖ ↘ Liv 3 → CV 22	Enters the 11th & 12th Vessel		

The 9th, 10th, 11th and 12th vessels in the charts above refer to four auxiliary extraordinary vessels that are commonly used by many acupuncturists in Japan. They are "extra" extraordinary channels and, as such, are typically paired with each other in a manner similar to the various pairings of the original eight extraordinary vessels. Different practitioners refer to these vessels in different ways, although they all use the same master and couple holes with little variation. The meridian style extraordinary vessel specialist Kazuto Miyawaki describes them in the following manner. The 9th extraordinary vessel in the chart above corresponds to the *zu yang ming mai* (foot *yang ming* vessel), the master hole of which is *Chong Yang* (St 42), and the couple hole of which is *He Gu* (LI 4). The 10th extraordinary vessel is the *shou da chang mai* (hand *yang ming* vessel), the master hole of which is LI 4, and the couple hole of which is St 42. The 11th extraordinary vessel is the *shou jue yin mai* (hand *jue yin* vessel), the master hole of which is *Tong Li* (Ht 5) and the couple hole of which is *Tai Chong* (Liv 3). The 12th extraordinary vessel is the *zu jue yin mai* (foot *jue yin* vessel), the master hole of which is Liv 3 and the couple hole of which is Ht 5.[6]

THE NEW CHANNEL DIVERGENCE TREATMENT METHOD[7]

Whatever the theoretical benefits of accessing acupuncture holes such as *Jing Ming* (Bl 1) and *Tong Zi Liao* (GB 1), the fact remains that the delicate regions of the face and neck upon which many of the channel divergence master holes lie can be difficult to needle. This is particularly the case when one considers stimulating these points with electricity, which was Seki's modality of choice. So we see that, in addition to a desire for greater clinical simplicity, there are some very practical reasons

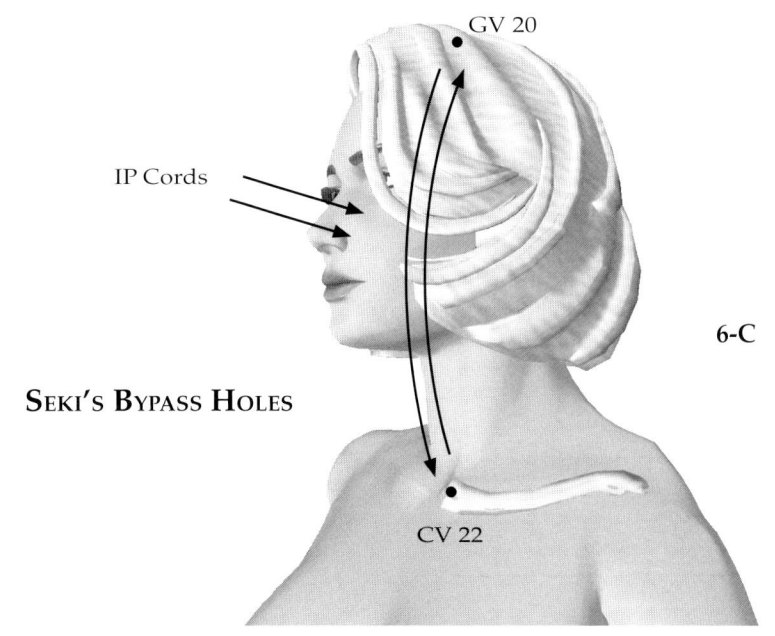

GV 20

IP Cords

6-C

SEKI'S BYPASS HOLES

CV 22

for refining the channel and network treatment strategy described above. We will now explore the last of Seki's channel divergence treatment strategies. This represents a synthesis of the material presented above. To do this, we must return to the notion of a bypass system.

The idea of an acupuncture hole with qualities complementary to GV 20 is not unique to Kodo Seki and is a notion that has been developed by a number of clinicians. The original insight apparently originated in the spring of 1949 when Yoshio Manaka was introduced to Mr. Kishi, a blind patient of an opthalmologist friend of his. It became immediately apparent that Mr. Kishi was extraordinarily sensitive to the sensation of the flow of qi through his body.[8] Manaka's book contains dramatic photographs of Mr. Kishi tracing the channels on his body while he is being needled. In his research with Manaka, it was Mr. Kishi who identified CV 22 as the complementary hole to GV 20. This makes a certain amount of sense. GV 20 is a meeting hole of all the yang channels, and it is located on the *du* vessel, the sea of yang. A complementary hole for the yin channels should, therefore, be located on the *ren* vessel which is the sea of yin. Practically speaking, the options for such a complementary hole occurring on the *ren* vessel on the head or neck are rather narrow. We are limited to *Cheng Jiang* (CV 24), *Lian Quan* (CV 23), or CV 22. CV 24 is an intersection hole of the *ren* vessel and *du* vessel as well as the stomach and large intestine channels, making it an obvious candidate for the job of complementary hole to GV 20. However, CV 24 is as painful to needle as any of the channel divergence master holes, making it a poor substitute for other tender areas. Finally, its status as a major intersection hole notwithstanding, CV 24 has predominantly local indications. CV 23 is a very good candidate because, in addition to being located at the extremity of the *ren* vessel, it is also an intersection hole of the *yin wei* vessel, thereby establishing a linkage with the reservoir of yin along two vectors. Unfortunately, however, it is difficult to get a real sense of this acupuncture hole. It has been our experience that, when practicing the *qigong* technique known as the microcosmic orbit, leading qi up the *du* vessel and down the *ren* vessel, nothing much happens at CV 23. We may feel the qi collect at GV 20, but it runs right past CV 23 down to CV 22. CV 22 is really the last "big" acupuncture hole on the *ren* vessel or, depending on one's perspective, the first real pooling place on the microcosmic orbit. Most people can feel something at CV 22. Anatomically, it is located directly anterior to *Da Zhui* (GV 14) which is a meeting hole of all the yang channels. There is a certain symmetry in the attribution of this hole as a meeting hole of all the yin. It is also recognized as having a distinctly downbearing quality, thereby drawing the qi back into the interior. Finally, we must simply acknowledge that CV 22 has proven its worth as a meeting hole of the yin over the course of two decades of clinical application by acupuncturists throughout Japan.

Seki essentially adopted GV 20 and CV 22 as the "master holes of the master holes." Ultimately, he simply omits traditional channel divergence master holes from his treatment strategies all together. If all of the channel divergence master holes possess internal connections to these two holes anyway and they are more convenient to needle and stimulate electrically, then why bother with the traditional master holes? In this simplified approach, we are instructed to needle both GV 20 and CV 22. In addition, we must then connect these two holes with ion pumping cords to reinforce the communication between them. Two cords are used such that the polarity runs both ways. (See 6-F, on page 115)

In simplifying his methodology, Seki reverts to his original strategy of using both the yin and yang source holes of the channel divergence confluence pair to access the qi on the level of the channel divergences. These holes are then connected to one of the bypass holes. A negative lead is attached to both of the source holes of the confluence pairs. The positive lead is then attached to one of the bypass holes depending on whether one wants to access the yin or yang channel of the confluence pair. In keeping with his earlier methodology, we make the connection with GV 20 if we wish to access the three paired yang channels of a confluence pair, and with CV 22 if we wish to access the yin channel of a confluence pair.

The polarity of the electrical stimulation for the channel divergences is reversed for the fourth, fifth, and sixth confluences, with bypass holes receiving the negative lead and the source holes receiving the positive lead. Again, we see a reversal in polarity between the first three confluences and the latter three confluences, and the rationale for this switch is essentially the same as we described in Seki's first treatment protocol. (See 6-D) Because the fourth, fifth, and sixth confluences all lie on the upper extremity, the charge must flow from the bypass holes which are essentially surrogate channel divergence master holes to the associated access hole. We may also infer that assigning the positive lead to the upper extremities in the case of the latter three confluences reinforces the fundamentally upbearing and exteriorizing functions of the channel divergences. Functionally, the channels on the upper extremities may be understood as being superior and exterior to the head. Whichever way the polarity of the charge is established, the stimuli is applied for 5-10 minutes at an amplitude of 10Hz.

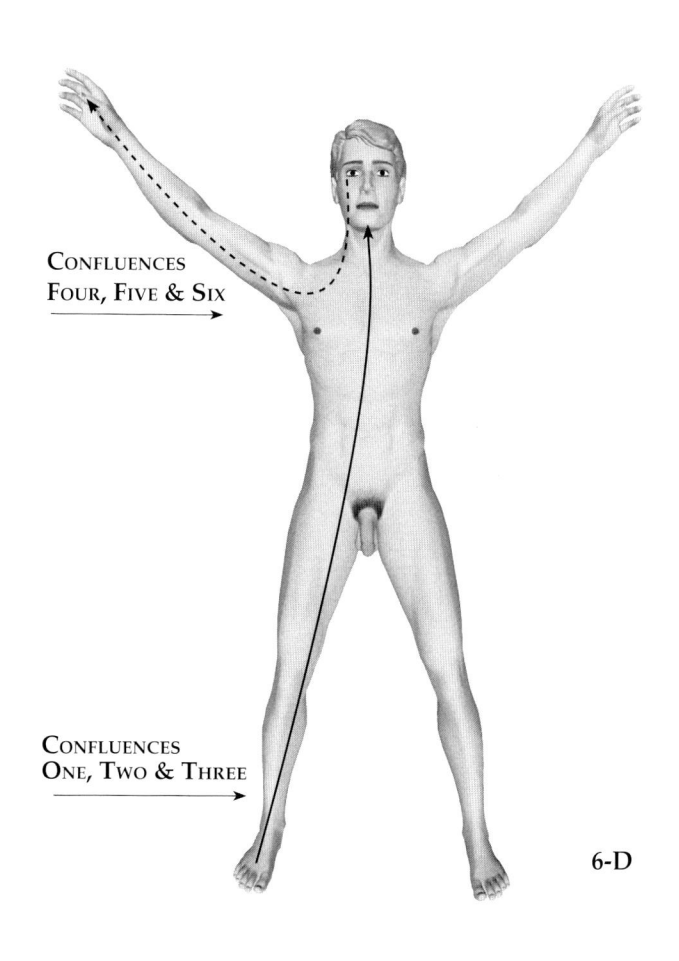

CONFLUENCES FOUR, FIVE & SIX

CONFLUENCES ONE, TWO & THREE

6-D

Seki's New Channel Divergence Treatment Method

Channel Divergence	Electrical Stimulation Positive	Electrical Stimulation Negative	Predominant Channel Producing Main Symptoms
First Confluence	Ki 3	GV 20	Yang channel
First Confluence	Bl 64	CV 22	Yin channel
Second Confluence	Liv 3	GV 20	Yang channel
Second Confluence	GB 40	CV 22	Yin channel
Third Confluence	Sp 3	GV 20	Yang channel
Third Confluence	St 42	CV 22	Yin channel
Fourth Confluence	GV 20	Ht 7	Yang channel
Fourth Confluence	CV 22	SI 4	Yin channel
Fifth Confluence	GV 20	Per 7	Yang channel
Fifth Confluence	CV 22	TB 4	Yin channel
Sixth Confluence	GV 20	Lu 9	Yang channel
Sixth Confluence	CV 22	LI 4	Yin channel

Seki refined this methodology one step further in a subsequent publication, adding a three bypass ion pumping cord and a second simple IP cord to his basic channel divergence hookup.[9] This arrangement simply amplifies the influence of the original protocol by shunting the electrical stimuli beyond the primary acupuncture holes in the circuit to the adjunctive points. (See 6-F.)

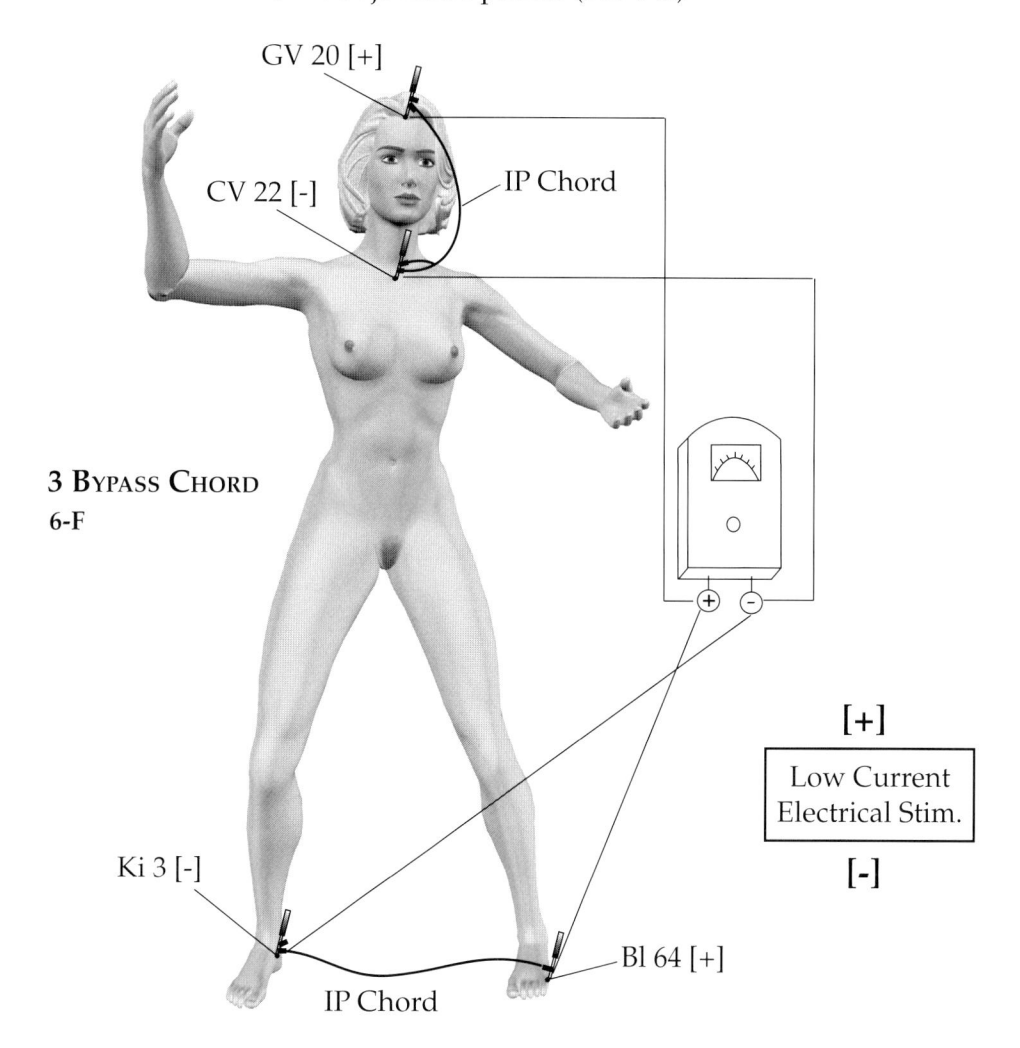

GV 20 [+]

CV 22 [-]

IP Chord

3 Bypass Chord
6-F

Ki 3 [-]

IP Chord

Bl 64 [+]

[+]
Low Current Electrical Stim.
[-]

Seki's treatment protocols open many doors to the application of the channel divergence system in modern clinical practice. However, the authors have primarily used Seki's methods as a springboard for our own investigations. For instance, we have found that the application of electrical stimulation of any kind must be applied judiciously to the channel divergences or the practitioner runs the risk of greatly aggravating the presenting complaint. It is our experience that this caveat extends even to the use of microcurrent, and, at this juncture, we are much more inclined to apply Seki's polarity-based principles within the context of gold and silver or stainless steel needles. Rather than using electrical stimulation, we prefer to use a gold needle where a positive (+) influence is indicated, and a silver or stainless steel needle where a negative (-) influence is indicated. This strategy is actually quite simple to apply clinically and is particularly appropriate for highly sensitive or severely depleted individuals.

The use of gold and silver needles in lieu of electrical stimulation or other polarity based treatment techniques such as ion pumping cords is a versatile and effective strategy that eliminates the need for a lot of elaborate equipment. When applied to Seki's ion pumping bypass strategy, however, a number of decisions must be made. Seki's bypass protocol, connecting GV 20 and CV 22, calls for the connection of two cords attached to these holes in opposing directions to effectively create a charge that moves in both directions. Such a connection cannot practically be created using gold and silver needles which require a definitive decision regarding which way we want a given influence to be directed. Thus, we must decide whether we want to direct the qi from CV 22 (-) to GV 20 (+) or from GV 20 (-) to CV 22 (+). Naturally, arguments can be made for either connection based on the specifics of the presenting condition. As a general rule, however, when using the bypass technique within the context of a channel divergence treatment, we prefer to needle GV 20 with a silver or stainless steel needle (-) and CV 22 with a gold (+) needle. Having already raised and exteriorized the qi into the head, it makes sense to then descend the qi back into the core, and we believe that needling the bypass holes in such a manner achieves this end. It is our opinion that it is always wise to root the qi.

In actuality, Miki Shima uses a different but complementary rationale for needling the bypass holes in the above-mentioned manner, one that is based on the most common state of the extraordinary vessels. It is his observation that, in most individuals, the *du* vessel is relatively replete, while the *ren* vessel is relatively vacuous. Take, for instance, the relationship between the heart and the kidneys. In Shima's experience, the heart is most often in a state of repletion and heat, while the kidneys are most often in a state of vacuity and cold. This pattern typically presents itself within the context of the extraordinary vessels as a repletion of the *du* vessel and a vacuity of the *ren* vessel. Given this assessment, it is only natural that one would treat GV 20 with a stainless steel needle and hence a negative influence, and CV 22 with a gold needle and a positive influence. Naturally, there are numerous exceptions to this rule. However, Shima finds it useful as a general rule of thumb.

While Seki's "new" channel divergence treatment protocol greatly simplifies his existing work on the treatment of the channel divergences and eliminates the need for needling painful regions of the face, in our clinical experience, this protocol represents a degree of refinement that comes at the expense of clinical efficacy. It's our opinion that the most indispensable component of any channel divergence strategy is the stimulation of the channel divergence master holes on the head and neck. GV 20 and CV 22 may be an invaluable adjunct to a channel divergence treatment strategy and may provide a convenient means of promoting communication between the main channels, the extraordinary vessels, and the channel divergences. Nevertheless, we do not believe that they are effective as an outright substitute for the channel divergence master holes.

CASE HISTORIES

CASE ONE[10]

On April 30, a 59 year-old female presented with a chief complaint of left knee pain. The patient reported that she had experienced pain in her right knee 2-3 years and had received two injections of a local analgesic which, to a certain degree, had taken care of the problem, although some pain remained. In addition, she had developed pain in her left knee as well. The Western medical diagnosis was deformation of the knee joint.

GV 20
TB 8 [-]   TB 8 [-]
No name [+]   No name [+]
                 6-G
GB 35 [+]   GB 35 [+]
Sp 6 [-]

Seki first administered the Normal Ion Pumping (NIP) Protocol #1 (see 6-G) with electrical stimulation. He followed this with the first confluence using IP cords. The therapy was completed with electrical stimulation on *a shi* points on the knee. (See Appendix 4 for description of NIP.)

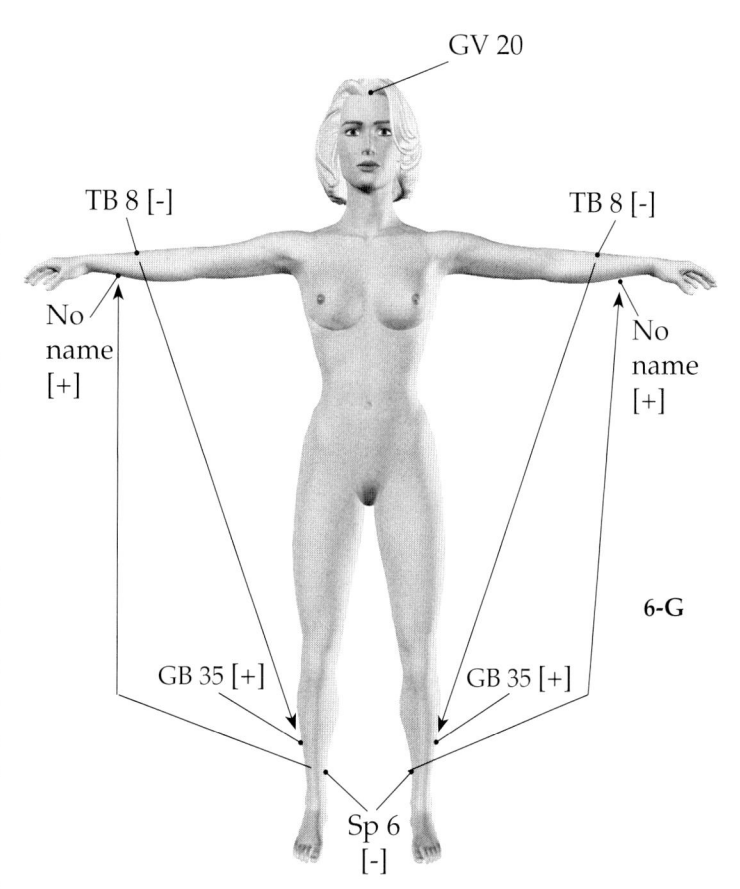

2ND TREATMENT

The patient returned two days later. Seki first administered the NIP Protocol #1 with electrical stimulation. He then treated the first and third confluences on the left leg only using IP cords and again completed the therapy with electrostimulation on *a shi* points on the knee.

3ʀᴅ Treatment

The patient returned one more time the next day. Seki once again administered NIP Protocol #1 with electrical stimulation. He then treated the first and third confluences on the left leg using bypass IP cords. Finally, he administered 3500 gauss magnets to *Yin Bai* (Sp 1) and *Gong Sun* (Sp 4) and sent the patient home. This treatment alleviated the knee pain completely.

Authors' Comment:

In this case Seki used the #1 NIP protocol, suggesting an assumption on his part, of vacuity. Shima has observed that the Japanese patient population is truly and fundamentally deficient. They tend to be overworked and undernourished. In light of this, the more supplementing NIP Protocol #1 is an obvious choice. Any of the first three confluences could conceivably have been chosen for a knee problem depending on the specific nature of the disorder. In the absence of more specific information regarding the knee beyond its obviously arthritic condition, Seki's use of the first confluence in this case suggests an assumption on his part that a 59 year-old female would benefit most from kidney supplementation. In this context, the treatment strategy may be understood as moving from general supplementation with the NIP protocol to more specific supplementation via the first (and third) confluences, culminating with a very specific and localized *a shi* therapy.

Within Japanese acupuncture, NIP and channel divergence strategies are typically combined with more localized forms of treatment, whether they be superficial needling of the channel sinews, interdermal (*hinaishin*) treatments, or rapid in-and-out (*tanshi*) needling of *a shi* points. Clearly, Seki prefers to administer these adjunctive therapies last. However, it must be understood that this is merely his personal preference. Shima, for instance, prefers to take the opposite approach, needling local *a shi* points first using the *tanshi* method and then moving on to more global therapies. This strategy ensures that the qi mobilized in the root treatment can reach the affected area because localized obstructions have already been removed.

As we have seen from the variety of channel divergence therapies developed by Seki himself, simply stating that he needled the first and third confluences leaves a lot of room for interpretation. In general however, Seki's channel divergence treatments were administered bilaterally, stimulating a yang channel on one side and a yin channel on the other. His choice of confluences was based primarily on basic symptom presentation.

Seki conceptualized the application of magnets in rather simple terms. He used them to make the qi flow. Clearly the patient's knee problem was located primarily on the spleen and bladder channels. His use of magnets on the spleen channel suggests that in this case he used the yin channel on the third confluence rather than the yang channel connection that is more typical for him. His basis for selecting holes on which to place the magnets was most probably palpation for point tenderness. From a more theoretical perspective, Sp 1 is the origin of the channel where the qi begins to flow, and Sp 4 is the network hole which is indicated for chronic obstructions. Whatever his rationale, Seki's choice of these distal holes served to mobilize the qi and push through the long-standing obstruction in the knee.

CASE TWO

On May 5, a 45 year-old male presented with the chief complaints of malaise, heaviness in the neck and shoulders, and back pain following a whiplash injury sustained eight years previously. He had been hospitalized for three months and had used a corset for one month.

Seki's initial treatment was as follows: *Shen Mai* (Bl 62) black to *Hou Xi* (SI 3) red and *Wai Guan* (TB 5) black to *Lin Qi* (GB 41) red needled ipsilaterally. He then treated the fourth confluence bilaterally, needling the yin channel on one side and the yang channel on the other, and administered electrical stimulation. The third component of the therapy involved his bypass treatment.

2ND TREATMENT
The patient returned on May 8, complaining of occipital headaches and spastic pressure pain lateral and inferior to the left scapula. Seki administered Bl 62 black to SI 3 red and TB 5 black to GB 41 red needled ipsilaterally. He then treated the fourth confluence bilaterally. In addition, he applied 3500 gauss magnets north to *Zan Zhu* (Bl 2) and south on *Mei Chong* (Bl 3) respectively. The magnets cleared the headaches.

3RD TREATMENT
The patient returned on May 13, two days subsequent to the previous treatment, the patient again experienced the neck pain and occipital headache. Bending his head backward caused pain at Bl 10. Seki administered 3500 gauss magnets in a supplementing manner on the urinary bladder channels. He followed this with Bl 62 black to SI 3 red and TB 5 black to GB 41 red needled ipsilaterally, Finally he needled the fourth confluence bilaterally. This treatment proved only mildly effective.

4TH TREATMENT
The patient returned on May 20, complaining of back pain with a heavy pressure sensation. Backward bending caused a sensation of blockage. Seki administered 3500 gauss magnets in a supplementing manner on the urinary bladder channels and then administered the NIP Protocol # 1 with electrical stimulation. His next step was to stimulate the first confluence bilaterally. He finished by applying *nen-shin* to *Kun Lun* (Bl 60) which produced excellent results.[11]

5ᵗʰ Treatment

On May 30, the patient returned complaining of a tight sensation in the upper part of the shoulders and the back of his neck. Seki administered 3500 gauss magnets in a supplementing manner on the urinary bladder channel and then administered the NIP Protocol # 1 with electrical stimulation. His next step was to stimulate the first confluence bilaterally.

6ᵗʰ Treatment

On June 5, the patient returned complaining of a painful feeling in the occipital area accompanied by spasms in his shoulders. However, he was still able to turn his neck. Seki administered Bl 62 black to SI 3 red, and TB 5 black to GB 41 red needled ipsilaterally. He then treated the second and fourth confluence bilaterally. This again produced an excellent result.

Authors' Comment:

The vagueness of the actual therapies notwithstanding, this is an honest case. There is clearly a great deal of trial and error going on here. Seki's approach to this patient illustrates the importance of administering the correct therapy in the right sequence at the correct time. His initial treatment strategy is obviously based on a combination of Manaka's whiplash treatment employing IP cords with the extraordinary vessels, and the channel divergences. This approach alone is insufficient in this case, however, and Seki casts about for the right adjunctive treatments. Although he uses his bypass strategy in the first treatment, he quickly switches to magnets.

While the magnets appear to have been somewhat helpful symptomatically in this case, they do not appear to be the central factor in an effective therapy. Nevertheless, we see Seki moving from using magnets locally in a draining, pain-relieving manner to using them in a vague but ostensibly more systemic and supplementing manner. This supplementation is moderately effective but is not sufficient to resolve the case. So he includes the NIP protocol which produced a fundamental shift in the therapy. Here again we see Seki's fondness for the NIP supplementing protocol in cases where a systemic supplementation is indicated. After three treatments, which achieved only marginal results, he added the NIP protocol and needle twirling *nenshin* technique to produce a definitive improvement.

Having found the missing piece in his therapy, Seki applied the NIP protocol again in the subsequent treatment but eliminated all but the channel divergence therapies. Once things were moving in the right direction, he then returned to his original treatment strategy, using the extraordinary vessels and the channel divergences.

Despite his obvious predilection toward electrical stimulation, Seki was actually quite adept at needle manipulation and even published on this topic. The *nenshin* needle twirling technique was a potent tool in his hands, particularly in the treatment of pain. He would stay with his patient, twirling the needle gently, 40-60 seconds a needle for extended periods of time. This technique may also have been a pivotal factor in the positive resolution of this case, and it is curious that he only used it once.

CASE THREE

A 64 year-old female presented on April 22, 1981 with back pain accompanied by an electrical sensation referring down her legs. Her medical history included a two-month hospitalization for a third-degree burn in 1980.[12] In March of 1981 the patient began experiencing occasional back pain accompanied by pain referring down the upper thighs accompanied by numbness on the posterior and lateral sides of the legs. Seki administered the NIP Protocol #1 with electrical stimulation. He then needled the first and second confluences bilaterally. He then administered a bypass cord to GV 20 and CV 22.

2ND TREATMENT
The patient returned on April 27, and the treatment was repeated.[13]

3RD TREATMENT
The patient returned the next day and the above treatment was repeated. In addition, electrical stimulation was applied to *a shi* holes on the lumbar region.

Following this course of three treatments the patient achieved a complete cure.

AUTHORS' COMMENT:

In this case Seki began with the NIP Protocol #1 administered in conjunction with the yang channel pairs of the first and second confluences, the bladder and gallbladder channel divergences. We surmise that the addition of the bypass therapy serves to both integrate and potentiate the effect of the other two facets of the treatment. The patient achieved some degree of improvement subsequent to the first two treatments but it isn't until a more local treatment is added utilizing electro-acupuncture on the *a shi* holes that the pain disappears completely. Clearly, a root treatment, regardless of whether it is a channel divergence or extraordinary vessel therapy, is sometimes insufficient to resolve a condition completely and in these instances a symptom relieving step is indicated. It is interesting to note, however, that Seki's first impulse was to see what the combined NIP/channel divergence protocol could achieve on its own.

CASE FOUR

A 41 year-old female presented on April 9, 1981. She reported having suffered from migraines since 1971, and from muscle spasms in her shoulders since 1980. Seki administered the NIP Protocol #1 with electrical stimulation. He then needled the second confluence on the right side with bypass cords.

2ND TREATMENT
The patient returned on April 23, 1981 and Seki administered the same treatment with the addition of 3500 gauss magnets applied to *Tong Zi Liao* (GB 1) north, and *Ting Hui* (GB 2) south.

3RD TREATMENT
The patient returned on May 5, 1981. Seki administered the NIP Protocol #1 with electrical stimulation. He then needled the second confluence on the right side with bypass cords.

4TH TREATMENT
The patient returned on May 13, 1981 and Seki administered the same treatment with the addition of 3500 gauss magnets applied to GB 1 north and GB 2 south.

5TH TREATMENT
The patient returned on May 19 and Seki administered the same treatment as the previous visit.

6TH TREATMENT
The patient returned on June 2 and Seki administered the same treatment but did not apply the magnets.

Subsequent to this course of six treatments, the patient no longer suffered from migraines or muscle spasms in her shoulders.

AUTHORS' COMMENT:

Once more we see the integration of magnets into a combined NIP and channel divergence protocol. Seki had no fixed criteria for when to use magnets and would assess the state of each patient's qi by palpation and determine on a case-by-case basis whether magnets were indicated. His choice of the north pole on GB 1 and the south on GB 2 was based in his intention of creating an initial momentum for the flow of qi in a downward direction.

ENDNOTES

[1] See Appendix 3 for a discussion of the Hirata Zones.
[2] Seki's *Modern Electro-acupuncture Therapeutics* states that the acupuncture hole *Da Zhong* (Ki 4) is the access hole for the kidney channel divergence. This is a typographical error as is evident from his many other publications that list *Tai Xi* (Ki 3) as the access hole of choice.
[3] Reader is referred to pages 37-38 for discussion of empirical basis of these therapies.
[4] Seki once mentioned to Shima that modern Japanese have too much yang qi in their head, and that, in his opinion, draining GV 20 worked well simply because it calmed people down. The same is probably true of Westerners.
[5] It must be acknowledged that, despite their obvious efficacy, nothing has been shown to move through IP cords when connected to needles without electrical stimulation. When the bias is greater than 0.4 volts in electro-acupuncture, electrons do flow through a diode in the manner specified by Seki.
[6] Miyawaki: 32
[7] Seki, 1986: 33
[8] Manaka, 1983: 39
[9] Seki, 1986-B: 33
[10] All case histories are taken from Seki: 1982
[11] *Nenshin* is defined as the very gentle consistent twirling of a needle to elicit a tingling sensation (*hibiki*) without the stronger *deqi* sensation of distending soreness. It is regarded as a central component of many Japanese acupuncture traditions and it is essential that an acupuncturist give good *nenshin*.
[12] This case history and those that follow are especially terse. For instance, Seki does not specify the location of the burn in this case, nor is any mention made of the patient's progress.
[13] The case history makes no mention of the patient's progress at this time.

7

Shigeji Naomoto's Biorhythmic Channel Divergence Pairings

Shigeji Naomoto rarely presented himself as a teacher. He preferred the role of compiler and synthesizer of the ideas of his more well-known peers despite the fact that he made some substantial contributions of his own to channel divergence therapy. Originally trained as an electrical engineer, Naomoto is, perhaps, best known as the man who actually built many of Yoshio Manaka's famous electrical acupuncture machines. He taught very little, giving only a few seminars in his lifetime. Naomoto died in 1987, and it was left to his son Shigeharu Naomoto to publish some of his father's work. Nevertheless, Naomoto incorporated some of the more interesting facets of acupuncture theory and diagnosis developed by others in the Topological Acupuncture Society into a remarkably effective channel divergence therapy. Primary among these innovations was channel pairing for the channel divergences based on the Chinese clock.

Diagnostic Parameters

Naomoto's diagnostic process began simply enough with a case history focusing on the relationship between the presenting complaint and the patient's personal and medical history. As a part of this process, he also performed Oda facial diagnosis. Like many of his peers in the Topological Society, Naomoto was enamored with novel diagnostic methods. His primary and, perhaps, most unique diagnostic method for the channel divergences was based on the five sounds of traditional Chinese musicology, one of which he attributed to each of the six confluences. A tuning fork tuned to each of the five sounds was placed on the patient's palm, and the patient was then evaluated as to his or her degree of resonance with the sounds.[1] While this style of channel divergence evaluation was the distinguishing feature of his diagnostic process, Naomoto cross-referenced his sonic findings with a wide variety of other diagnostic methods, some traditional and some developed by others in the Topological Acupuncture Society.

Foremost among Naomoto's secondary diagnostic methods was Man's Prognosis/Wrist Pulse (*ren ying-cun kou*) diagnosis. This method of pulse diagnosis, based on Chapter 48, *Jin Fu* "On Prohibiting [Access of Information] to the Unworthy," of the *Divine Pivot*, is still commonly used in Japan and involves a comparison of the Man's Prognosis (*ren ying*) pulse at the carotid artery and the "inch mouth" (*cun kou*) pulse at the wrist.[2] Naomoto also made extensive use of abdominal diagnosis, focusing on the *mu* alarm holes and Manaka's reflex holes. Among the more modern diagnostic methods Naomoto used were Oda facial observation, bi-digital O-ring testing on source holes, range of motion testing on the extremities, the Ito triceps-balancing test system, and electrical measurement using a diode ring. In this last method, a diode was applied to the yin channel of each confluence pair, and the amperage was determined by electrical measurement. The site of the lowest amperage determined the most imbalanced channel divergence. It is worth noting that, while many channel divergence specialists explicitly or implicitly placed greater importance on the yang channel of each confluence pair, Naomoto's diagnostic and treatment style evidences a clear preference for the yin channels.

The prospect of trying to make sense of the information gleaned from all of the diagnostic methods Naomoto appears to have used is a daunting task. He offered little guidance in choosing between these methodologies. He did, however, state a preference for using patient histories and a range of motion evaluation for motor disorders, while viscera and bowel disorders required some combination of the above-mentioned methods. Naomoto was no more specific than this.

Treatment strategies

Although Naomoto referred to his treatment approach as a midday-midnight point selection method (*zi wu liu zhu liao fa*), implying stem and branch related acupuncture hole selection with all its attendant charts and calculations, his method is more accurately understood simply as a midday-midnight needling method. His essential idea was to maximize the influence of a channel divergence treatment by creating a bias or polarity between a confluence pair and its opposing channel on the Chinese clock. At first sight, his treatment protocol looks rather complex. However, in actuality, it is quite simple. The two channels in each confluence pair are seen as a single functional entity. However, in picking an opposing channel, Naomoto assigns a clear predominance to the yin channel of a confluence pair. For instance, in the case of the first confluence, the urinary bladder or kidney channels are needled along with the large intestine channel, which opposes the kidney on the Chinese clock. Naomoto was also careful to time the administration of his treatments in accordance with the relevant phases of the Chinese clock. It is worth noting that there is little in Naomoto's protocols to actually suggest a channel divergence influence. They appear to be channel divergence treatments simply by virtue of the fact that they involve the use of yin-yang channel pairs. His basic biorhythmic channel divergence pairings are as follows:

BIORHYTHMIC CHANNEL DIVERGENCE PAIRINGS ACCORDING TO NAOMOTO		
First Confluence	Kidney Urinary Bladder	Large Intestine
Second Confluence	Liver Gallbladder	Small Intestine
Third Confluence	Spleen Stomach	Triple Warmer
Fourth Confluence	Heart Small Intestine	Gallbladder
Fifth Confluence	Pericardium Triple Burner	Stomach
Sixth Confluence	Lung Large Intestine	Urinary Bladder

Naomoto was rather specific in his selection of acupuncture holes for his biorhythmic treatments. He specified that the network hole should be used for the yang channel of the confluence pair and the confluence hole should be used for the yin channel of a confluence pair. The opposing channel should then be needled at the source hole. However, having said this, Naomoto suggested that the channels should be palpated and that the optimal acupuncture hole is best determined by pressure pain reactivity. He typically offered alternative hole options for the yang channel of the confluence pair. Thus, he provides us with a concrete conceptual framework from which to work but ultimately leaves the decision-making process up to the practitioner.

Because some sort of polarity-based bias is essential to his treatment strategy, we are faced with the question of how to direct the charge. When it comes to this, Naomoto follows the basic principles established by Irie. For the first three confluences, the current is directed from the confluence pair of channel divergences [-] to their opposing channel [+]. However, for the fourth, fifth, and sixth confluences, the pattern is reversed and the flow is directed from the opposing channel [-] to the designated confluence pair [+]. Examples of these are given below.

Needling & Polarity Pattern for Confluences One, Two & Three

[-] Yang Channel Network/(Source) ──┬── [+] Opposing Channel Source

[-] Yin Channel Confluence ─────────┘

Needling & Polarity Pattern for Confluences Four, Five & Six

[+] Opposing Channel Source ────┬── [-] Yang Channel Network Source

                                                └── [-] Yin Channel Confluence

\multicolumn{3}{c}{**BASIC BIORHYTHMIC CHANNEL DIVERGENCE PAIRINGS ACCORDING TO NAOMOTO**}
First Confluence	Bl 58 [-] Ki 10 [-]	[+] LI 4
Second Confluence	GB 37 (GB 35) [-] Liv 8 [-]	[+] SI 4
Third Confluence	St 40/St 41 [-] Sp 9 [-]	[+] TB 4
Fourth Confluence	SI 6 [+] Ht 3 [+]	[-] GB 40
Fifth Confluence	TB 5 [+] Per 3 [+]	[-] St 42
Sixth Confluence	LI 6 [+] Lu 5 [+]	[-] Bl 64

Like Irie, Naomoto strove to create unified treatment patterns, and, toward this end, he devised specific hand and foot confluence pairings. His primary means of creating a polarity was with electrical stimulation which he applied at an intensity of 1-6Hz for a maximum of 10 minutes. According to Naomoto, however, it was Yoshio Manaka's belief that his ion beam machine created the same effect.[3] This observation of Manaka's opened up the potential for more subtle means of activating his treatments, and Naomoto also administered his biorhythmic treatments using three bypass ion pumping cords. We have also found his treatment strategies to be quite effective when applied using bi-metal needles or simple cords. Naomoto's primary confluence pairings are as follows:

Naomoto's Biorhythmic Dual Confluence Pairings

Fourth Confluence & Second Confluence

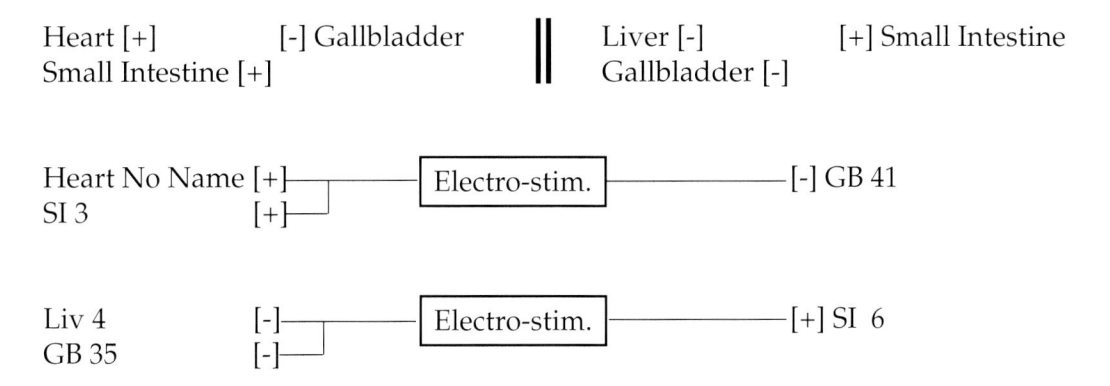

Heart [+]   [-] Gallbladder   ‖   Liver [-]   [+] Small Intestine
Small Intestine [+]   Gallbladder [-]

Heart No Name [+]⎯⎯⎯| Electro-stim. |⎯⎯⎯[-] GB 41
SI 3   [+]⎯⎯

Liv 4   [-]⎯⎯| Electro-stim. |⎯⎯⎯[+] SI 6
GB 35   [-]⎯⎯

Sixth Confluence & First Confluence

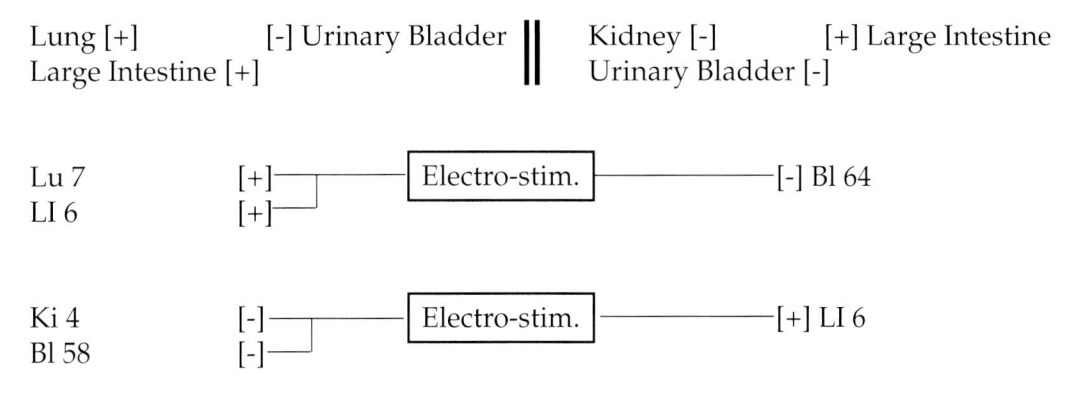

Lung [+]   [-] Urinary Bladder   ‖   Kidney [-]   [+] Large Intestine
Large Intestine [+]   Urinary Bladder [-]

Lu 7   [+]⎯⎯| Electro-stim. |⎯⎯⎯[-] Bl 64
LI 6   [+]⎯⎯

Ki 4   [-]⎯⎯| Electro-stim. |⎯⎯⎯[+] LI 6
Bl 58   [-]⎯⎯

Fifth Confluence & Third Confluence

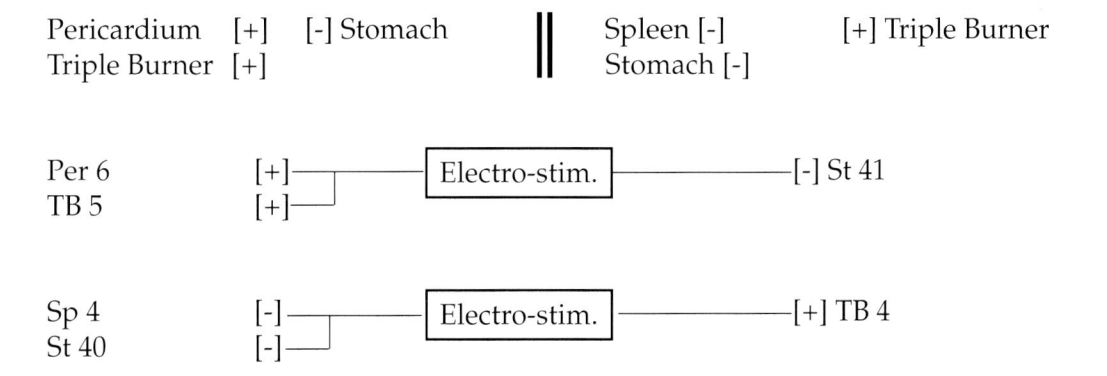

Pericardium   [+]   [-] Stomach   ‖   Spleen [-]   [+] Triple Burner
Triple Burner [+]   Stomach [-]

Per 6   [+]⎯⎯| Electro-stim. |⎯⎯⎯[-] St 41
TB 5   [+]⎯⎯

Sp 4   [-]⎯⎯| Electro-stim. |⎯⎯⎯[+] TB 4
St 40   [-]⎯⎯

Naomoto's Biorhythmic Confluence Pairings Incorporating a Bypass Cord

The three bypass ion pumping cord was a technological innovation adopted by many acupuncturists associated with the Topological Acupuncture Society, and it remains a popular treatment tool even today.[4] Where a regular ion pumping cord is a single length of wire containing a diode to induce an electrical bias, the bypass cord has a Y-configuration that allows three acupuncture holes to be incorporated into a single connection. Like the standard IP cords, the alligator clips on the three bypass cord are color-coded. In this case, the red clip is designated the positive [+] pole, the green clip is designated the negative [-] pole, and the third black clip is seen as a ground.

Three Bypass Ion Pumping Cord

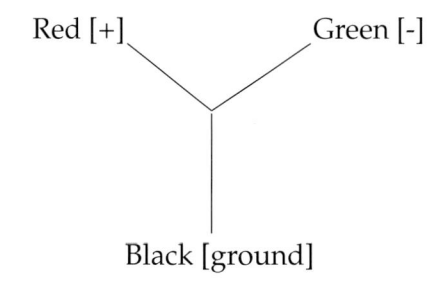

```
    Red [+]           Green [-]
         \           /
          \         /
           \       /
            \     /
             \   /
              \ /
               |
               |
               |
          Black [ground]
```

Although its scope of application is fairly broad, most clinicians employ the three bypass cord as part of a branch treatment to address a specific set of symptomatic complaints, such as shoulder pain, sciatica, or insomnia. Interestingly, Kawai uses the three bypass cord in his own adaptation of Seki's bypass strategy connecting *Bai Hui* (GV 20) and *Tian Tu* (CV 22) that we discussed in Chapter 6. For Naomoto, however, the three bypass cord was an obvious tool for connecting the master and access holes of the channel divergences with their biorhythmic correlates.

In Shigeji Naomoto's scheme, the channel divergence is accessed via the confluence hole on the yin channel of the confluence pair and the network hole of the yang channel of the confluence pair. The ground is attached to the source hole on the channel biorythmically opposite to the yin channel of each confluence pair. For imbalances that primarily afflict the yang channel of a confluence pair, the red [+] clip is attached to the yin channel and the green [-] clip is attached to the yang channel. This connection is reversed for disorders focusing on the yin channel of each confluence pair. For instance, in the case of sciatica afflicting the second confluence, the connection would be:

Liv 8 {G}[-]   GB 37 {R}[+]   SI 4{B}

However, in the case of hepatitis the connection would be:

Liv 8 {R}[+]   GB 37 {G}[-]   SI 4{B}

These pairings are summarized below.

NAOMOTO'S CHANNEL DIVERGENCE BYPASS PAIRINGS			
First Confluence	Ki 10 {G}[-]	Bl 58 {R}[+]	LI 4{B}
Second Confluence	Liv 8 {G}[-]	GB 37 {R}[+]	SI 4{B}
Third Confluence	Sp 9 {G} [-]	St 40/St 43 {R}[+]	TB 4{B}
Fourth Confluence	Ht 3 {G} [-]	SI 6 {R} [+]	GB 40{B}
Fifth Confluence	Per 3 {G} [-]	TB 5 {R} [+]	St 42{B}
Sixth Confluence	Lu 5 {G} [-]	LI 6 {R} [+]	Bl 64{B}

Naomoto did not administer his channel divergence treatments alone. He found he obtained the best results when combining the channel divergences with the extraordinary vessel master holes related to the channel divergences he was activating. For this, he used ion pumping cords. He made frequent use of the NIP protocols as well. His integration of these treatment modalities is illustrated in the case histories below.

NAOMOTO'S CASE HISTORIES

CASE ONE [5]

A 63 year-old male suffered from wind pathogen syndrome as a young man. He had been shot in the left thigh during his military service. Six years previous to his initial visit, he had fallen off a cot while sleeping. This had caused him to develop severe pain in the right side of his lower back. The patient underwent orthopedic surgery and traction. After the surgery, he developed an extreme sensitivity to variances in temperature. When he sat in an air-conditioned room, he would have severe spasms in his right leg, and, when he sat cross-legged on the floor, he would experience pain referring down the right lateral aspect of his lower leg. At the time of his visit, the pain and numbness had become so severe that he could barely walk. The sonic test resonated most strongly with the tones associated with the spleen (*gong*) and lungs (*shang*).[6] Abdominal diagnosis revealed pressure pain on right *Zhong Fu* (Lu 1) and *Da Heng* (Sp 15).

Naomoto's treatment was divided into two stages. In stage one, a channel divergence pairing employing the third and sixth confluences was administered in the following manner:

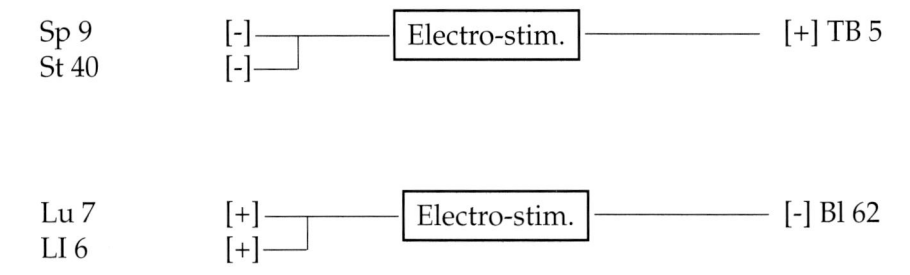

```
Sp 9      [-]┐
St 40     [-]┴───── Electro-stim. ───── [+] TB 5


Lu 7      [+]┐
LI 6      [+]┴───── Electro-stim. ───── [-] Bl 62
```

Electrical stimulation was applied at an appropriate voltage at 5Hz for six minutes. In addition, a bypass ion pumping cord treatment was administered with the black clip attached to *Bai Hui* (GV 20), the red clip attached to *Wai Guan* (TB 5), and the green clip attached to *Shen Mai* (Bl 62).

This initial phase of treatment was followed by the balancing NIP Protocol #1 administered in the following manner:

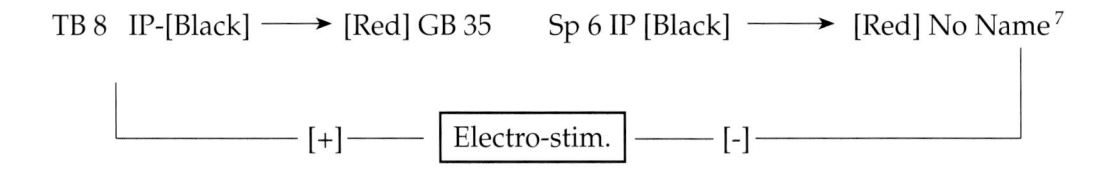

```
TB 8  IP-[Black] ──▶ [Red] GB 35    Sp 6 IP [Black] ──▶ [Red] No Name[7]
       └──────────── [+] ─── Electro-stim. ─── [-] ────────────┘
```

The black clip of the IP chord was attached to the side of the greatest electrical sensation elicited by the electro-acupuncture unit, and the red clip was attached to the side of the least electrical sensation.

2ND TREATMENT

The patient reported an 80% improvement immediately following therapy. The next day, Mr. Naomoto again administered Seki's NIP Protocol #1 as a follow-up treatment, and the patient achieved a complete recovery.

AUTHORS' COMMENT:

Here we see Naomoto administering his channel divergence treatment according to his basic methodology with one major exception. The triple burner hole should be *Yang Chi* (TB 4), the source hole, and the urinary bladder hole should be *Jing Gu* (Bl 64), again the source hole. Naomoto's choice of TB 5 and Bl 62 may have simply been a result of their greater reactivity, since he allowed for this consideration in his methodology. In any case, the selection of these two holes is fortuitous in that they allow for the skillful integration of the channel divergences with the extraordinary vessels. The inclusion of a bypass connection between TB 5, Bl 62, and GV 20 links the third and sixth confluences with the *yang wei* and *yang qiao* vessels respectively. This is particularly useful since the patient's main complaint was musculoskeletal pain in his lower extremities, a condition very amenable to treatment with these extraordinary vessels.

Having addressed the core condition using a combination of channel divergence and extraordinary vessel strategies, Naomoto completed his treatment with some generalized supplementation using the NIP Protocol #1. Naomoto's choice of where to attach the black and red clips of the IP cord was based on the degree of electrical sensation elicited at each hole. Theoretically at least, the black clip conducts the charge from the area of repletion, in this case, the site of the greatest electrical sensation, to the red clip that is attached to the area of vacuity where there is the least electrical sensation. Apparently, a repeat of the NIP portion of this treatment the following day to consolidate the treatment effect was the only further intervention that was required to effect a recovery.

CASE TWO

A 13 year-old male had suffered damage to his optic nerve. Two months previously he had been hit on the left side of his face by a tennis ball. He consulted an ophthalmologist who diagnosed his situation as a minor trauma to the optic nerve that should recover shortly. Nevertheless, the patient was left with frequent left-sided headaches, vertigo, and photophobia. When he suffered from these episodes, he would also have pain in the upper epigastric area, and there was some conjecture among his physicians that he might be suffering from Meniere's disease. There was also tenderness upon palpation at *Ju Que* (CV 14), *Shang Wan* (CV 13), and right *Jian Jing* (GB 21).

As in the above case, Naomoto's treatment was divided into two stages. In stage one, the fourth and second confluence pairings were treated in the following manner with 5Hz of electrical stimulation at weak voltage for five minutes:

Heart No Name [+] ─┬─ | Electro-stim. | ── [-] GB 41
SI 3   [+] ─┘

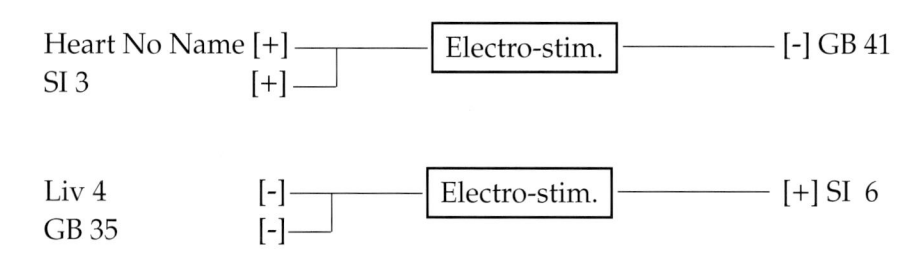

Liv 4   [-] ─┬─ | Electro-stim. | ── [+] SI 6
GB 35   [-] ─┘

In addition, an extraordinary vessel bypass ion pumping chord treatment was administered with the black clip attached to GV 20, the red clip attached to *Yang Lao* (SI 6), and the green clip attached to *Lin Qi* (GB 41).

In stage two, the initial treatment was followed by a more balancing ion pumping extraordinary vessel treatment. Five Hz of electrical stimulation was also administered at this time for a duration of five minutes. The treatment was administered in the following manner:

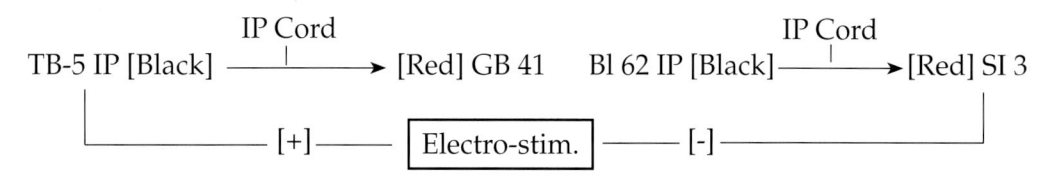

```
              IP Cord                              IP Cord
TB-5 IP [Black] ──┬──→ [Red] GB 41    Bl 62 IP [Black] ──┬──→ [Red] SI 3
    └────── [+] ──── | Electro-stim. | ──── [-] ──────────┘
```

The black clip of the IP chord was attached to the side of the greatest electrical sensation elicited by the electro-acupuncture unit, and the red clip was attached to the side of the least electrical sensation. After three treatments, the patient reported that most of the discomfort had disappeared.

AUTHORS' COMMENT:

In case two, we again see that the master holes on the opposing channels have been selected with secondary extraordinary vessel connections in mind. An auxiliary bypass hookup is incorporated in the channel divergence connection, and this is followed in the second phase of treatment by a more straightforward extraordinary vessel connection.

CASE THREE

A patient of indeterminate age and sex suffered from pain in the root of their tooth and, for this, Naomoto administered a symptomatic treatment. Diagnosis was based on sonic evaluation and muscular range of motion tests pertaining to the various channels. The first confluence was needled and activated with the negative leads of an electro-acupuncture unit. This was combined with the ninth extraordinary vessel, the large intestine vessel, using a combination of electrical stimulation and IP cords. Three to five Hz of electrical stimulation was applied for six minutes.

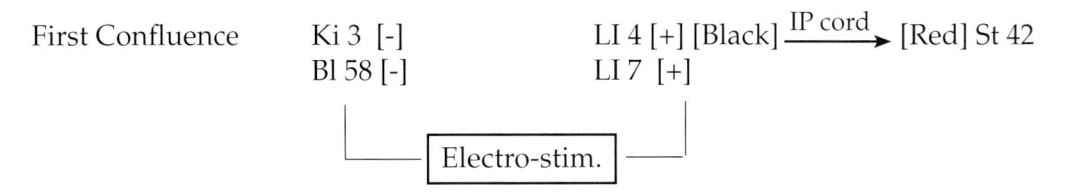

First Confluence   Ki 3 [-]   LI 4 [+] [Black] $\xrightarrow{\text{IP cord}}$ [Red] St 42
                       Bl 58 [-]   LI 7 [+]
                                           | Electro-stim. |

Using this treatment, the patient was cured.

AUTHORS' COMMENT:

Like the first case, this case is an example of the skillful integration of a variety of treatment strategies. The rationale for using the first confluence is apparently based solely on "objective" findings, such as sonic evaluation and muscular range of motion tests. Nevertheless, it must be remembered that the kidneys govern the bones and the teeth are the surplus of the bones. Naomoto's channel divergence strategy links the kidneys with the large intestine channel, a channel which directly links to the teeth. It is again curious that he uses the network hole for his connection as opposed to the source hole. The reason for this may simply be palpatory reactivity, or it may be that Naomoto wished to reserve *He Gu* (LI 4) for his secondary connection with the stomach. Regardless of the rationale, the end result was an elegant treatment.

ENDNOTES

[1] A further discussion of *Suihara* sound diagnosis appears in Appendix 3.
[2] A further discussion of this diagnostic method appears in Appendix 3.
[3] Naomoto: 5
[4] Kiiko Matsumoto regularly presents the three bypass treatment protocols of Kawai in her seminars.
[5] All case histories are derived from Naomoto: 1985-B.
[6] A further discussion of *Suihara* sound diagnosis appears in Appendix 3.
[7] The no name hole is located on the heart channel, 5 *cun* proximal to Ht 7 (Seki, 1982: 27). Manaka asserted that it is the correlated hole to *Yang Jiao* (TB 8), serving as an intersection point for all of the hand yin channels just as *Yang Jiao* functions as an intersection point for all of the hand yang channels.

8

MIKI SHIMA'S APPROACH TO CHANNEL DIVERGENCE THERAPY

We have now covered the treatment strategies of some of the seminal developers of channel divergence therapy. Many of these approaches are similar in some respects, even as they differ greatly in others. At this juncture, it is fruitful to look at how an experienced acupuncturist practicing in the West has made sense of all this information over the course two decades of clinical experience. Miki Shima's approach to channel divergence therapy represents a conceptual synthesis of many of the ideas we have explored thus far. In the process of his own investigation, Shima has extracted what he has found to be the most useful ideas advanced by Irie, Seki, and Naomoto. The end result for Shima is a versatile methodology that is both easy to administer and clinically effective. In addition, Shima's style of practice opens a window to a deeper understanding of how the channel divergences may be used in the larger context of an overall treatment strategy. We will first outline the basic tenants of Shima's approach and then take an in-depth look at his diagnostic and treatment process using a number of his case histories.

Shima's own development as an acupuncturist closely parallels the development of channel divergence therapy in Japan, and, like most of the other Japanese channel divergence specialists, Shima's approach to the channel divergences has gone through successive stages of refinement and development. He has benefited greatly from a cross-fertilization of ideas among fellow practitioners in both the United States and Japan as he evolved his own unique approach to the channel divergence system. Shima's interest in acupuncture began in 1967 when he received acupuncture for exhaustion resulting from overwork. After his recovery, he began an apprenticeship with Shoji Nakamura, a well-known Japanese acupuncturist, and the herbalist Tsuneo Mizuno. In addition, he developed an interest in Chinese literature and linguistics. Having finished an apprenticeship in acupuncture and herbal medicine in Japan, Shima came to the United States in 1974.

Shima's interest in the channel divergences began in 1978 when he read Irie's articles in the journals of the *Ido-no-Nippon-Sha (The Journal of Japanese Acupuncture and Moxbustion)*.[1] In 1979, Tadashi Irie's first book established itself as the definitive text on the channel divergences and defined the standard master holes on the head. Shima immediately adopted this methodology. In 1982, Shima brought Irie to teach a two-week seminar in the U.S. During this visit, Shima expressed his frustration to Irie over the lack of a satisfactory means of diagnosing the channel divergences. Encouraged by Irie, Shima developed the channel divergence interpretation of the Akabane test. Shima was also influenced by the writings of other channel divergence investigators in Japan and began combining channel divergences and extraordinary vessel treatments together during this time.

By 1983, Seki's ideas on the channel divergences were becoming more widely known in Japan. Although intrigued by Seki's conceptual ideas, Shima was less interested in his predilection toward technology and emphasis on Western medical models. During this time, Naomoto was also integrating auriculotherapy with channel divergence treatments, an innovation that would become a cornerstone of Shima's own approach. When Irie began using magnets and the bi-digital O-ring test (developed by Yoshiaki Omura, M.D.) diagnostically in 1985, Shima found that he preferred the Akabane methodology he had developed years earlier and struck out on his own. He began teaching his own approach to the channel divergences at this time as well. By 1986, it became clear to him that he obtained the most consistent results using the confluence (*he*) holes as access holes and began using these holes exclusively.

In 1990, the legal climate in California made it difficult to use IP cords, magnets, or electricity in acupuncture therapy, thus prompting Shima to begin using gold, silver, or stainless needles in his channel divergence treatments, a practice the he continues to the present.[2] It was also in 1990 that Terry Oleson's works on auriculotherapy provided Shima with a vehicle for refining his own integration of body and ear acupuncture, which he calls Somato-Auricular Therapy (SAT).[3]

Access Holes

Shima's approach to channel divergence therapy has a number of distinguishing features. The most immediate characteristic of his treatment of the channel divergences is his standardization of the access holes on the extremities. Shima exclusively uses the confluence holes on the knees and elbows as his access holes, combining these with Irie's standard set of master holes on the head. There are a number of rationales for his choice of confluence holes, the first and foremost being that Shima simply finds them the most clinically effective. This choice of access holes also makes a great deal of sense when one considers that the confluence holes are the points along the trajectory of the channel where the qi goes deep and this is just what the channel divergences themselves do. Shima is not alone in his clinical application of the confluence holes to deep organ problems. One of his primary influences, the abdominal diagnosis master Shoji Kobayashi also uses the confluence holes diagnostically to detect imbalances specifically on the level of the viscera and bowels, although his treatment approach does not involve the channel divergences *per se*.[4] Finally, the confluence holes at the elbows and knees share the same designation as confluences as do the six confluences of the channel divergences.

In Chapter 1, we presented the textual argument for understanding all the channel divergences as diving deeply at the confluence holes. On theoretical grounds, Shima reasons that source holes exert less of an influence on the viscera or bowels but more strongly convey the influence of the original qi within the channel. While they certainly influence the interior, according to the 66th difficult issue of the *Nan Jing (Classic of Difficult Issues)*, source holes are the primary means of transmitting source qi to the channels in the periphery. Given the strong viscera and bowel influence conferred by the channel divergences, such an interpretation makes the source holes a poor choice for universal access holes. Because of their strong indications for resolving stagnation resulting from acute pain patterns the cleft holes typically exert their influence most prominently on the channel sinew. Similarly, network holes tend to have a more superficial influence overall which is out of character with the deep trajectories of the channel divergence.[5] Moreover, the network holes specifically access the network channels, thus at least conceptually muddying their influence on other layers of the channel and vessel system. To further complicate matters, many of the network holes have been co-opted as master and couple holes of the extraordinary vessels. Shima is quick to admit however, that, when all is said and done, such conjecture only serves as a prop or guide for careful observation, and, in his clinical experience, the access hole of choice is the confluence hole. The following table summarizes Shima's choice of access and master holes for the channel divergences.

CHANNEL DIVERGENCE ACCESS AND MASTER HOLES ACCORDING TO SHIMA		
First Confluence-Urinary Bladder/Kidney	Bl 40 & Ki 10 [-]	Bl 11 [+] / Bl 1 [+]
Second Confluence-Gallbladder/Liver	GB 34 & Liv 8 [-]	GB 1 [+]
Third Confluence-Stomach/Spleen	St 36 & Sp 9 [-]	St 1 [+]
Fourth Confluence-Small Intestine/Heart	SI 8 & Ht 3 [+]	Bl 1 [-]
Fifth Confluence-Triple Burner/Pericardium	TB 10 & Per 3 [+]	GB 12 [-]
Sixth Confluence-Large Intestine/Lung	LI 11 & Lu 5 [+]	St 12 [-]

140   The Channel Divergences

Acupuncture Location of Zu San Li (St 36)

Moxibustion Location of (St 36)

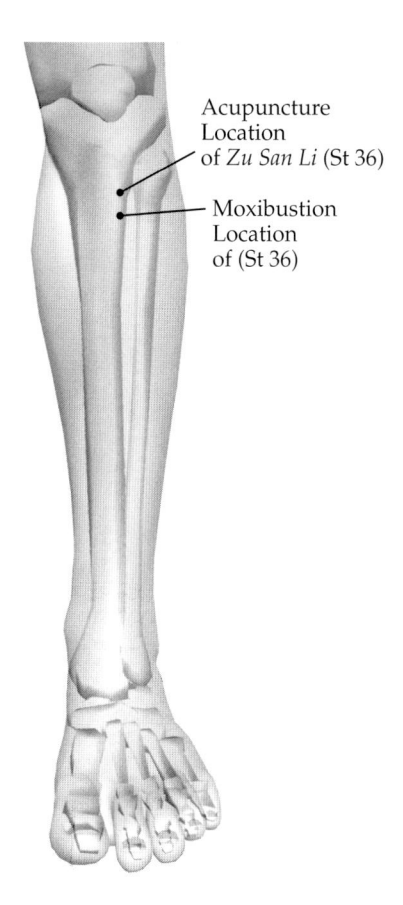

Any discussion of acupuncture hole locations in the context of Japanese acupuncture must be prefaced by the caveat that Japanese acupuncturists are taught that standardized locations are merely places to begin looking for acupuncture holes. Acupuncture holes are located by palpation and may move depending on the condition of the patient. Acupuncture holes are relatively more superficial on men than they are in women and overall, the weaker or more vacuous a patient is, the deeper the hole will be found. Acupuncture holes also tend to migrate towards the torso as people weaken. Moreover, the modality being applied influences the location of acupuncture holes and needling locations typically differ from moxibustion locations.[6] Roughly speaking, moxibustion holes tend to be especially tender to deep pressure. A superior way of locating a moxa hole, however, is to pass an incense or moxa stick over the general area. The spot that the patient reports as responding most comfortably to the heat is the spot that should be moxaed. Shima is fond of saying that, "There is no hole until you find it." The reader is encouraged to keep this perspective in mind when reviewing the following hole locations.

Jing Ming (Bl 1) is a challenging hole to needle. If needled improperly, it can be painful and may result in a black eye. It is needled shallowly and perpendicularly 0.1 *cun* superior to the inner canthus of the eye. The lid is closed and the acupuncturist uses his or her finger to both shield the eyeball and gently push it aside. For most of the master holes, the needle is best taped firmly in place with micropore tape. The difficulty of needling Bl 1 was probably a factor in the development of alternate master holes, such as *Da Zhu* (Bl 11) which Shima frequently uses as the master hole for the first conflu-

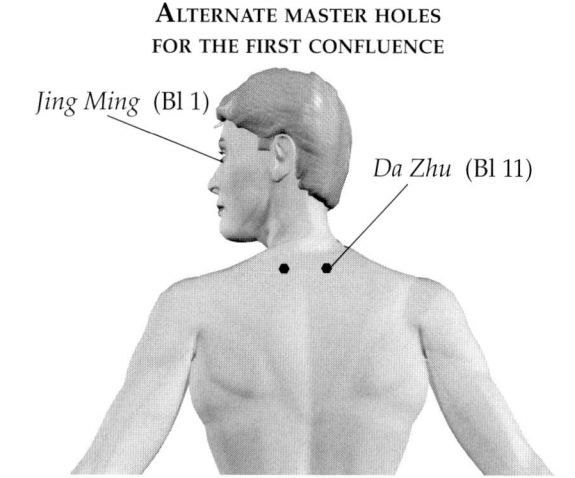

ALTERNATE MASTER HOLES FOR THE FIRST CONFLUENCE

Jing Ming (Bl 1)

Da Zhu (Bl 11)

ence. When Bl 11 is used as a master hole, it is needled toward the spine, reinforcing the strong affinity the channel divergences have for the spine.

Japanese acupuncturists often find acupuncture holes in slightly different places than their standard Chinese locations, and some of the access and master holes of the channel divergences reflect these idiosyncrasies. The following are the "Japanese" locations of some of these major channel divergence holes:

Tong Zi Liao (GB 1) is often needled slightly posterior to its standard Chinese location in an indentation in the orbital ridge but not quite on *Tai Yang*. It is needled in a latero-posterior direction.

Cheng Qi (St 1) is needled just over the edge of the orbital ridge into the space between the ridge and the eyeball.

Zu San Li (St 36) is located as much as one *cun* lower than the standard Chinese location, still lateral to the tibia, but in a depression in the fleshy part of the muscle.

Yin Ling Quan (Sp 9) may be needled in the standard Chinese location and in the direction of the channel flow. For patients suffering from hypertension, Sp 9 may be located in a slightly higher position on a sore spot approximately 1-2 *cun* above its standard location.

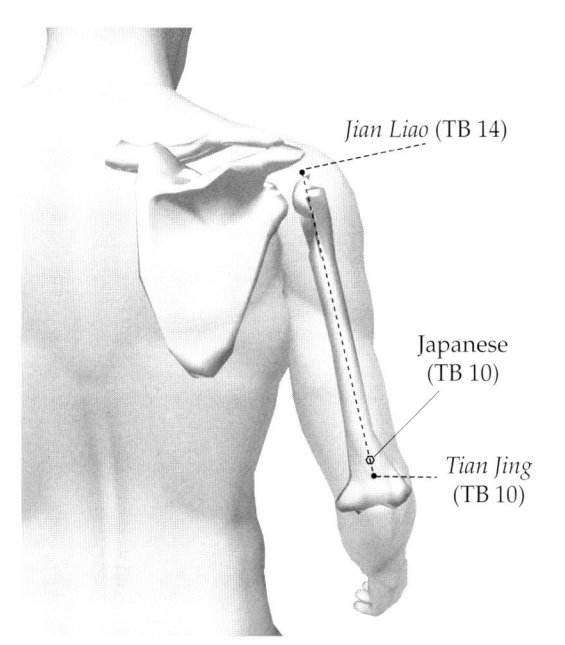

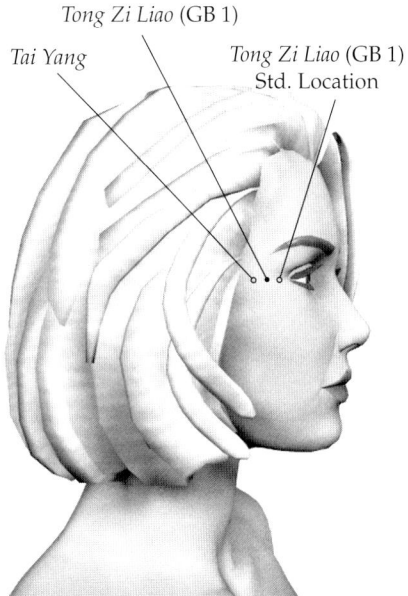

JAPANESE LOCATION OF *TONG ZI LIAO* GB 1

Xiao Hai (SI 8) is located approximately 0.5 *cun* superior to its standard Chinese location and closer to the heart channel.

Wan Gu (GB 12) is needled toward the top of the head.

Tian Jing (TB 10) is needled approximately 0.5 *cun* proximal to its standard Chinese location and in a more prominent depression.

Finally, *Que Pen* (St 12) is needled by finding the deepest part of the supraclavicular fossa and inserting the needle posteriorly toward *Jian Jing* (GB 21).

AKABANE TESTING

The next feature of note in Shima's overall channel divergence methodology is his frequent reliance on Akabane testing as his primary diagnostic modality. Shima does not invariably use the Akabane technique, nor does he apply his Akabane findings in a rigid manner. He also makes extensive use of pulse, abdomen, tongue, and questioning examinations, often constructing an acupuncture treatment plan on this information alone. Overall, however, it is fair to say that he he places great emphasis on his Akabane findings. For instance, we will see in three of the cases that follow that Shima's acupuncture treatment is guided almost exclusively by his Akabane methodology.

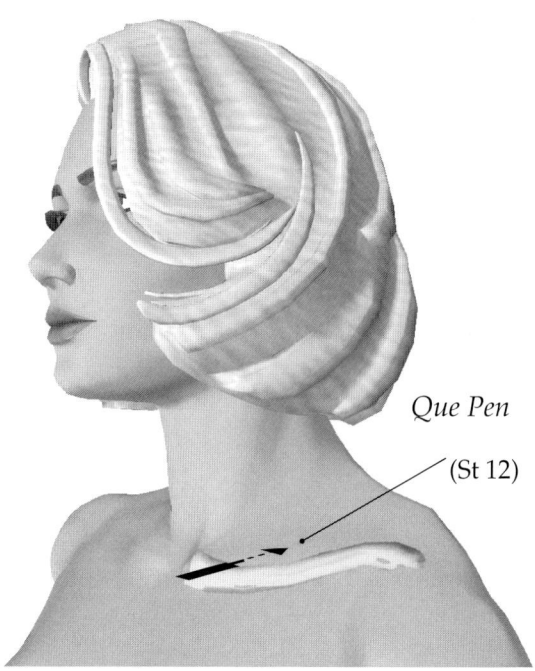

POSTERIOR INSERTION OF QUE PEN (ST 12) FROM THE HOLLOW OF THE SUPRACLAVICULOR FOSSA

One of the reasons Shima is so drawn to the Akabane method as a diagnostic modality is its relevance to the Japanese idea of *hie* 冷. *Hie* is a general idea conveying a feeling of cold. This may be a generalized sense of cold or it may be a cold body part. *Hie* begins in the toes and moves toward the body. It is one of the six pathogenic factors responsible for the retardation of the flow of qi and blood locally on the level of the channels, the viscera, or in any combination thereof. Therefore, it is a key etiological factor in a variety of cardiovascular diseases including coronary heart disease and stroke.

Although *hie* may or may not be experienced by the patient, the evaluator's objective experience of cold somewhere on the patient's body is of primary importance. *Hie* is closely akin to the principle that all disease is, at its core, due to the presence of cold or yang vacuity. Although all pathodynamics tend to transform into heat, cold is the primordial pathogen. *Hie* is often identified even in cases where there are clear signs of heat, and, in some instances, it may be of even greater importance than other contradictory symptoms that are much more pronounced. Thus we may understand Akabane testing in one context as a means of evaluating the relative degree of *hie* in each of the channels. Conversely, another way of stating this is to say that Akabane testing is a means of evaluating the relative state of the yang in each of the channels. Because the channel system in general and the extraordinary vessels and channel divergences in particular all exert a direct influence on the state of the yang in the body, Akabane testing is an obvious diagnostic criteria for decision-making on this level.

We have briefly discussed the specific methodology for determining the most imbalanced channel divergences in Chapter 3. We will now discuss this technique in greater depth and focus our attention on how to apply the information gained from Akabane testing. Akabane testing as used by Shima provides the core information necessary to determine the two or three most imbalanced channels and the most relevant extraordinary vessel pairings. While these findings must naturally be cross-referenced with other palpatory findings and the patient's history, Shima places the greatest diagnostic weight on the Akabane findings that appear most consistently over the course of regular testing.

The basic Akabane method involves the tabulation of the number of strokes required to elicit a heat response at each of the well *jing* holes. Shima adds the stroke counts from the left and right side to yield a total, and also calculates the difference between the left and right stroke counts to yield a deviation.

TABLE 1: LATERAL POLARIZATIONS

FOOT					HAND				
Channel	R	L	Tot.	Dev.	Channel	R	L	Tot.	Dev.
Spleen	5	9	14	4	Lung	6	5	11	1
Liver	7	9	16	2	L. Intestine	6	11	17	5
Stomach	12	12	24	0	Pericardium	4	4	8	0
Gallbladder	15	22	37	7	Triple Burner	5	9	14	4
Kidney	14	13	27	1	Heart	15	8	23	7
Bladder	14	42	56	28	S. Intestine	4	5	9	1

The totals for each channel are noted again in Table 2 where they are arranged into yin-yang confluence pairs. The difference between each of these pairs is tabulated as the deviation. The channels with the greatest deviations are selected for treatment. In the table below, we see that the first and second confluences reflect the greatest deviations.

TABLE 2: CHANNEL DIVERGENCE POLARIZATIONS

	Tot.	Dev.		Tot.	Dev.		Tot.	Dev.
Ki	27	29	Sp	14	10	Per	8	6
Bl	56		St	24		TB	14	
Liv	16	21	Ht	23	14	Lu	11	6
GB	37		SI	9		LI	17	

144 The Channel Divergences

Shima's choice of whether to access the yin or yang channel pair of a given channel divergence, and on which side to needle a given hole is most often dictated by his Akabane findings as well. In the example above we would needle the yang channel of the first confluence bladder channel because it shows itself to be the weakest of the first confluence pair with a stroke total of 56. Shima then refers back to the left-right findings in Table 1 and selects the side to treat the bladder channel based on whichever side has the highest stroke total. In the above example, we would treat the left side because it has a stroke total of 42 as compared to a stroke total of 14 on the right.

GENERAL PREFERENCES

Shima is particularly fond of using the Akabane method when he perceives that a patient's qi is stagnant, and that the qi in the channels and networks is simply not flowing. He is more likely to employ Akabane when someone is extremely fatigued, and he conceptualizes it as jump starting the flow of qi so that he can more effectively administer the rest of the acupuncture treatment. Akabane is to be avoided, however, when a patient presents with hot hands and feet, a frank fever, or other overt heat signs.

Since Akabane findings do not always dictate the form an acupuncture treatment will take, over the years Shima has developed some general rules of thumb that guide his decision making. Having determined the most imbalanced confluences by whatever means, Shima prefers to work first on the level of the yang channels and only uses the yin channels if his initial results are unsatisfactory. This is particularly the case in pain conditions where he finds that the yang channels produce a more rapid response.

Shima often needles the channel divergences bilaterally, using a yang channel on one side and a yin channel on the other. This is a strategy pioneered by Seki. In this case, he may needle the master holes bilaterally or he may only use the master hole on the head on the side of the yang channel being needled, again showing his overall preference for the yang channels. For instance, if he were stimulating the second confluence, he might needle *Yang Ling Quan* (GB 34) on the left and *Qu Quan* (Liv 8) on the right. In this example, he would then

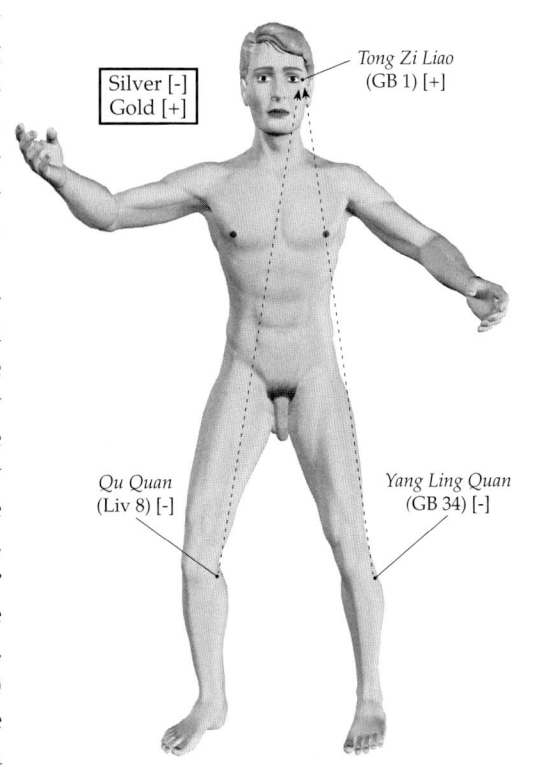

Silver [-]
Gold [+]

Tong Zi Liao (GB 1) [+]

Qu Quan (Liv 8) [-]

Yang Ling Quan (GB 34) [-]

needle *Tong Zi Liao* (GB 1) on the left. Like Irie and Seki, Shima also frequently combines pairs of channel divergences such that two, and occasionally three confluence pairs are stimulated at the same time in a single treatment.

AN INTEGRATED APPROACH TO DIAGNOSIS

It would be disingenuous to flatly state that Shima practices acupuncture and herbal medicine in the Japanese style. As with most clinicians who have been in practice for quite some time, his approach to healing has benefited from many influences. His fairly extensive Western medical training is no less important to him than his training in the *Kanpo* style of herbal medicine, nor is his training in more TCM modes of thought. Moreover, each of these ways of thinking are reflected in his case records, although the unique circumstances of each patient interaction cause him to emphasize some aspects of diagnosis over others. Sometimes Shima bases his treatment strategy on his Akabane findings, and sometimes on the pulse and abdomen. Sometimes the biomedical diagnosis will influence his treatment decisions and Shima will administer auriculotherapy, or body acupuncture to achieve some specific hormonal, neurological, or immunological effect.

Shima typically begins each patient visit with an evaluation of their status from a biomedical perspective and he performs a brief physical exam, taking blood pressure, and listening to heart sounds etc. Is the patient stable? Is lab work required to clarify the clinical picture? Does this patient require a referral? During this time he has also gathered most of the verbal information for the patient that he requires. Next, he examines the tongue, and palpates the pulse and abdomen. Finally, he performs the Akabane technique and tallies his findings.

Shima's acupuncture prescribing may be based exclusively on his Akabane findings, or he may rely on more conventional means for determining which confluences to treat. His herbal prescribing is based largely on his abdominal and pulse diagnosis.

THE RIGHT TOOLS FOR THE JOB

Virtually all of the other Japanese channel divergence specialists we have discussed thus far have at some time in their practice relied heavily on electrical stimulation to initiate the qi-bias that is an essential principle of Japanese channel divergence therapy. Shima is no different in this regard. However, he equally often adopts more "low-tech" strategies for both diagnosis and the modalities he uses to produce a qi-bias. The decision to use one type of stimulation or another is based largely on the nature of the problem he is treating and the person who is receiving the treatment.

Because Shima's practice is focused quite heavily on internal medicine, his application of the channel divergences is directed toward patients who tend to be physically debilitated and/or hypersensitive. Electrical stimulation is often too strong for many of these patients even though it may be essential in achieving a satisfactory result in others. For instance, patients who are not hypersensitive but present with profound kidney vacuity, regardless of whether it is a vacuity of yin, yang, or qi, often benefit from electrical stimulation of the channel divergences using the kidney return treatment discussed below. Therefore, Shima's application of electrical stimulation is based entirely on empirical grounds. However, Shima conceptualizes the kidney qi and original qi (*yuan qi*) as being inherently sluggish in nature. When this level of qi becomes deeply debilitated, a strong stimulus may be required to get things flowing again. Hence, his use of electricity with the channel divergences.

Shima also has some more general criteria for determining whether or not to use electricity, the most important of which is the patient's overall constitution, which he decides is either fundamentally vacuous or fundamentally replete. He is more inclined to use electrical stimulation on stronger individuals. Nevertheless, some patients are extremely sensitive to electrical stimulation and cannot tolerate it regardless of their constitutional type. Conversely, he finds that some patients respond well to electrical stimulation and actually request it even though they are quite weak.

Shima's electro-acupuncture device of choice is the Electro-Stimulator 4-C produced by Pantheon Research.[8] For purposes of supplementation, Shima tends to use a constant waveform at 2Hz, while for drainage, he prefers a mixed waveform at 10 or more Hz. For the kidney return protocol in particular, Shima uses settings of 1Hz 5-10 milliamperes at nine volts for 10 minutes.

Shima typically uses a bi-metal needle technique for most of his patients, the efficacy of which he believes is superior to virtually all other needling modalities, including the use of ion pumping cords. It is likely that Shima's success with bi-metal needles is as much a result of his needle technique as the modality itself. Although the efficacy of IP cords is greatly enhanced by precise point location, the practitioner still fundamentally relies on the cord to get the job done. This phenomena may ultimately serve as a disincentive to developing one's own needle technique.

THE QUESTION OF DIRECTIONALITY

Whenever one is using a stimulation technique involving bias, regardless of whether the stimulus involves electricity, ion pumping cords, bi-metal needles, or magnets, a decision must be made regarding the direction of the qi flow. As we have already seen, this is a topic of considerable debate. In this, Shima most often follows the general protocols originally advanced by Irie. That is, access holes are negative and master holes are positive for the first three confluences. Access holes are positive and master holes are negative for the fourth, fifth, and sixth confluences. In general, Shima first stimulates the negative pole with a silver or stainless steel needle and, only after obtaining the qi at this location, will he then needle the positive pole with a gold needle. The rationale for this is based on the supposition that a silver needle sends the qi away, whereas a gold needle attracts or accumulates the qi.

Shima is quick to point out that Irie's directional protocols are just rules of thumb and that the practitioner must always decide on the direction of a given treatment for themselves. The astute reader will have noticed that the channel divergences in general, and the protocols utilizing Irie's polarity schema in particular direct a great deal of qi upward in the body, specifically into the head. Given that many conditions are already characterized by an ascending counterflow of qi, such an upbearing strategy may strike many as ill-advised. Although there are certainly conditions where the standard polarity protocols are indeed contraindicated, these protocols are valid much more often than one might initially think. This may be explained in a number of ways.

We must first consider that the overall flow of qi through the channel divergences is decidedly upward. This is once again assuming that qi flows through the channels in the direction of its stated trajectory. In light of this, Irie's polarity protocols are consistent with this general trend. His methodology brings qi upward from below in the case of the first three confluences, and conducts qi from the head even further distally into the hands in the case of the latter three confluences.

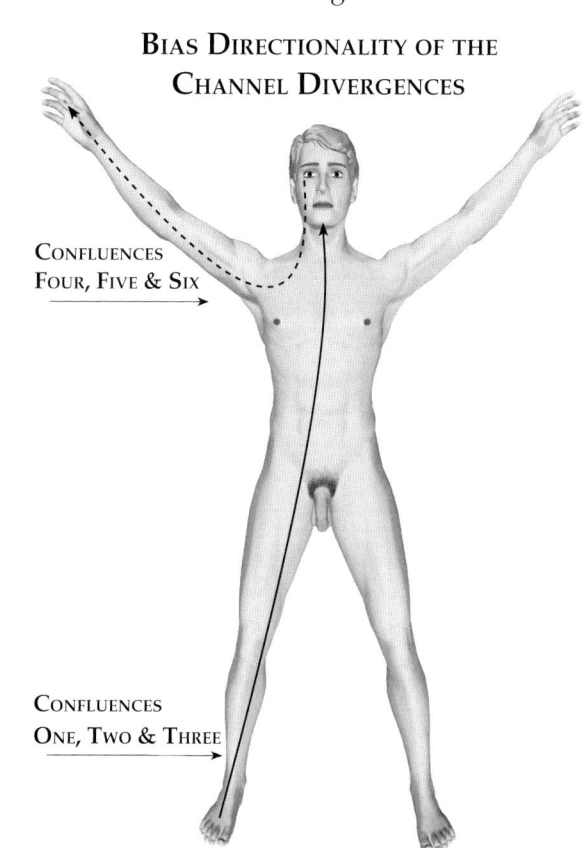

BIAS DIRECTIONALITY OF THE CHANNEL DIVERGENCES

CONFLUENCES FOUR, FIVE & SIX

CONFLUENCES ONE, TWO & THREE

Given the intimate relationship of the channel divergences to the gathering or ancestral qi and the close relationship between gathering qi and clear yang, we may hypothesize that an essential function of the channel divergences is the upbearing and exteriorization of clear yang within the body. In accessing the channel divergences, we are promoting this core physiological function and we can let the counterflow take care of itself.[9]

We must also consider the channel divergences within the larger context of their relationship with the main channels. Although the bias for the first three confluences is directed toward the head in Irie's system, all of these channel divergences terminate at or near the origins of their paired yang channel, (*i.e.* at Bl 1, GB 1, and St 1), and the qi of the three foot yang channels runs downward. This may create a built-in system of qi return. Admittedly, this return circuit may not always be sufficient to accommodate every contingency. However, it does seem to work in many cases of counterflow.

The bias-induction from the head to the upper extremities in the case of the latter three confluences may also be interpreted as draining qi congestion away from the head even as it further upbears and exteriorizes the qi. Understood in this way, Naomoto's confluence pairings make a great deal of sense in promoting a healthy and generalized circulation of qi. Regardless of the channels one selects, the combination of a lower limb confluence with an upper limb confluence enhances qi circulation throughout the entire body. Of course, this is only theory. When all is said and done, the only definitive thing that can be said is that, in Shima's experience, Irie's standard polarity protocol is appropriate about 80% of the time. There are some obvious exceptions to this rule, however.

Let us take, for example, the case of migraine headaches due to ascendant liver yang hyperactivity. In this example, the second confluence is a likely candidate for a channel divergence treatment. Shima's standard protocol calls for the bias to be directed from the access holes GB 34 or Liv 8 toward the head at GB 1. This would seem to be exactly the opposite direction that one would want to direct the qi in such a case, but there are a number of things to take into consideration. If the patient in our example was suffering from an acute migrainous episode, then downbearing the qi would likely be a prudent choice. In this instance, the force of the counterflow is so pronounced that only direct subduing or suppression will suffice. In the remission phase of the illness, however, the standard upbearing directionality can probably be used as long as the qi is redirected downward by some other facet of the treatment. One possible strategy is to modulate the strength of the bias being induced by taking into consideration the type of needles one uses. Although the direction of the bias is an essential component of any bias induction technique, it is Shima's experience that unwanted counterflow is much less of a concern when using gold and silver bi-metal needle techniques, because this produces a much weaker bias. In our example of a migraine patient, the gentler gold and silver technique may be desirable.

Whatever the method of bias-induction, channel divergence therapies are potent and can backfire if one fails to pay attention. This can occur quite rapidly, often in 30-60 seconds. There are no hard and fast rules that apply in every case, and readers are cautioned to integrate any of the treatment strategies discussed in this book into their acupuncture practices in a gradual manner, expanding their scope of application as they gain experience with these new tools. Shima has observed that the channel divergences have markedly detoxifying properties, and this may be a function of their deep trajectories through the viscera and bowels. Whatever the reason, Shima finds that the channel divergences are even more useful than the extraordinary vessels for patients on toxic medications. This detoxifying influence, however, may temporarily exacerbate symptoms or otherwise disrupt things. In light of this, when deciding on a method for stimulating the channel divergences, it is important to consider the robustness of a patient's overall constitution, their specific disease presentation, and any other medication they may be taking. It may, in fact, be wise to forgo the use of the channel divergences in especially sensitive patients until they are stronger and one has become more familiar with how they tend to react.

One way of testing the proper direction of treatment is to first apply magnets to the holes that are to be treated. The north pole of a magnet is placed on the hole with the negative charge, and the south pole of another magnet is placed on the hole with a positive charge. The practitioner then evaluates changes in the pulse and abdomen and receives feedback from the patients regarding any uncomfortable sensations. Unlike many of his mentors, Shima uses magnets only as a means of testing the direction of a treatment and chooses not to use them as therapy in and of themselves. He has found that his patient population is often too sensitive for magnet therapy. It is his experience that magnets will, as often as not, produce more symptoms than they relieve.

Overall Treatment Strategy & Extraordinary Vessel Combinations

It is important to understand that for Shima, like most of the other Japanese acupuncturists presented in this book, a channel divergence therapy is only one, albeit essential, part in an overall treatment strategy. Either sequentially or simultaneously addressing the channel sinews and especially the extraordinary vessel layers may act as a modulating factor in preventing unwanted side effects in his channel divergence treatments. People suffering from more severe illnesses such as cancer, naturally tend to have deeper constitutional weaknesses. In such cases, Shima first applies moxibustion to the back transport holes on the side shown to be the weakest by Akabane testing. Otherwise, he generally begins with some sort of channel sinew therapy. This may involve needling localized areas of stagnation or *kori*, but more often consists of manual massage. According to Shima, this opens up the superficial layers of the channel and network vessel system and, in so doing, reduces the likelihood of the qi becoming stuck and producing unwanted side effects. Next, Shima proceeds to the simultaneous treatment of the channel divergences and the extraordinary vessels.[10]

We have already seen how Seki and Naomoto actively combined channel divergence strategies with extraordinary vessel protocols, activating these layers of the channel and network vessel system either simultaneously or sequentially. Shima typically combines the channel divergences and the extraordinary vessels in a single treatment step. Although he sometimes relies on other diagnostic criteria, Akabane testing is his primary means of determining which channel divergence and extraordinary vessel connections to use.

Shima's approach to the extraordinary vessels is similar to that of a many Japanese acupuncturists in that he tends to conceptualize them not so much as eight completely separate channels but as four composite pairs. For instance, rather than accessing the *du* vessel or the *yang qiao* vessel he thinks of stimulating the *du/yang qiao* connection. The thing that determines whether a treatment is a *du* vessel treatment *per se*, is really the placement of the gold needle or positive pole on *Hou Xi* (SI 3), the master hole of the *du mai*. This conceptualization of the extraordinary vessels as functional pairs is also reflected in his Akabane methodology.

Table 3 summarizes the stroke totals from each of the channels arranged by extraordinary vessel master-couple hole pairs. The extraordinary vessel pair possessing the greatest difference or deviation between stroke count totals is selected for treatment. In the example below, we see that the small intestine (SI 3) and bladder (Bl 62) channels, with stroke counts of 9 and 56 respectively, have the greatest deviation. The *yang qiao/du* connection is therefore selected for treatment. We know that Bl 62 is going to be designated as the master hole because with a stroke count of 56, it has the highest tally of the pair.

TABLE 3: EXTRA CHANNEL POLARIZATIONS

	Tot.	Dev.		Tot.	Dev.		Tot.	Dev.
SI 3	9	(47)	Lu 7	11	16	Lu 7	11	3
Bl 62	(56)		Ki 6	27		Sp 4	14	
GB 41	37	(23)	Per 6	8	6	Ht 5	23	4
TB 5	14		SP 4	14		Ki 6	27	
LI 5	17	7	Per 6	8	8			
St 40	24		Liv 4	16				

Except when referring to specific pulses associated with each individual extraordinary vessel, we will refer to the extraordinary vessels as functional pairs in this chapter, first citing the master vessel and then citing the couple vessel. For instance a *du mai/yang qiao* connection implies that *Hou Xi* (SI 3) is master hole and a gold needle or positive pole is applied there, while a silver or stainless needle, or negative pole is applied to *Shen Mai* (Bl 62). Conversely, a *yang qiao/du mai* connection implies that Bl 62 is the master hole and a gold needle is applied there, while a silver, or stainless needle is applied to SI 3.

As with the channel divergences, Akabane testing also dictates which side a given hole is needled on. We next refer back to the left and right stroke tallies for the bladder and small intestine channels in Table 1 (page 143) to determine on which sides Bl 62 and SI 3 are going to be needled. Since the bladder channel on the left side is weakest with a stroke tally of 42, Bl 62 is needled with a gold needle on the left side. Since the small intestine channel on the right side is the strongest with a stroke tally of 4, SI 3 is needled on the right side with a silver or stainless steel needle.

Because Shima does not rely exclusively on the Akabane technique, he also has some more general preferences that often guide his use of the extraordinary vessels. When treating chronic conditions, he generally needles both the master and couple holes of a given extraordinary vessel on a single side. For instance, he might needle *Hou Xi* (SI 3) and *Shen Mai* (Bl 62) on the right and *Wai Guan* (TB 5) and *Lin Qi* (GB 41) on the left. If this proves unsatisfactory, he will then cross the connection needling SI 3 and GB 41 on the right and TB 5 and Bl 62 on the left. Shima also finds this contralateral crossing of master and couple holes especially effective in treating acute conditions. The integration of the channel divergences and the extraordinary vessels is a particularly potent combination that will typically elicit some immediate change within five to ten minutes. If there has not been an improvement in symptoms, pulse, tongue or abdomen in this time, or if the patient reports an increase in her discomfort, then Shima will often switch his extraordinary vessel connections.

CONTRALATERAL NEEDLING OF EXTRAORDINARY VESSELS IN CONCERT WITH CHANNEL DIVERGENCE THERAPY

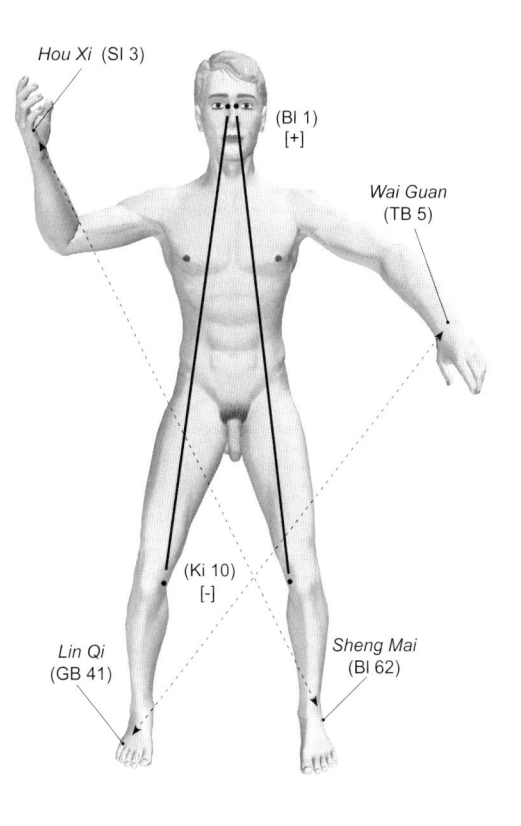

Hou Xi (SI 3)
(Bl 1) [+]
Wai Guan (TB 5)
(Ki 10) [-]
Lin Qi (GB 41)
Sheng Mai (Bl 62)

Although an optional step for him, Shima may elect to follow-up this stage of treatment with another set of acupuncture holes, utilizing the three yin and three yang channels as a means of balancing the main channels. In addition, he almost invariably compliments this combination of extraordinary vessel and channel divergence strategies with extensive use of auriculotherapy. It is Shima's experience that the integration of the three modalities of the channel divergences, the extraordinary vessels, and auriculotherapy yield a therapeutic result that is substantially greater than the sum of its parts. Finally, Shima is careful to direct his needle insertions for the channel divergences at a 45° angle with the flow of the channel. He bases this practice on the research done by Hikoichi Kanari demonstrating that a needle insertion at this angle optimizes the effect of the needle stimulation.[11]

Shima's selection of extraordinary vessel connections in conjunction with the channel divergences is typically based on Akabane findings, pulse and abdominal presentations, and only incidentally on the patient's presenting symptoms. Having said this, however, he finds that certain combinations of extraordinary vessels and channel divergences are especially effective. Such cookbook combinations may be particularly useful for practitioners who are just beginning to integrate channel divergence and extraordinary vessel therapies into their clinical practice. As we have already seen in Chapter 6, modern Japanese acupuncturists have invented a number of auxiliary extraordinary vessel connections and Shima makes extensive use of these. A comprehensive listing of these auxiliary pairings appears in the Akabane chart at the end of Chapter 3 and in the case histories later in this chapter. Confluence pair and extraordinary vessel combinations are summarized as follows:

Confluence Pair	Extraordinary Vessel Combinations
First Confluence	*Chong/yin wei, ren/yin qiao* and *du/yang qiao* connections
Second Confluence	*Dai/yang wei, ren/yin qiao* and *gan/yin wei* connections[12]
Third Confluence	*Chong/yin wei, ren/yin qiao* and *wei/da chang* connections[13]
Fourth Confluence	*Du yang/qiao, ren/yin qiao* and *xin/shen* connections[14]
Fifth Confluence	*Yin/wei chong* and *yang wei/da* connections
Sixth Confluence	*Ren/yin qiao* and *chong/yin wei* connections

The Kidney Return Protocol

It is not uncommon to encounter patients who, for whatever reason, appear to have little or no qi with which to work. Before one can even begin to treat such patients effectively, an acupuncturist must first rally whatever reserves of kidney qi remain. By their very nature, the channel divergences access very deep layers of visceral qi, and it makes sense that they might be used to "jump-start" patients whose kidney qi is in a profound state of depletion. The Kidney Return Protocol was developed precisely for this purpose.

Tadashi Irie originally developed the Kidney Return Protocol and transmitted it to Shima during an early visit to the United States. Regardless of its origin, the Kidney Return Protocol serves as one of the most immediate applications of Shima's own approach to channel divergence therapy and provides an ideal starting point for acupuncturists who wish to begin incorporating channel divergence therapies into their practice. The basic protocol consists of three acupuncture holes, *Wei Zhong* (Bl 40), *Shen Shu* (Bl 23), and *Da Zhu* (Bl 11). Bl 40 is needled with a negative [-] bias, while Bl 23, and Bl 11 are needled with a positive [+] bias, using either bi-metal needles, ion pumping cords, or electrical stimulation. Electrical stimulation should be applied at 1Hz, 3 volts, and 3-5 milliamperes for five to ten minutes.

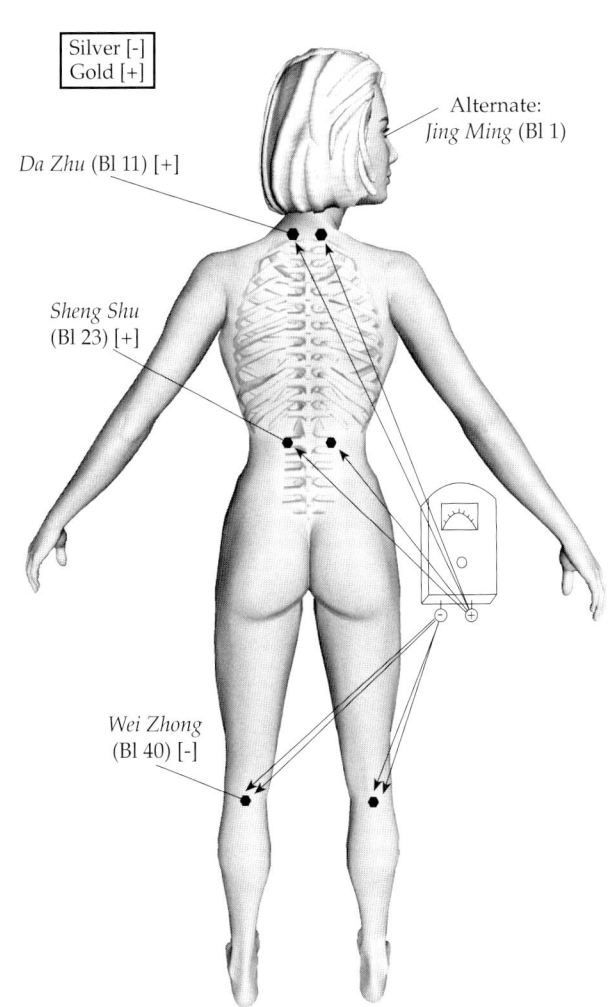

A number of variations on this theme are possible. As we have seen, Shima prefers to begin treatment using the yang channel of a confluence pair. Nevertheless, it is often necessary to bring the yin channels into play, either substituting *Yin Gu* (Ki 10) for Bl 40 or using both acupuncture holes together. In either case, a [-] bias is applied to these access holes of the first confluence in keeping with rules outlined above.

Some patients cannot lie prone, making it necessary to construct a treatment strategy that does not require the use of back transport holes. In this case, *Jing Ming* (Bl 1) may substituted for Bl 11 [+] and *Qi Hai* (CV 6) may be substituted for Bl 23. In cases characterized by kidney vacuity and an insufficiency of clear yang ascending to the head, such as vertigo in a geriatric patient, Bl 1 may be a superior choice to Bl 11 even if the patient can lie prone comfortably.

KIDNEY RETURN PROTOCOL

Shima typically uses the Kidney Return Protocol as part of a more comprehensive needling strategy. He may administer it first as a separate step, or he may combine it with the extraordinary vessels in a single stage of treatment. Applied in this manner, the Kidney Return Protocol specifically rallies the kidney qi and, therefore, facilitates the rest of the treatment. Shima is quick to acknowledge that, while he finds this integration of therapies most effective, it is really a matter of personal preference. The Kidney Return Protocol may be used by itself as a first or second step in a sequenced treatment and, when used in this manner, it is generally applied for 10 minutes before moving on to the next step in the treatment plan. We will now examine a number of Shima's case histories in detail so that we may gain a clearer sense of how Shima actually works.

CASE HISTORIES

The following five cases are representative of Shima's approach to channel divergence therapy. Three of these cases reflect Shima's reliance on Akabane findings as the primary criteria for determining which channel divergences and extraordinary vessels to treat as well determining on which side to needle individual holes. All three cases illustrate how the Akabane methodology is applied in internal medicine and gynecology. The final two cases reflect a more conventional approach to constructing a treatment plan. Because Shima typically prescribes herbal medicine in concert with his acupuncture therapies, we have also included this facet of the therapy in the case reports.

Our goal here is to provide the reader with a sense of the variety of ways in which the channel divergences can be approached in a clinical setting. Shima does not rigidly adhere to any one set of ideas concerning the channel divergences and we will see that he occasionally breaks his own rules, just as most clinicians do. These cases reflect how Shima actually practices as opposed to an idealized version of how he might practice. Throughout this book we have attempted to provide the reader with a variety of approaches to the channel divergences so that he or she can choose which perspective integrates most effectively with their own practice. In presenting the variety of perspectives Shima himself employs when working the channel divergences, we hope to reinforce the point that there is no single best method of channel divergence therapy.

The reader will find that only four of the cases reflect outcomes that might be considered cures. One patient presents with severe cervical dysplasia, one presents with infertility, while another presents with uterine fibroids and a constellation of attendant symptoms. The dysplasia resolves, the patient conceives, the fibroids shrink and the symptoms disappear. These cases proceeded in the orderly fashion of typical textbook case histories. However, many of the illnesses we are called upon to treat present with diseases that are not going to go away. Moreover a patient's lifestyle choices often predispose them to problems that we as clinicians have little influence over and can only hope to ameliorate. In light of this, we have also included two cases profiling Shima's treatment of disorders that are not really curable *per se*. One of the patients presents with insulin dependent diabetes, while the other develops throat cancer over the course of her treatment. While we see an overall improvement in the health of both patients, these two cases reflect situations that are more accurately understood in the context of the goal of disease management as opposed to cure.[15]

Since the fundamental criteria dictating the selection of acupuncture holes is often the Akabane findings, one might conclude that the rest of the information presented in the four Akabane cases is essentially irrelevant. However, such a perspective creates a rather distorted understanding of Shima's diagnostic and treatment process. Akabane technique plays only a small role in Shima's herbal prescribing, which is informed primarily by abdominal and pulse diagnosis. Like many clinicians trained in Japanese styles of practice, Shima is mainly concerned with the information he receives from the pulse, abdomen and Akabane findings. Nevertheless, a patient's symptom presentation does play a secondary role in guiding all facets of treatment. For instance, in one case Shima choses to ignore the predominant Akabane finding because, in his opinion, the secondary Akabane finding more accurately reflects the presenting pattern as evidenced by the signs and symptoms. More often than not, however, the reader will notice that the other diagnostic parameters, reflect the major Akabane findings.

The herbal prescribing presented below is based on the *Kanpo Yaku* style of herbal medicine, which relies heavily on the integration of abdominal diagnosis with other presenting symptoms. While Shima uses much of the terminology of the Traditional Chinese Medicine style of herbal medicine he is definitively not a TCM practitioner and the reader is encouraged to keep this in mind when reading the following cases.

CASE ONE

Susan G., a 53 year-old Caucasian, right-handed female was first seen on September 3, 1993. The patient's chief complaint was fatigue. In addition, she complained of left hip pain when she failed to walk regularly. She experienced hot flashes with neck and shoulder aches and occipital headaches. Ms. G. had experienced occasional migrating pains that were worse on the right earlier in 1993. Some of this was pain from a previous fractured first metatarsal that radiated to the ankle and then to the knee in the spring of 1995. Her concentration and memory were poor, and her sleep was disturbed by heat sensations at night, although she did not have night sweats. She described a sensation of achy intestines in her lower right quadrant.

The patient suffered from asthma from the time of her adolescence until she was 44 or 45 years old. When she was 19, she sustained a trauma to her sternum. At age 31, she contracted hepatitis A in New York City. Ms. G. reported that she had been diagnosed with anemia, however, she could not be more specific. She had developed chest pain the previous autumn and was evaluated at Kaiser Permanente at that time. Both electrocardiogram and chest x-rays were normal, and she was diagnosed with arthritis of the sternum probably related to the injury she had in her teenage years. Ms. G. had treated this condition with an herbal preparation she had prescribed for herself and recovered.

The patient's face was sallow and livid with a background darkness, and her sclera were mildly bloodshot. Her tongue was large and damp with thin white fur and some mild cracking in the area corresponding to the middle burner. Ms. G.'s pulse was wiry and choppy overall, particularly in the *chi* position, which was also bilaterally weak and sunken. In addition, the *guan* positions were bilaterally weak, suggesting an insufficiency of middle qi. Manual examination of her back revealed a generalized state of muscle spasm. Abdominal diagnosis revealed subcostal tension suggestive of liver qi stagnation, *spleen shaku*[16] and dampness in the stomach suggestive of spleen vacuity and dampness, areas of hardness in the right and left lower quadrants suggestive of blood stasis and lower abdominal flaccidity suggestive of kidney weakness.

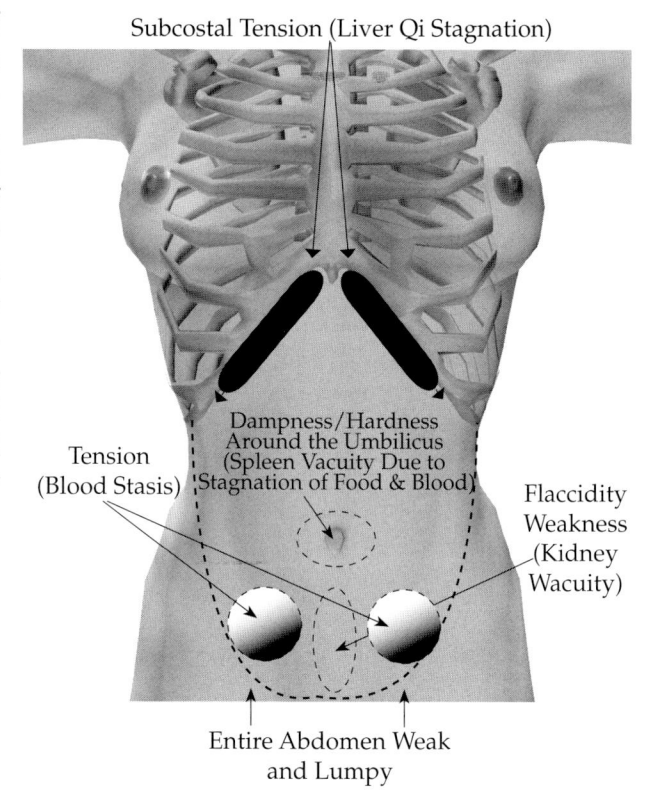

Subcostal Tension (Liver Qi Stagnation)

Tension (Blood Stasis)

Dampness/Hardness Around the Umbilicus (Spleen Vacuity Due to Stagnation of Food & Blood)

Flaccidity Weakness (Kidney Wacuity)

Entire Abdomen Weak and Lumpy

The Akabane readings were as follows:

TABLE 1: LATERAL POLARIZATIONS

FOOT

Channel	R	L	Tot.	Dev.
Spleen	5	9	14	4
Liver	7	9	16	2
Stomach	12	12	24	0
Gallbladder	15	(22)	37	7
Kidney	14	13	27	1
Bladder	14	(42)	56	(28)

HAND

Channel	R	L	Tot.	Dev.
Lung	6	5	11	1
L. Intestine	6	11	17	5
Pericardium	4	4	8	0
Triple Burner	(5)	9	14	4
Heart	15	8	23	7
S. Intestine	(4)	5	9	1

Table 2: Channel Divergence Polarizations

	Tot.	Dev.		Tot.	Dev.		Tot.	Dev.
Ki	27	(29)	Sp	14	10	Per	8	1
Bl	(56)		St	24		SI	9	
Liv	16	(21)	Ht	23	14	Lu	11	6
GB	(37)		SI	9		LI	17	

Table 3: Extra Channel Polarizations

	Tot.	Dev.		Tot.	Dev.		Tot.	Dev.
SI 3	9	(47)	Lu 7	11	16	Lu 7	11	3
Bl 62	56		Ki 6	27		Sp 4	14	
GB 41	37	(23)	Per 6	8	6	Ht 5	23	4
TB 5	14		Sp 4	14		KI 6	27	
LI 5	17	7	Per 6	8	8			
St 40	24		Liv 4	16				

The Akabane findings confirmed both the liver and kidney weakness suggested by the pulse and abdomen. However, the tongue and pulse patterns suggestive of a middle burner weakness were not reflected in the Akabane findings.

TREATMENT:

1) General *Sesshokushin*
   Shima first administered *Sesshokushin* to relieve the muscle spasm in Ms. G.'s back as a means of facilitating the rest of the treatment. *Sesshokushin* is a general term for a variety of superficial needling techniques. Shima's application of *Sesshokushin* in this case involved deep palpation for sore and reactive *Hua Tuo Jia Ji* holes along the spine and on the general level of the channel sinews. These were then needled lightly using the supplementation technique described in Difficult Issues 78 and 80 of the *Classic of Difficult Issues*.

2) Moxibustion on left *Pang Guang Shu* (Bl 28)
   Moxibustion with soft, large cones of aged moxa applied to the transport holes on the back is a key step in resolving the left-right imbalances identified by the Akabane diagnosis. This moxibustion technique was in the primary therapy that Akabane himself used in treating patients. With an Akabane finding of 42, Ms. G.'s left bladder channel was the weakest of all the channels, and therefore moxibustion on left Bl 28 is the first step in rectifying this situation.

3) Channel divergence treatment was administered to the first and second confluences using gold and silver needle technique. This was combined with an extraordinary vessel treatment utilizing the *yang qiao/du* and *dai/yang wei* connections. These channels were treated in the following pattern:

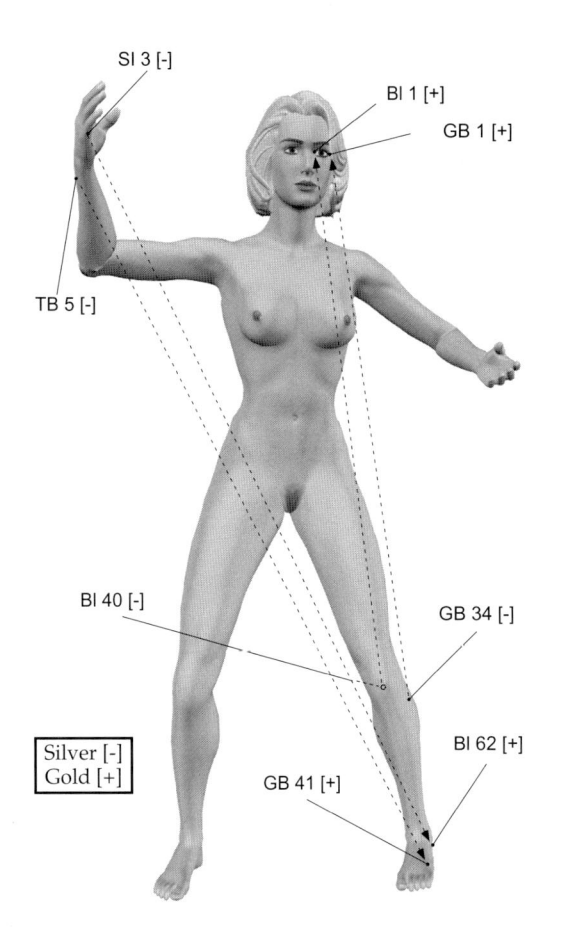

The unilateral selection of holes was determined exclusively by the Akabane findings. We see from the tallies in Table 2 pertaining to the channel divergences, that the first and second confluences reflect the greatest imbalances, with total deviations of 29 and 21 respectively. Table 2 also tells us that the yang channels reflected the greatest imbalances, with totals of 56 and 37 respectively, so Shima needled the yang channel of each confluence pair. Finally, he needled the bladder and gallbladder channel divergences on the left side because these channels were both weakest on the left.

Shima applied the same rationale to his selection of extraordinary vessels. With total deviations of 47 and 23 respectively tallied in Table 3, the *yang qiao/du* and *dai/yang wei* connections reflected the greatest imbalances. The gold needle was placed on the master hole of the weakest channel in each extraordinary vessel pairing. Since the bladder channel required 56 strokes, it was considerably weaker than the small intestine channel that only required 9 strokes. Bl 62 was designated the "master hole" and was needled with a gold needle. It was needled on the left side because the left side showed higher Akabane findings than the right reflecting a weaker condition. Its coupled hole, SI 3 was needled with a silver needle on the right side because the Akabane finding of 4 on the right showed that the right small intestine channel was stronger than the left.

4) Finally, Shima needled Omura's Thymus holes:
Omura's Thymus holes are *Xuan Ji* (CV 21) and any of the sore points in the subclavicular area.[17] These holes were needled because they function to boost the immune response. Ms. G. received no auriculotherapy because she was too weak to tolerate it.

2ND TREATMENT

Ms. G. returned two weeks later on September 17, to report that she was feeling better overall. Much of the pain she had been experiencing had diminished. Her appetite had improved, and her bowel movements were regular, despite the fact that this aspect of her situation had not been addressed directly. She still complained of a subjective sense of tightness in her abdomen, which Shima attributed to liver qi depression although her abdomen was flaccid upon palpation.

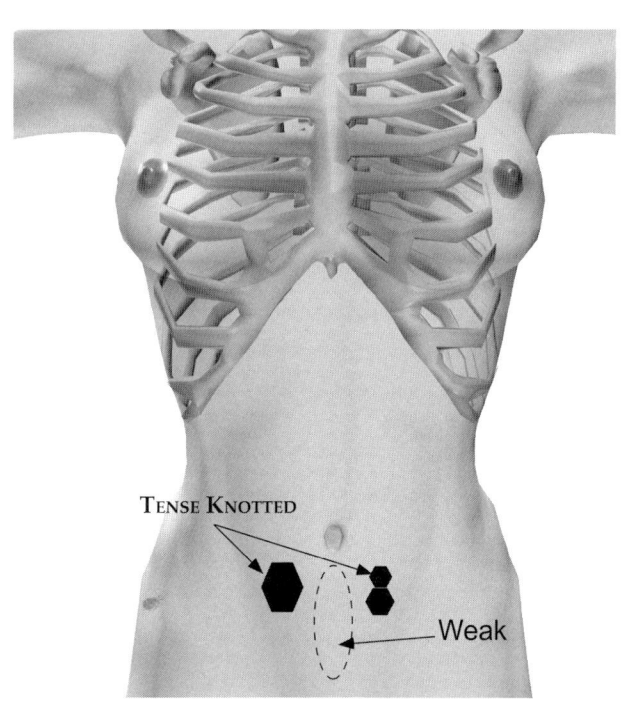

Ms. G.'s pulse was generally stronger. However, the right *chi* position was still profoundly weak, both deep and superficially. This reflected a persistent vacuity of the kidney and bladder.

THE AKABANE READINGS WERE AS FOLLOWS:

TABLE 1: LATERAL POLARIZATIONS

FOOT

Channel	R	L	Tot.	Dev.
Spleen	9	9	18	0
Liver	7	14	21	7
Stomach	6	9	15	3
Gallbladder	(19)	19	38	0
Kidney	11	11	22	0
Bladder	16	(28)	44	(12)

HAND

Channel	R	L	Tot.	Dev.
Lung	14	14	28	0
L. Intestine	7	11	18	4
Pericardium	18	7	25	11
Triple Burner	(4)	8	12	4
Heart	9	5	14	4
S. Intestine	9	(5)	14	4

TABLE 2: CHANNEL DIVERGENCE POLARIZATIONS

	Tot.	Dev.		Tot.	Dev.		Tot.	Dev.
Ki	22	㉒	Sp	18	3	Per	25	13
Bl	㊹		St	15		TB	12	
Liv	21	⑰	Ht	14	0	Lu	28	10
GB	㊳		SI	14		LI	18	

TABLE 3: EXTRA CHANNEL POLARIZATIONS

	Tot.	Dev.		Tot.	Dev.		Tot.	Dev.
SI 3	14	㉚	Lu 7	28	6	Lu 7	28	10
Bl 62	44		Ki 6	22		Sp 4	18	
GB 41	38	㉖	Per 6	25	7	Ht 5	14	8
TB 5	12		Sp 4	18		Ki 6	22	
LI 5	18	3	Per 6	25	4			
St 40	15		Liv 4	21				

Once again the Akabane findings confirmed the bladder and kidney weakness suggested by the pulse and the presence of liver qi suggested by the abdomen.

TREATMENT:

1) Moxibustion was administered to right *Pang Guan Shu* (Bl 28). Bl 28 is the back transport hole of the bladder and it was treated to correct the channels reflecting the most profound left-right imbalance. With a stoke tally of 28, the left side was shown to be weaker than the right.

2) A channel divergence treatment was administered to the first confluence on the left and

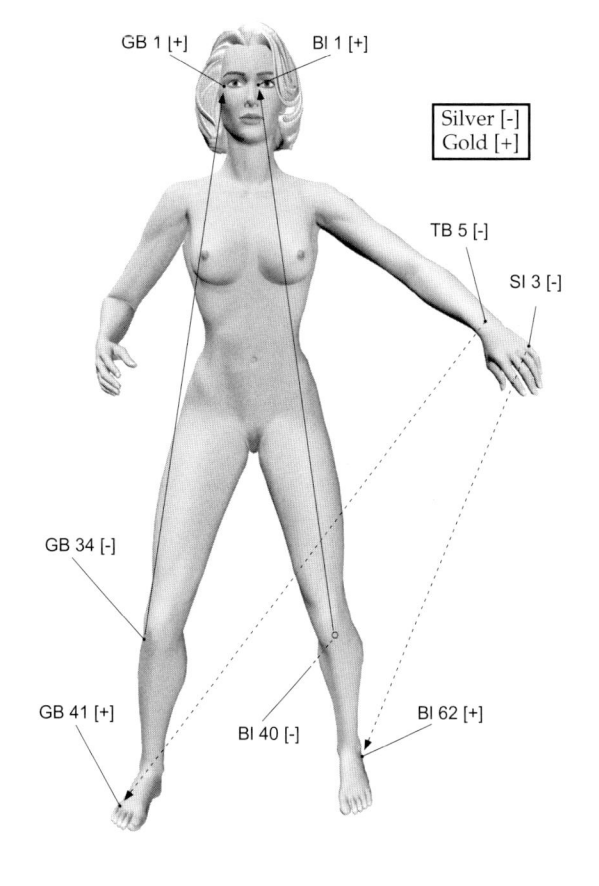

GB 1 [+]
Bl 1 [+]
Silver [-]
Gold [+]
TB 5 [-]
SI 3 [-]
GB 34 [-]
GB 41 [+]
Bl 40 [-]
Bl 62 [+]

the second confluence on the right. Extraordinary vessel treatment was administered using the *dai/yang wei* and *yang qiao/du* connections.

The yang channels of both the first and second confluence were weaker than their paired yin channels so Shima needled the yang channel of each confluence. The Akabane findings indicated that the first confluence should be needled on the left because the left side was the weakest as evidenced by its higher number of strokes. Although the left-right Akabane readings for the gallbladder were the same, Shima treated the second confluence on the right simply to balance out the treatment. This rationale extended to his selection of sides for the *dai/yang wei* as well. GB 41 could have been needled on either side. However, needling it on the right created a greater sense of balance.

Ms. G. responded well to these initial treatments and continued to see Shima regularly. Treatment proceeded much as described above with minor variations based on her symptoms and Akabane findings.

20TH TREATMENT

On December 22, 1995, Ms. G.'s pulse was uniformly deep and weak, suggesting to Shima a vacuity of the *chong* and *ren mai*. However, the left *chi* position was the weakest, reflecting a vacuity of the bladder and kidneys. The tongue coat was thick and moist in the areas corresponding to the middle burner and heart. The abdomen reflected subcostal tightness suggesting liver qi stagnation, epigastric spasm suggesting obstruction of heart qi, spleen *shaku* suggesting spleen vacuity and dampness, lower abdominal flaccidity suggesting kidney vacuity, and knots of hardness suggesting blood stasis in the lower burner.

Subcostal Tension (Liver Qi Stagnation)
Spleen *Shaku*
Blockage of Heart Qi
Blood Stasis
Lower Abdominal Flaccidity

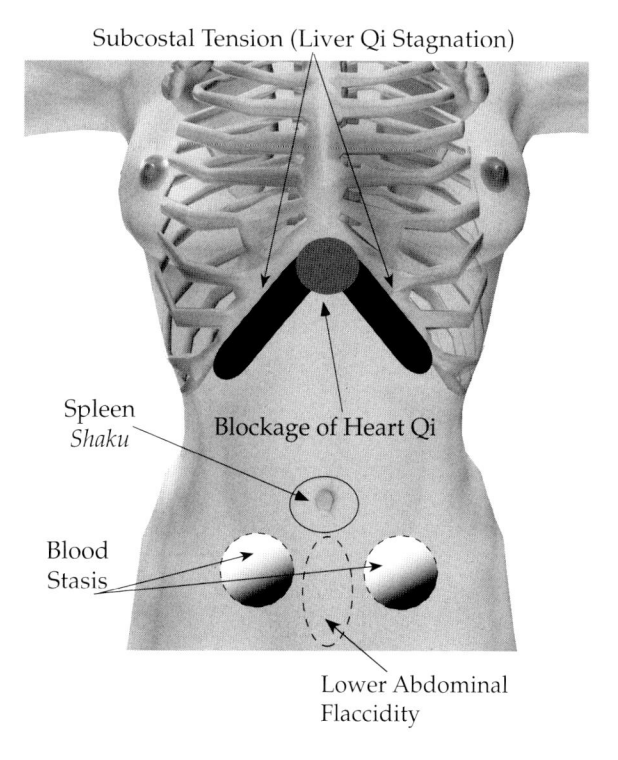

The Akabane readings were as follows:

Table 1: Lateral Polarizations

FOOT

Channel	R	L	Tot.	Dev.
Spleen	18	26	44	8
Liver	30	36	66	6
Stomach	19	(47)	66	(28)
Gallbladder	(40)	39	79	1
Kidney	23	19	42	4
Bladder	18	(43)	61	(25)

HAND

Channel	R	L	Tot.	Dev.
Lung	(36)	14	50	(22)
L. Intestine	14	15	29	1
Pericardium	14	7	21	7
Triple Burner	14	(10)	24	4
Heart	13	7	20	6
S. Intestine	(11)	13	24	2

Table 2: Channel Divergence Polarizations

	Tot.	Dev.		Tot.	Dev.		Tot.	Dev.
Bl	61	19	GB	79	13	Ht	20	4
Ki	42		Liv	66		SI	24	
St	(66)	(22)	Per	21	3	Lu	(50)	(21)
Sp	44		TB	24		LI	29	

Table 3: Extra Channel Polarizations

	Tot.	Dev.		Tot.	Dev.		Tot.	Dev.
SI 3	24	(37)	Lu 7	50	8	Lu 7	50	6
Bl 62	61		Ki 6	42		Sp 4	44	
GB 41	79	(55)	Per 6	21	23	Ht 5	20	22
TB 5	24		Sp 4	44		KI 6	42	
LI 5	29	37	Per 6	21	2			
St 40	66		Liv 4	23				

Here we see that the Akabane findings now emphasize the middle burner on the level of the channel divergences while also reflecting an imbalance of the sixth confluence despite the absence of any other confirmatory signs or symptoms. Interestingly, the Akabane results did not reflect a primary kidney involvement on the level of the channel divergences, nor did they concur on the *chong mai* involvement.

Miki Shima's Approach

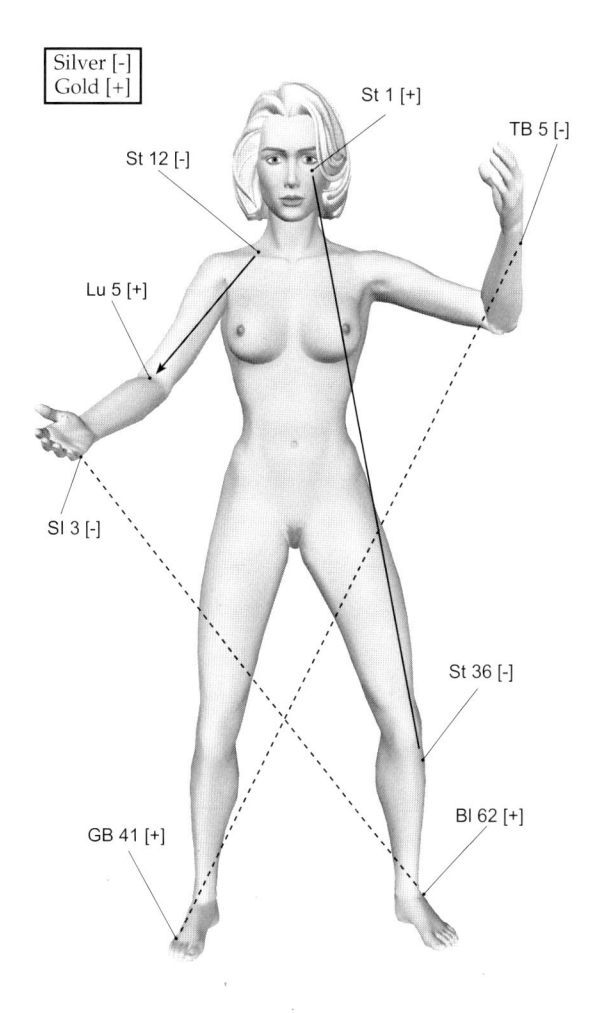

Silver [-]
Gold [+]

St 1 [+]
St 12 [-]
TB 5 [-]
Lu 5 [+]
SI 3 [-]
St 36 [-]
GB 41 [+]
Bl 62 [+]

Treatment:

1) Moxibustion on Bl 13 right, Bl 21 left, and Bl 28 left. These holes were needled to correct the channels reflecting the most profound left-right imbalances as recorded in the deviation column.

2) Shima then needled the third confluence on the left and the sixth confluence on the right side. Extraordinary vessel treatment was administered using the *dai/yang wei* and the *yang qiao/du* connections.

Here we see that the third and sixth confluences reflect the greatest imbalances, with total deviations of 22 and 21 respectively.

The yang channel of the third confluence with at stroke tally of 66 and the yin channel of the sixth confluence with a totals of 50 tabulated in Table 2, reflected the greatest imbalances so Shima needled these channels. Finally, he needled the stomach channel on the left and the lung channel on the right because these channels were both weakest on the left and because the stroke tally was highest on these sides.

As for the extraordinary vessels, with total deviations of 37 and 55 respectively, the *yang qiao/du* and *dai/yang wei* connections reflected the greatest imbalances.[18] The gold needle was placed on the master hole of the weakest channel in each extraordinary vessel pairing. For instance, since the gallbladder channel had a stroke tally of 79 strokes, it was considerably weaker than the triple burner channel that only required 24 strokes. Therefore, GB 41 was designated as the master hole and was needled with a gold needle. It was needled on the right side because the original stroke tally tabulated in Table 1 showed that the right side was weakest with 40 strokes. Its coupled hole, TB 5, was needled with a silver needle on the left side because the Akabane finding of 10 on the left as compared to 14 on the right showed that triple burner channel was stronger on the left.

27th Treatment

Shima's treatment of Ms. G.'s case was a long-term project. However, she made steady progress. By March 14, 1996, Ms. G. was doing well overall. She was walking every day, and her bowel movement and urination were normal. Her appetite was good, although she craved sweets. Ms. G.'s sleep was interrupted, and she would awaken gasping for air, but she felt she was getting enough rest. Shima referred her to an ear, nose, and throat (ENT) specialist. She was mildly depressed and complained of occasional lower back pain. Ms. G.'s pulse on the right side was floating and tight, reflecting a *du mai/yang qiao mai* vacuity. Her abdomen again showed liver qi stagnation, blockage of heart qi, spleen *shaku*, and blood stasis in the lower abdomen.

The Akabane readings were as follows:

Table 1: Lateral Polarizations

FOOT

Channel	R	L	Tot.	Dev.
Spleen	10	8	18	2
Liver	8	8	16	0
Stomach	12	8	20	4
Gallbladder	(20)	17	(37)	3
Kidney	(19)	14	(33)	5
Bladder	16	16	32	0

HAND

Channel	R	L	Tot.	Dev.
Lung	6	(6)	12	0
L. Intestine	5	9	14	4
Pericardium	13	6	19	(7)
Triple Burner	7	(7)	14	0
Heart	6	6	12	0
S. Intestine	5	12	17	7

Table 2: Channel Divergence Polarizations

	Tot.	Dev.		Tot.	Dev.		Tot.	Dev.
Bl	32	2	GB	(37)	(21)	Ht	12	5
Ki	33		Liv	16		SI	17	
St	20	2	Per	19	5	Lu	12	2
Sp	18		TB	14		LI	14	

Miki Shima's Approach

TABLE 3: EXTRA CHANNEL POLARIZATIONS

	Tot.	Dev.		Tot.	Dev.		Tot.	Dev.
SI 3	17	15	Lu 7	12	(21)	Lu 7	12	6
Bl 62	32		Ki 6	33		Sp 4	18	
GB 41	37	(23)	Per 6	19	1	Ht 5	12	21
TB 5	14		Sp 4	18		Ki 6	33	
LI 5	14	6	Per 6	19	3			
St 40	20		Liv 4	16				

Note that the pulse matched neither the abdominal nor the Akabane findings.

TREATMENT:

1) Three cones of soft direct moxa were applied to *Jue Yin Shu* (Bl 14) right, *Dan Shu* (Bl 19) right, *Shen Shu* (Bl 23) right, and *Pang Guang Shu* (Bl 28) right. As always, the Akabane findings dictated Shima's choice of back transport holes. With total stroke tallies of 37 and 33, the gallbladder and kidney channels were shown to be the weakest. Since the gallbladder and kidney were weakest on the right side, and the tallies were the same on both bladder channels, Shima moxaed the right side.

2) A channel divergence treatment was administered to the second confluence on the right. In addition, the *dai/yang wei* and *ren/yin qiao* connections were stimulated in the manner depicted in the graphic:

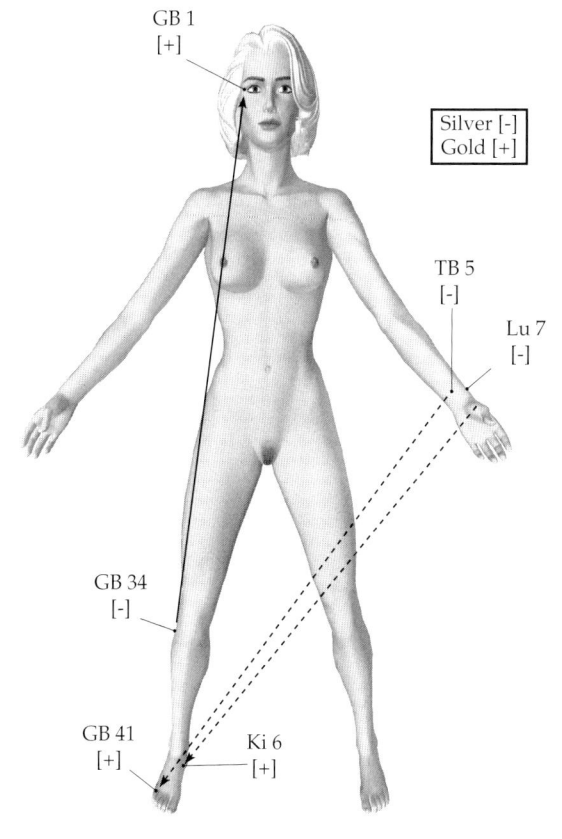

The needles were retained for 30 minutes.

With a total deviation of 21 tallied in Table 3, the second confluence was Shima's choice for a channel divergence treatment. The gallbladder channel was obviously the weakest, with a stroke tally of 37 compared to a stroke tally of 16 for the liver. He needled the gallbladder on the right side because the right side required 20 strokes while the left side only required 17 (Table 1).

As for the extraordinary vessels, with total deviations of 23 and 21 respectively, the *dai/yang wei* and *ren/yin qiao* connections reflected the greatest imbalances. With a stroke tally of 37 strokes, the gallbladder was once again considerably weaker than the triple burner channel that only required 14 strokes. Therefore, GB 41 was designated as the master hole and was needled with a gold needle. It was needled on the right side because the original stroke tally tabulated in Table 1 showed that the right side was weakest with 20 strokes. The Akabane values for the triple burner and the lungs were the same on both the right and left sides at 7 and 6 respectively, (Table 1). Therefore, the extraordinary vessel pairings could be connected either ipsilaterally or contralaterally. Shima chose contralateral or crossing connections because the triple burner and lung involvement were new in her case and he prefers contralateral connections in more acute conditions. No auricular therapy was administered.

Ms. G. was then given a combination of *You Gui* and *Zuo Gui Wan* (Right & Left Return [the Kidneys] Pills) for one month.[19,20,21]

31ST TREATMENT

Later in the spring Ms. G. was diagnosed with throat cancer. It is interesting to note that although she had complained about her throat being dry and she would gasp for air during her sleep, she never said her throat was actually sore. From a Chinese medical perspective, her primary problem was clearly a kidney and urinary bladder vacuity, which showed up consistently in her Akabane tests. It is likely that the enduring kidney vacuity failed to nourish the lungs for such a long time that the lung yin became desiccated and predisposed her to a malignancy in the tissues associated with the lungs.

On March 14, 1997, it was determined that Ms. G. had responded to local radiation therapy for her cancer and continued to feel well. She experienced no further problems with her throat. She was sleeping through the night in spite of the dryness of the air, and her appetite was returning. In addition to the *Zuo You Gui Tang* (Left and Right Return [the Kidneys] Decoction) prescribed by Shima, she had been taking an herbal prescription from Kee Lai, a local Chinese herbalist.[22] Finally, she was instructed to take 30 grams of powdered *Dong Chong Xia Cao* (Cordyceps Sinensis) per day.

At this examination, Ms. G.'s pulse was weak in the left *chi*, right *guan*, and left superficial *guan* positions, reflecting to Shima a vacuity of the kidneys, spleen, and gallbladder. In addition, Ms. G.'s pulse was overly strong in the left *chi* position, suggesting to Shima repletion in the heart and small intestine. In addition, her tongue was swollen and moist in the areas corresponding to the middle burner and the heart. The tongue had no coat, and there was a crack in the middle. Abdominal diagnosis reflected the continued presence of blood stasis and ongoing kidney vacuity.

The Akabane readings were as follows:

TABLE 1: LATERAL POLARIZATIONS

FOOT

Channel	R	L	Tot.	Dev.
Spleen	12	26	38	(14)
Liver	14	14	28	0
Stomach	8	10	18	2
Gallbladder	35	13	(48)	(22)
Kidney	16	18	34	2
Bladder	33	(34)	(67)	1

HAND

Channel	R	L	Tot.	Dev.
Lung	7	12	19	5
L. Intestine	14	13	27	1
Pericardium	12	12	24	0
Triple Burner	17	17	34	0
Heart	9	6	15	3
S. Intestine	10	14	24	4

TABLE 2: CHANNEL DIVERGENCE POLARIZATIONS

	Tot.	Dev.		Tot.	Dev.		Tot.	Dev.
Bl	67	(33)	GB	48	(20)	Ht	15	9
Ki	34		Liv	28		SI	24	
St	18	(20)	Per	24	10	Lu	19	18
Sp	38		TB	34		LI	37	

TABLE 3: EXTRA CHANNEL POLARIZATIONS

	Tot.	Dev.		Tot.	Dev.		Tot.	Dev.
SI 3	24	(43)	Lu 7	19	15	Lu 7	19	19
Bl 62	67		Ki 6	34		Sp 4	38	
GB 41	48	14	Per 6	24	14	Ht 5	15	19
TB 5	34		Sp 4	38		Ki 6	34	
LI 5	27	9	Per 6	24	4			
St 40	18		Liv 4	28				

TREATMENT:

1) Moxibustion on left *Pi Shu* (Bl 20) and right *Dan Shu* (Bl 19). This was administered to correct the channels reflecting the most profound left-right imbalance as indicated by the channels with the greatest numerical deviations in the Akabane test. (Table 1)

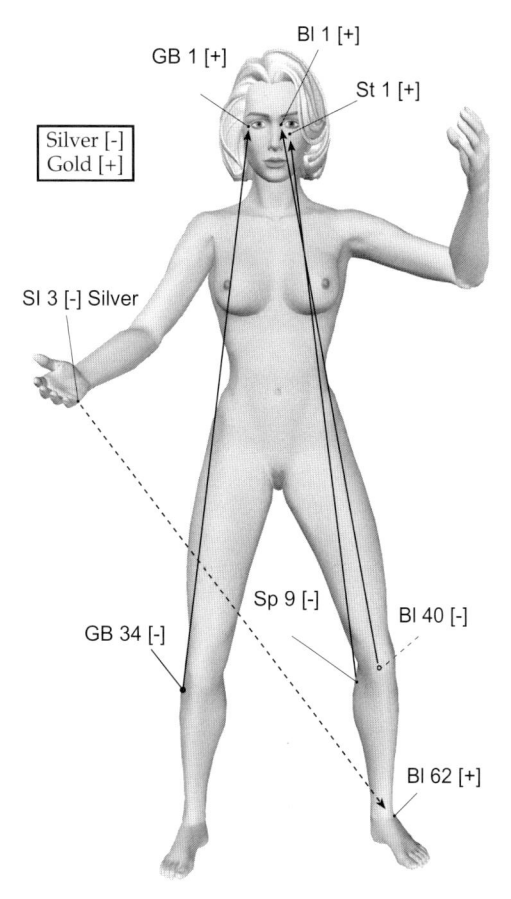

2) A channel divergence treatment was administered to the first and third confluences on the left and the second confluence on the right. An extraordinary vessel treatment was administered contralaterally to the *du/yang qiao* connection.

With deviations of 33, 20, and 20 tallied in Table 2, Shima selected the first, second and third confluences for treatment. The yang channels of the first and second confluence, and the yin channel of the third confluence were the weakest so Shima treated these.

Shima selected only the *yang qiao/du* connections from his extraordinary vessel tabulations. With a stroke tally of 67, Bl 62 was selected as the master hole and was needled on the left side because this side was incrementally weaker (Table 1). SI 3 was needled on the right side because this side had a lower stroke tally.

MIKI SHIMA'S COMMENTARY:

Ms. G. has continued to do well since her treatment for throat cancer. She has some fluctuations, but they are minor. She tends to be over-stressed most of the time due to her busy practice. She also takes care of her 81 year-old mother whom I also see as a patient. Ms. G. takes *You Gui Wan* (Restore the Right [Kidney] Pills) and *Zuo Gui Wan* (Restore the Left [Kidney] Pills) along with Cordyceps Extract from Meditalent Co. She eats very well but sleeps poorly. She is so emotionally sensitive that she tends to be excessively concerned about things at night.

As we can see from her Akabane results, she frequently requires correction of the *du/yang qiao* and *dai/yang wei* vessels and the first and second confluences. These are basically kidney-bladder and liver-gallbladder imbalances. They are truly chronic problems caused by excessive taxation of her body and mind. Aside from Ms. G.'s own battle with throat cancer, her mother has a severe pulmonary condition as well. By far, the weakest facet of her channel system is the kidney-bladder confluence, and I think it has drained so much qi from her lungs that it caused her throat cancer. I have her throat rechecked every six months and, so far, it has yet to recur.

Over the years, Ms. G. has cut down on her work and has begun walking an hour a day. She has also begun eating more animal protein, including red meats, which has fortified her lungs and kidneys very much. She avoids cold vegetables and fruit most of the time. She also meditates regularly now, as a means of improving her insomnia, and this has been having some positive effect of late. I continue to monitor the status of her throat cancer quite carefully because this type of cancer has a tendency to recur even after many years. Radiation is often only ameliorative, not curative, and, if the cancer recurs, her only other option is a continuous course of chemotherapy for the rest of her life just to keep it under control.

The Cordyceps Extract from Meditalent has been very good for Ms. G. and other lung cancer patients in my practice. I use very large dosages (30-60g per day), and it appears to supplement the lungs as well as the kidneys.

I counseled Ms. G. to reduce her work schedule by 50% until all of her Akabane readings have normalized. However, she says that this is financially impossible for her. This is unfortunate because a recurrence of throat cancer would have an extremely poor prognosis.

I often check the overall total tabulations and the tabulations of left-right deviations on the channel divergence system because I am curious about not only the yin-yang deviations but also the total vacuity of channel divergence. If two pairs of confluences have the same deviation, I pick the one with greater total vacuity.

Case Two

Sally O. was a 38 year-old, Caucasian female who presented on April 21, 1999 with insulin dependent diabetes mellitus (IDDM1) which was diagnosed at age 26. Her chief complaints were a tendency to fatigue and foggy headedness, chronic, low-grade headaches, and neck pain. Ms. O. experienced premenstrual syndrome, dysmenorrhea and irregular menstruation with dark red blood and clots in her menstuate. Her libido was low, and she experienced cravings for chocolate and barbecue-flavored potato chips. She reported a sensitivity to wheat and experienced fatigue when she ate it. Ms. O. consumed approximately 70g of protein per day. The patient reported that she required a total of 60 units of insulin per day, administered by pump at a rate of approximately 2.5 unit per hour, per 10 grams of carbohydrates. Over the course of a day, she would consume 60 units. Her glucose average was 200mg/dl. All other vital signs were normal. Her pulse was wiry, tight, and strong. Ms. O.'s abdomen showed subcostal tension indicative of liver qi stagnation, a generalized sense of cold, phlegm and dampness, and sub-umbilical hardness reflecting blood stasis.

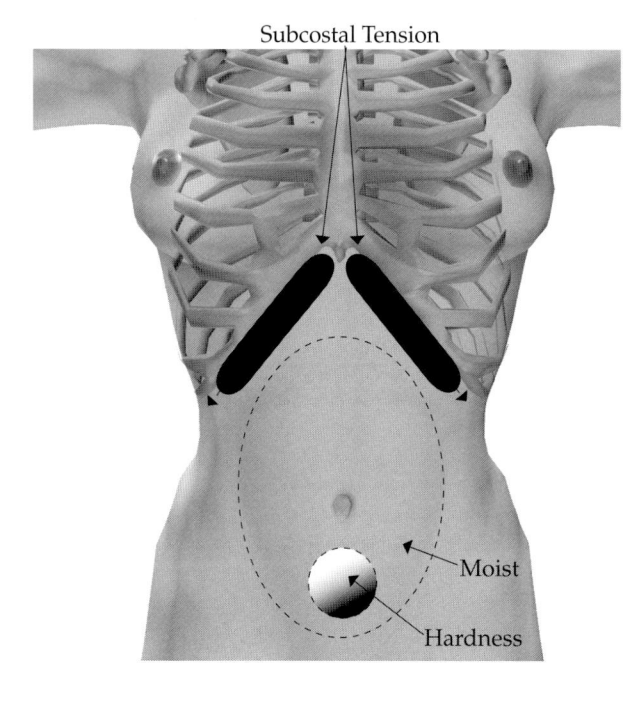

Shima took no Akabane readings on this initial visit. The patient was given the following Chinese herbal formulas in bulk herb decoctions based on her symptoms, menstural history and abdominal conformation. They were phased to her menstrual cycle with the intention of supplementing the spleen, quickening the blood, and coursing the liver.

For days 1-5 of her menstrual cycle Ms. O. received a decoction of *Tao Hong Si Wu Tang* (Peach Kernel and Carthamas Four-Agents Decoction), one cup, twice daily. It contained the following ingredients: *Tao Ren* (Semen Pruni Persicae) 6g, *Hong Hua* (Flos Carthami Tinctorii), 6g, *Shu Di Huang* (Radix Rehmanniae Glutinosae Conquitae) 3g, *Dang Gui* (Radix Angelicae Sinensis) 6g, *Bai Shao* (Radix Paeoniae Lactiflorae) 3g, and *Chuan Xiong* (Radix Ligustici Wallichii) 6g. This addressed the blood stasis producing clotting and dysmenorrhea.

For days 5-15 of her menstrual cycle, Ms. O. received the following in desiccated extract form: *Ba Zhen Tang* (Eight Gem Decoction), 35g,[23] *You Gui Wan* (Right Restoring [Life-gate] Pills), 35g, *Zuo Gui Wan* (Left Restoring [Life-gate] Pills), 35g, *Tu Su Zi* (Semen Cuscutae Chinensis), 5g, *Che Qian Zi* (Semen Plantaginis) 10g, *Xian Ling Pi* (Herba Epimedii), 10g. Five grams of this formula was taken twice daily for 12 days. This addressed the vacuities of qi, blood, kidney yin during the follicular phase.

For days 16-30 of her menstrual cycle received the following modification of *Gui Zhi Fu Ling Tang* (Cinnamon & Hoelen Decoction). *Gui Zhi* (Ramulus Cinnamomi Cassiae) 6g, *Fu Ling* (Sclerotium Poriae Cocos) 6g, *Tao Ren* (Semen Pruni Persicae) 6g, *Bai Shao* (Radix Paeoeniae Lactiflorae) 6g, and *Mu Dan Pi* (Cortex Moutan Radicis) 6g, *Tao Ren* (Semen Pruni Persicae) 6g, *Hong Hua* (Flos Carthami Tinctori), 6g, *Shu Di Huang* (Radix Rehmanniae Glutinosae Conquitae) 3g, *Dang Gui* (Radix Angelicae Sinensis) 6g, *Bai Shao* (Radix Paeoniae Lactiflorae) 3g, and *Chuan Xiong* (Radix Ligustici Wallichii) 6g, *Xiang Fu* (Rhizoma Cyperi Rotundi), 15g, *Wu Yao*

(Radix Linderae Strychnifoliae), 10g, and *Zhi Ke* (Fructus Citri Aurantii), 10g. Once again, one cup was taken twice daily, for 15 days. Acupuncture was prescribed on a once monthly basis, although none was administered the first visit. The following office visits are representative of Ms. O.'s overall progress.

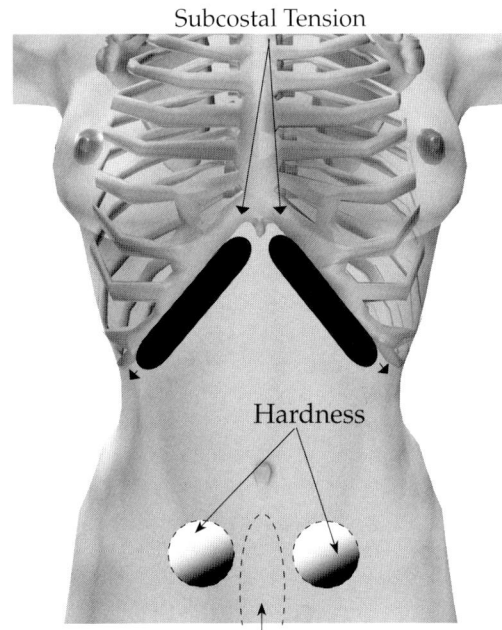

Subcostal Tension

Hardness

Lower Abdominal Weakness

Third Treatment[24]

On July 9, 1999, Ms. O. reported that she was doing well, although she was putting in long hours setting up her business and felt that she was on the verge of burning out. She reported that she was walking 20-30 minutes 3-4 days per week. Her last menstruation was only slightly painful and slightly heavy, lasting a little longer than usual at four days. Finally, she reported that she was experiencing some pain in her Achilles tendon. Her left pulse was a *du* pulse and stronger than the right, while the right pulse was a *ren* pulse. Ms. O.'s abdomen exhibited subcostal tension suggestive of liver qi depression, tension in the lateral abdominal area suggestive of blood stagnation and weakness along the centerline just above the pubic bone reflecting kidney vacuity.

Akabane findings were as follows:

TABLE 1: LATERAL POLARIZATIONS

FOOT				
Channel	R	L	Tot.	Dev.
Spleen	19	11	30	8
Liver	13	33	46	(20)
Stomach	36	18	54	(18)
Gallbladder	(40)	40	80	0
Kidney	(38)	10	48	(28)
Bladder	16	20	36	4

HAND				
Channel	R	L	Tot.	Dev.
Lung	18	20	38	2
L. Intestine	15	25	40	10
Pericardium	14	19	33	5
Triple Burner	10	(16)	26	6
Heart	6	(6)	12	0
S. Intestine	8	8	16	0

TABLE 2: Channel Divergence Polarizations

	Tot	Dev.		Tot.	Dev.		Tot.	Dev.
Bl	36	⑫	GB	80	㉞	Ht	12	4
Ki	48		Liv	46		SI	16	
St	54	㉔	Per	33	7	Lu	38	2
Sp	30		TB	26		LI	40	

TABLE 3: Extra Channel Polarizations

	Tot.	Dev.		Tot.	Dev.		Tot.	Dev.
SI 3	16	20	Lu 7	38	10	Lu 7	38	8
Bl 62	36		Ki 6	48		Sp 4	30	
GB 41	80	㉞	Per 6	33	3	Ht 5	12	㊲
TB 5	26		Sp 4	30		Ki 6	㊽	
LI 5	40	14	Per 6	33	13			
St 40	54		Liv 4	46				

Ms. O.'s Akabane findings on the level of the channel divergences were consistent with both her pulse and abdomen.

TREATMENT:

1) Moxibustion on *Gan Shu* (Bl 18) left, *Wei Shu* (Bl 21) right, and Bl 23 right. These holes were moxaed to to correct the channels reflecting the most profound left-right imbalance as indicated by the channels with the greatest numerical deviations in the Akabane test. (Table 1)

2) Miki Shima treated the first, second, and third confluences and the *dai/yang wei* and *xin/shen* connections.

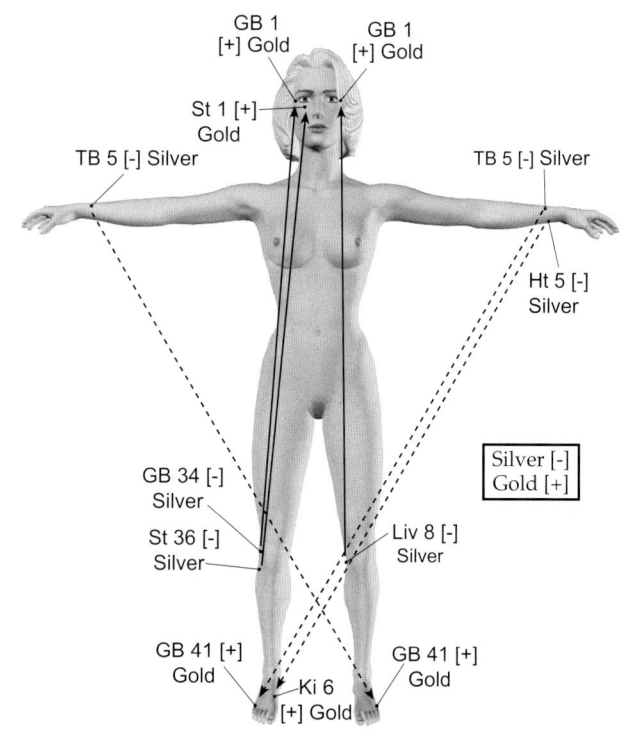

With deviations of 12, 24 and 34 tallied in Table 2, Shima selected the first, second and third confluences for treatment. The yang channels of both the confluence pairs were still the weakest so he treated these. In the case of the second confluence, the left-right values for the gallbladder channel were the same. Here Shima deviated from his usual methodology. Rather than needling the gallbladder channel bilaterally, he needled the liver channel on the left, its weakest side, and the gallbladder on the right.

Shima selected only the *dai/yang wei*, and *shen/xin* connections from his extraordinary vessel tabulations in Table 3. With a stroke tally of 80, GB 41 was selected as the master hole and because the left-right stroke tally was the same he needled it bilaterally (Table 1). With the greatest stroke total of 48 on the right, Shima needled Ki 6 on the right. Ht 5 was needled on the left side, because the heart qi is usually stronger on the left.

He did not administer *sesshokushin* or auriculotherapy.

4ᵀᴴ Treatment

On August 13, 1999, Ms. O.'s overall health continued to improve. Her glucose levels remained at 130 mg/dl. per hour while resting and at 230-250 mg/dl per hour after eating, which was still too high. She was endeavoring to lose some weight by reducing her carbohydrate intake. She reported that her Achilles tendinitis had improved greatly. Ms. O.'s menstrual flow continued to run abnormally longer than in the past, and she was experiencing chronic mild headaches. Her pulses were bilaterally wiry and tight, and her left pulse continued to be markedly stronger than the right. Ms. O.'s abdominal pattern remained the same.

The Akabane readings were as follows:

TABLE 1: LATERAL POLARIZATIONS

FOOT				
Channel	R	L	Tot.	Dev.
Spleen	19	11	30	⑧
Liver	8	15	23	7
Stomach	4	8	12	4
Gallbladder	13	20	33	7
Kidney	25	9	34	⑯
Bladder	13	7	20	6

HAND				
Channel	R	L	Tot.	Dev.
Lung	12	14	26	2
L. Intestine	13	15	28	②
Pericardium	8	9	17	2
Triple Burner	2	9	11	7
Heart	7	7	14	0
S. Intestine	6	6	12	0

Table 2: Channel Divergence Polarizations

	Tot.	Dev.		Tot.	Dev.		Tot.	Dev.
Bl	20	(14)	GB	33	10	Ht	14	2
Ki	34		Liv	23		SI	12	
St	12	(18)	PC	17	6	Lu	26	2
Sp	30		TB	11		LI	28	

Table 3: Extra Channel Polarizations

	Tot.	Dev.		Tot.	Dev.		Tot.	Dev.
SI 3	12	8	Lu 7	26	8	Lu 7	26	4
Bl 62	20		Ki 6	34		Sp 4	30	
GB 41	33	(22)	Per 6	17	13	Ht 5	14	(20)
TB 5	11		Sp 4	30		Ki 6	34	
LI 5	28	16	Per 6	17	6			
St 40	12		Liv 4	23				

1) Moxibustion was first applied to Bl 23 right, and Bl 20 right, these being the most imbalanced in the Akabane testing.

2) Next, Shima needled the first and third confluences and the extraordinary vessel *dai/yang wei* and *shen/xin* connections in the following pattern:

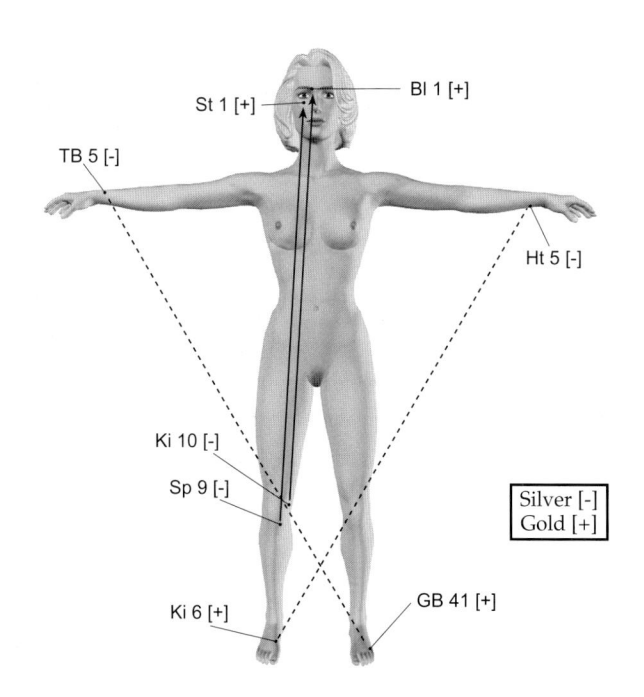

Bl 1 [+]
St 1 [+]
TB 5 [-]
Ht 5 [-]
Ki 10 [-]
Sp 9 [-]
Ki 6 [+]
GB 41 [+]

Silver [-]
Gold [+]

With deviations of 14 and 18 tallied in Table 2, Shima selected the first and third confluences for treatment. In this case, the yin channels of each pair were the weakest with totals of 34 and 30 respectively. The right kidney and spleen channels were the weakest with stroke counts of 25 and 19 respectively, tallied in Table 1 so Shima needled each of these confluences on the right side.

Shima again selected the *dai/yang wei* and *shen/xin* connections from his extraordinary vessel tabulations. With a stroke tally of 33, GB 41 was selected as the master hole and it was needled on the left side with a gold needle because this side was weaker (Table 1). TB 5 was needled on the right side with a silver needle because this side had the lowest right-left stroke tally. Using the same rationale, Ki 6 was selected as the master hole and was needled on the right side with a gold needle while Ht 5 was needled on the left with a silver needle.

3) Finally, he needled the left Kidney, Heart, Point Zero, and *Shen Men* ear points.

5ᵀᴴ TREATMENT

On September 24, 1999, Ms. O. reported that her headaches had disappeared and her last menstruation had been regular and easy. Her menses were due again any day. Her left pulse was a *yang qiao* pulse and her right pulse was a *yang wei* pulse. The weakness in Ms. O.'s lower abdomen had gone. Otherwise her abdominal pattern remained the same.

Akabane findings were as follows:

TABLE 1: LATERAL POLARIZATIONS

FOOT

Channel	R	L	Tot.	Dev.
Spleen	23	28	51	5
Liver	15	18	33	3
Stomach	25	28	53	3
Gallbladder	33	(40)	73	7
Kidney	17	18	35	1
Bladder	30	23	53	7

HAND

Channel	R	L	Tot.	Dev.
Lung	30	(31)	61	1
L. Intestine	10	20	30	10
Pericardium	15	29	44	(14)
Triple Burner	19	25	44	6
Heart	9	13	22	4
S. Intestine	(6)	12	18	6

176 The Channel Divergences

Table 2: Channel Divergence Polarizations

	Tot.	Dev.		Tot.	Dev.		Tot.	Dev.
Bl	53	18	GB	(73)	40	Ht	22	4
Kl	35		Liv	33		SI	18	
St	53	2	Per	44	0	Lu	(61)	(31)
Sp	51		TB	44		LI	30	

Table 3: Extra Channel Polarizations

	Tot.	Dev.		Tot.	Dev.		Tot.	Dev.
SI 3	18	35	Lu 7	61	26	Lu 7	62	11
Bl 62	(53)		Ki 6	35		Sp 4	51	
GB 41	73	29	Per 6	44	7	Ht 5	22	13
TB 5	44		Sp 4	51		Ki 6	35	
LI 5	30	23	Per 6	44	11			
St 40	53		Liv 4	33				

Despite the pulse findings, Shima needled the extraordinary vessel connections based on the Akabane results.

TREATMENT:

1) During this session, Shima needled the second and sixth confluences and the *yang qiao/du, dai/yang wei* and *ren/yin qiao* extraordinary vessel pairs in the following pattern:

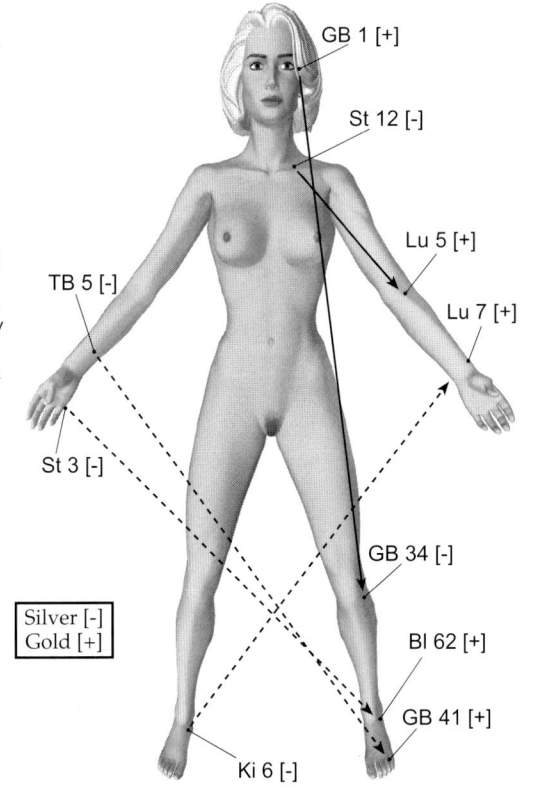

GB 1 [+]
St 12 [-]
Lu 5 [+]
Lu 7 [+]
TB 5 [-]
St 3 [-]
GB 34 [-]
Silver [-]
Gold [+]
Bl 62 [+]
GB 41 [+]
Ki 6 [-]

With deviations of 40 and 31 tallied in Table 2, Shima selected the second and sixth confluences. The gallbladder was the weakest of the second confluence pair with a stroke total of 73, while the lung was the weakest of the sixth confluence pair with a stroke tally of 61. Both were needled on the left side because this was the weakest.

Shima selected the *yang qiao/du*, *dai/yang wei* and *ren/yin qiao* from his extraordinary vessel tabulations. With a stroke tally of 53, Bl 62 was therefore selected as the master hole and was needled on the left side with a gold needle because this side was incrementally weaker (Table 1). SI 3 was needled on the right side because this side had a lower stroke tally. The same rationale was applied to the other two extraordinary vessel connections.

2) Finally, he needled the Gallbladder, Liver, Lung 1 and Lung 2, Large Intestine, *Shen Men*, Point Zero, and Uterus auricular points.

6ᵀᴴ TREATMENT

On December 10, 1999, Ms. O. returned to report that her insulin requirements had been cut in half and that her glucose levels were stable at 180 mg/dl per hour or less despite the fact that she was working 12 hours per day. She was limiting her carbohydrate intake to 40g per day. Her kidney function had improved, and she was continuing to exercise a bit. Ms. O.'s menstruation was ten days late this month and, when it came, was accompanied by cramps. Finally, she complained of a recent deep cough. Her pulse was wiry, tight, and weak.

Akabane findings were as follows:

TABLE 1: LATERAL POLARIZATIONS

FOOT

Channel	R	L	Tot.	Dev.
Spleen	14	29	43	15
Liver	30	18	48	12
Stomach	21	17	38	4
Gallbladder	26	(64)	90	38
Kidney	19	20	39	1
Bladder	30	28	58	2

HAND

Channel	R	L	Tot.	Dev.
Lung	17	30	47	(13)
L. Intestine	20	17	37	3
Pericardium	15	20	35	5
Triple Burner	18	15	33	3
Heart	8	13	21	5
S. Intestine	15	14	29	1

178   The Channel Divergences

TABLE 2: CHANNEL DIVERGENCE POLARIZATIONS

	Tot.	Dev.		Tot.	Dev.		Tot.	Dev.
Bl	58	19	GB	90	(42)	Ht	21	8
Kl	39		Liv	48		SI	29	
St	38	5	Per	35	2	Lu	47	10
Sp	43		TB	33		LI	37	

TABLE 3: EXTRA CHANNEL POLARIZATIONS

	Tot.	Dev.		Tot.	Dev.		Tot.	Dev.
SI 3	29	(29)	Lu 7	47	8	Lu 7	42	1
Bl 62	(58)		Ki 6	39		Sp 4	43	
GB 41	90	(57)	Per 6	35	8	Ht 5	21	18
TB 5	33		Sp 4	43		Ki 6	39	
LI 5	37	1	Per 6	35	13			
St 40	38		Liv 4	48				

TREATMENT:

1) Based on the above findings, Shima needled the second confluence and the *yang qiao/du* and *dai/yang wei* connections in the following pattern:

With a deviation of 42 tallied in Table 2, Shima selected only the second confluence for treatment. Shima needled the yang channel of the pair on the left side.

Shima elected the *du/yang qiao* and *dai/yang wei* connections from his extraordinary vessel tabulations. With a stroke tally of 58, Bl 62 was selected as the master hole and was needled on the right side because this side was incrementally weaker (Table 1). SI 3 was needled on the left side because this side had a lower stroke tally.

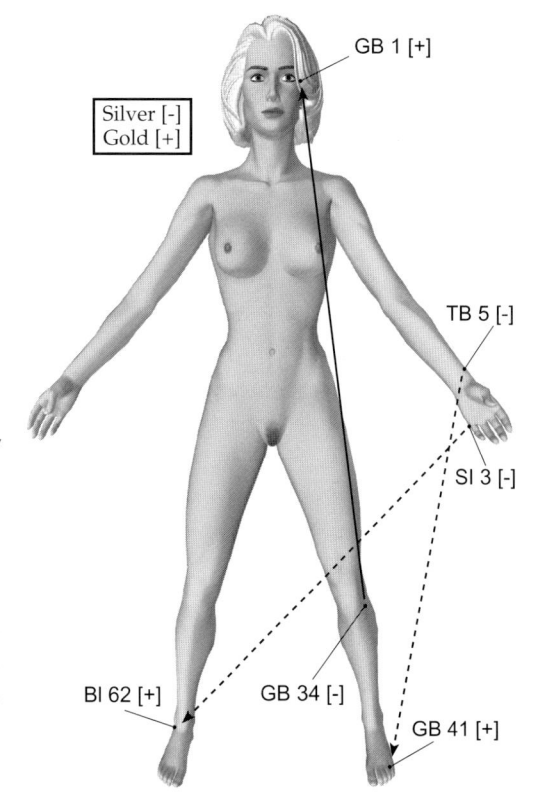

GB 1 [+]
Silver [-]
Gold [+]
TB 5 [-]
SI 3 [-]
Bl 62 [+]
GB 34 [-]
GB 41 [+]

Miki Shima's Commentary:

As of this writing, Ms. O. has lost 15 pounds in the past two months by changing her diet and exercising regularly. Her overall health and Akabane findings are greatly improved. However, a second confluence channel divergence imbalance and *dai/yang wei* imbalance persists. Her premenstrual syndrome, another expression of her liver-gallbladder imbalance, persists. At 8.3%, her glycosylated hemoglobin A1C on December 10, 1999 was still outside the reference ranges of 6.3-7.3% suggesting she is not properly controlling her diabetes.

Case 3

On January 7, 1999, Jane S., a 39 year-old female, presented with a chief complaint of dysmenorrhea and dysfunctional uterine bleeding due to uterine fibroids, which had first been diagnosed in May of 1998. Ultrasound confirmed a four-centimeter pedunculated fibroid on the anterior wall of the uterus and a number of smaller fibroids scattered throughout the uterus. The patient reported experiencing pressure and fullness in her abdomen around the time of her menstruation, and in the last 3-4 months she would experience pain with ovulation. Ms. S.'s menarche occurred at age 10 and she currently had a 25-day menstrual cycle. In general, the color of her menstruate was red, which became somewhat darker at the end of her flow during which time there was also some minor clotting.

The patient also reported feeling fatigued, and complained of large dark bags under her eyes. She bruised easily. She believed that her appetite was excessive and she would feel weak and fatigued if she missed a meal. She had injured her back many years previously and the area around the injury often felt cold. In addition, she had an aversion to cold in general. There was a family history of colon cancer on her mother's side and heart disease on her father's side.

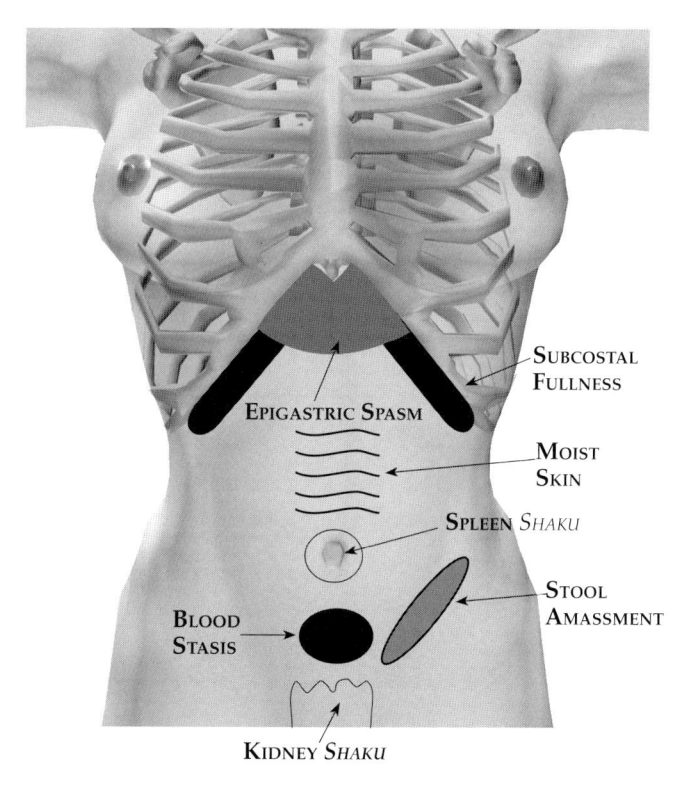

Ms. S.'s vital signs were normal. Abdominal examination revealed epigastric spasm, moist abdominal skin, spleen *shaku*, subcostal spasms, congealed blood, stool stagnation, and the presence of a uterine mass interpreted as kidney *shaku* and running piglet (*ben tun*).[25] Her pulse was sunken and weak.

The Akabane findings were as follows:

Table 1: Lateral Polarizations

FOOT

Channel	R	L	Tot.	Dev.
Spleen	8	3	11	5
Liver	⑫	11	23	1
Stomach	10	7	17	3
Gallbladder	6	3	9	3
Kidney	10	10	20	0
Bladder	18	20	38	2

HAND

Channel	R	L	Tot.	Dev.
Lung	10	⑥	16	4
L. Intestine	11	7	18	4
Pericardium	8	6	14	2
Triple Burner	10	9	19	1
Heart	8	⑥	14	2
S. Intestine	5	6	11	1

Table 2: Channel Divergence Polarizations

	Tot.	Dev.		Tot.	Dev.		Tot.	Dev.
Bl	38	⑱	GB	9	⑭	Ht	14	3
Ki	20		Liv	23		SI	11	
St	17	6	Per	14	5	Lu	16	2
Sp	11		TB	19		LI	18	

Table 3: Extra Channel Polarizations

	Tot.	Dev.		Tot.	Dev.		Tot.	Dev.
SI 3	11	㉗	Lu 7	16	㉒	Lu 7	16	5
Bl 62	38		Ki 6	20		Sp 4	11	
GB 41	9	10	Per 6	14	3	Ht 5	14	14
TB 5	19		Sp 4	11		Ki 6	28	
LI 5	18	1	Per 6	14	9			
St 40	17		Liv 4	23				

The herbal diagnosis was uterine fibroids, corresponding to the Chinese medical disease categories of kidney *shaku* running piglet and accumulations, gatherings and lump glomus *(ji ju pi kuai)*. This condition was the result of damp heat and congealed blood, spleen yang vacuity, and liver qi stagnation.

Although Shima prescribed an herbal preparation based on the above diagnosis, his acupuncture strategy was based primarily on his Akabane findings.

TREATMENT:

1) Shima needled the yin channel on the second confluence on the right side, and the *yang qiao/du* and *yin qiao/ren* extraordinary vessel connections on the left side, all with silver and gold needles.

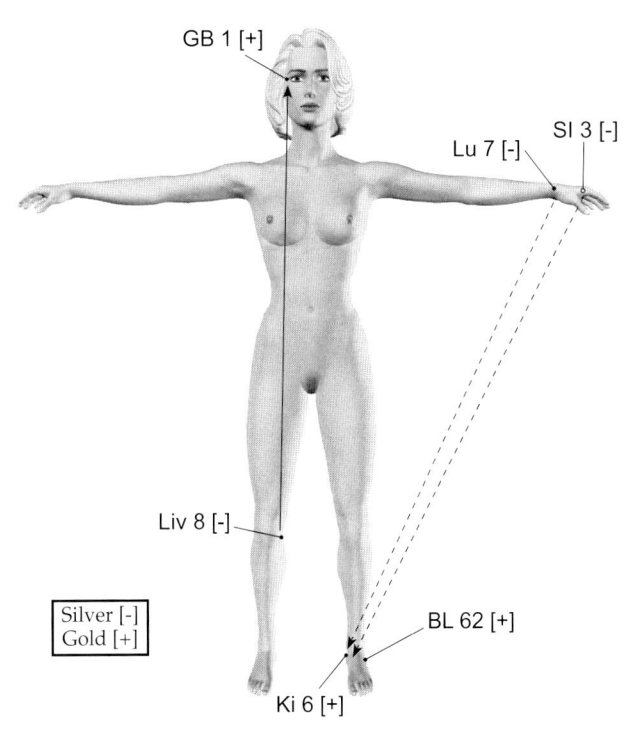

Despite the fact that the first confluence showed the greatest deviation in the Akabane findings, Shima elected to needle the second confluence only because he believed that Ms. S.'s liver pathology was of greater importance than her kidney weakness at this time. Of all the diagnostic tools at his disposal, Shima gives greatest weight to the Akabane findings, often constructing acupuncture treatments based almost soley on these findings. In this case, however, with only one set of Akabane readings to make a clinical decision, Shima's treatment strategy was heavily influenced by the overall clinical presentation.

2) Auriculotherapy was administered to Kidney 1 and Kidney 2, Uterus, *Shenmen*, and Point Zero, all on the right side.

In addition to once monthly acupuncture, Ms. S. was given the following herbal formulas.

Gui Zhi Fu Ling Tang (Cinnamon Twig and Poria Decoction), 2 capsules, twice daily between meals. This was administered empirically to address uterine fibroids due to blood stagnation and middle burner dampness.

Wen Jing Tang (Menses-Warming Decoction), 2 capsules, three times per day after meals.[26] This was also prescribed to address the blood stagnation, the cold, damp abdomen and weak pulse.

Yi Gan Ji Jia Chen Pi and *Ban Xia* (Liver Repressing Formula with additions of Orange Peel and Pinellia), 2 capsules twice daily before meals.[27] This was administered to address the epigastric and subcostal spasm, spleen *shaku* and liver qi stagnation.

The patient was also instructed to take 1 Tbs. of bran 2 times per day and was told to walk for an hour daily. Finally, she was taught to stimulate her well *jing* holes daily with an incense stick using the Akabane technique.

2ND TREATMENT

Ms. S. returned a month later on Feburary 15, and reported that she was doing well. Her last period had been mild although it remained somewhat clotty. Her pulse was wiry and strong.

The Akabane findings were as follows:

TABLE 1: LATERAL POLARIZATIONS

FOOT

Channel	R	L	Tot.	Dev.
Spleen	6	⑱	24	⑫
Liver	9	9	18	0
Stomach	5	6	11	1
Gallbladder	6	3	9	3
Kidney	⑬	8	21	5
Bladder	3	3	6	0

HAND

Channel	R	L	Tot.	Dev.
Lung	⑬	7	20	⑥
L. Intestine	7	6	13	1
Pericardium	9	6	15	3
Triple Burner	6	5	11	1
Heart	7	6	13	1
S. Intestine	5	3	8	2

TABLE 2: CHANNEL DIVERGENCE POLARIZATIONS

	Tot.	Dev.		Tot.	Dev.		Tot.	Dev.
Bl	6	⑮	GB	9	9	Ht	13	5
Ki	21		Liv	18		St	6	
St	11	⑬	Per	15	4	Lu	20	7
Sp	24		TB	11		LI	13	

Miki Shima's Approach

TABLE 3: EXTRA CHANNEL POLARIZATIONS

	Tot.	Dev.		Tot.	Dev.		Tot.	Dev.
SI 3	8	2	Lu 7	20	1	Lu 7	20	4
Bl 62	6		Ki 6	21		Sp 4	24	
GB 41	9	2	Per 6	15	⑨	Ht 5	13	8
TB 5	11		Sp 4	㉔		Ki 6	21	
LI 5	13	4	Per 6	15	3			
St 40	17		Liv 4	18				

Despite the fact that the presenting signs and symptoms tend to suggest that the liver involvement is still primary in this case, the Akabane results point more strongly to a kidney vacuity.

TREATMENT:

1) Shima began this treatment with moxabustion on the Bl 13 right and Bl 20 left. Shima applied moxibustion here and not in the first treatment, because the first set of Akabane findings revealed no right-left deviation greater than 10.

2) He then needled the yin channels of the first confluence on the right and the third confluence on the left, followed by stimulation of the *chong/yin wei* connection on the left.

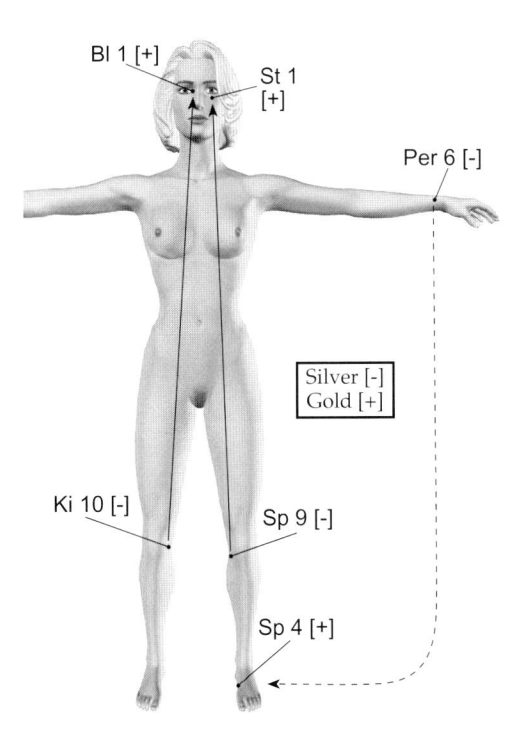

Bl 1 [+]
St 1 [+]
Per 6 [-]
Silver [-]
Gold [+]
Ki 10 [-]
Sp 9 [-]
Sp 4 [+]

As we can see, the first confluence had the greatest overall deviation of 15, followed by the third confluence, with a deviation of 13. Because the left-right totals of spleen and kidney, 24 and 21 respectively, were higher than their yang paired channels, Shima needled the yin channel pairs of the third and first confluences. He needled the third confluence on the left because the spleen channel was weakest on the left with a total of 18, as compared to a total of 6 on the right. By contrast, the kidney channel was needled on the right because the Akabane findings found it to be weakest on the right with a total of 13 as compared to a total of 8 on the left.

3) Auriculotherapy was administered to Kidney 1 and Kidney 2, Uterus, *Shen-Men*, and Point Zero, all on the right side.

3ʳᴅ Treatment:

Ms. S. returned a month later on March 8, and reported that her last period had been the easiest menses ever. However, her flow remained fairly heavy on the second day and she still experienced some left breast pain on day 17. Her pulse reflected a Ki, GB, and Bl vacuity and heat, small intestine and triple burner repletion.

Akabane findings were as follows:

Table 1: Lateral Polarizations

FOOT

Channel	R	L	Tot.	Dev.
Spleen	4	5	9	1
Liver	5	4	9	1
Stomach	4	5	9	1
Gallbladder	3	4	7	1
Kidney	3	3	6	0
Bladder	3	3	6	0

HAND

Channel	R	L	Tot.	Dev.
Lung	4	3	7	1
L. Intestine	4	4	8	0
Pericardium	5	3	8	2
Triple Burner	3	3	6	0
Heart	3	3	0	0
S. Intestine	3	3	6	0

Table 2: Channel Divergence Polarizations

	Tot.	Dev.		Tot.	Dev.		Tot.	Dev.
Bl	6	0	GB	7	2	Ht	6	0
Ki	6		Liv	9		St	6	
St	9	0	Per	8	2	Lu	7	1
Sp	9		SI	6		LI	8	

Table 3: Extra Channel Polarizations

	Tot.	Dev.		Tot.	Dev.		Tot.	Dev.
SI 3	6	0	Lu 7	7	1	Lu 7	7	2
Bl 62	6		Ki 6	6		Sp 4	9	
GB 41	7	1	Per 6	8	1	Ht 5	6	0
TB 5	6		Sp 4	9		Ki 6	6	
LI 5	8	1	Per 6	8	1			
St 40	9		Liv 4	9				

TREATMENT:

1) Because the Akabane findings reflected a relatively balanced condition Shima administered the NIP Protocol #2 with gold and silver needles and elected not to treat the channel divergences at all.

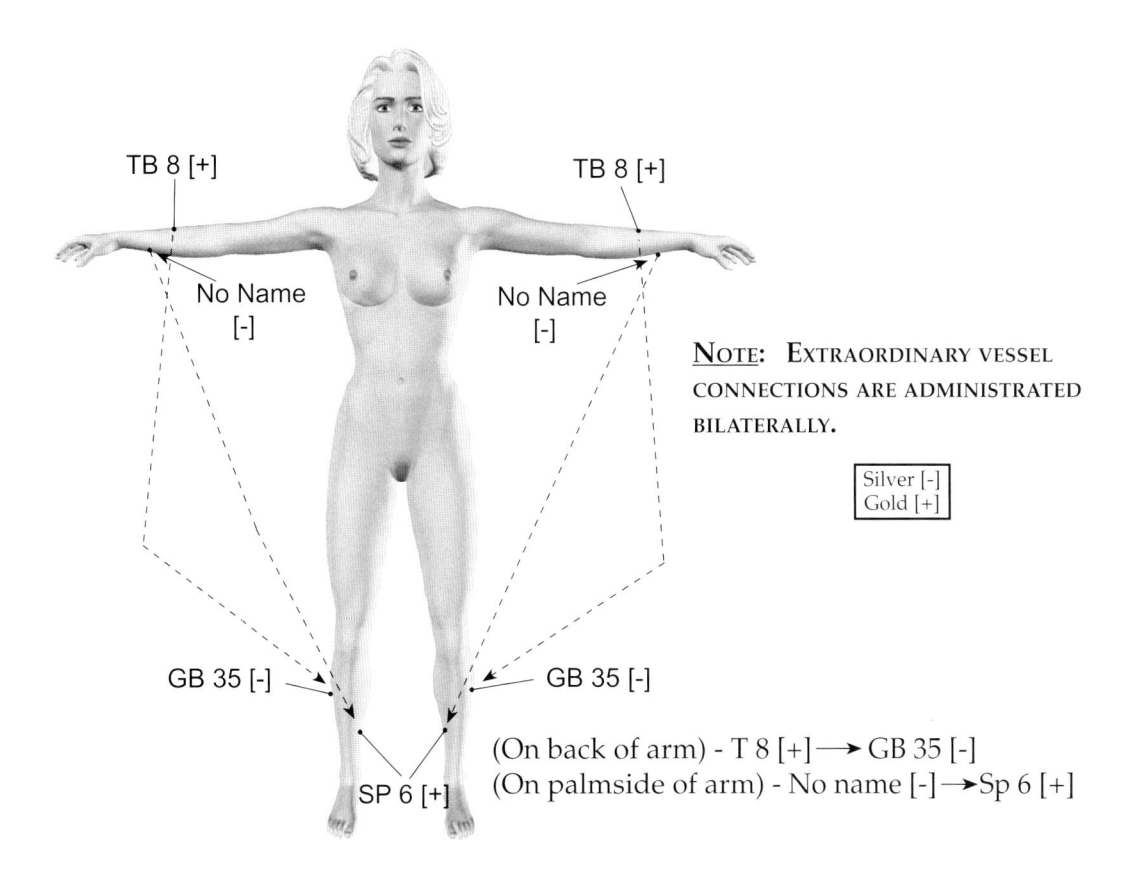

TB 8 [+]

TB 8 [+]

No Name [-]

No Name [-]

NOTE: EXTRAORDINARY VESSEL CONNECTIONS ARE ADMINISTRATED BILATERALLY.

Silver [-]
Gold [+]

GB 35 [-]

GB 35 [-]

SP 6 [+]

(On back of arm) - T 8 [+] → GB 35 [-]
(On palmside of arm) - No name [-] → Sp 6 [+]

Once again, we see the primacy accorded to the Akabane findings by Shima. At this juncture he had a few Akabane readings for this patient and they had consistently moved toward a state of balance. Despite the apparent imbalances in Ms. S.'s pulses, Shima placed greater trust in the Akabane findings than the pulse and based his acupuncture strategy on it.

2) Auriculotherapy was administered to Kidney 1 and Kidney 2, Uterus, *Shen-Men*, and Point Zero, all on the right side.

Over the next 2 months Ms. S.'s condition continued to improve. Except for some mild breast pain, she no longer experienced any menstrual or ovulatory discomfort. Her gynecologist performed a follow-up bimanual pelvic exam and found that the fibroids had substantially diminished in size. Since her Akabane findings remained quite balanced Shima elected not to needle the channel divergences and instead focused on a more generalized balancing strategy with the NIP protocol. Acupuncture was discontinued after a total of 5 treatments, although Ms. S. intermittently continued to take the herbal preparation Shima had prescribed whenever she experienced any menstrual discomfort.

MIKI SHIMA'S COMMENTARY:

Ms. S. made a fairly rapid recovery as evidenced by her symptomatic improvement, the follow-up pelvic exam, and the normalization of her Akabane findings. This was due, at least in part, to her daily self-administered Akabane treatments. This case raises the issue of how one should proceed once the Akabane findings have normalized making it difficult to discern a definite pattern. Sometimes the imbalances revealed by the Akabane findings are so minor as to be essentially irrelevant. How can we keep things moving in the right direction? One very basic approach that I applied here was to simply administer the NIP protocol in an effort to affect a generalized balancing of the channel system.

Of course, we also have a variety of other diagnostic tools at our disposal besides the Akabane method. When the Akabanes are normal or unremarkable, my next diagnostic priority for both acupuncture and herbal prescribing is the abdomen. Occasionally, I will see patients whose Akabanes are pretty much normal, but abdominal diagnosis reveals imbalances of the viscera and bowels but these cases are very rare.

I actually perform two different styles of abdominal diagnosis. First I'll do the relatively light style of abdominal diagnosis known as *Fukushin*, to determine which herbal formulas to prescribe. Next, I'll do a deeper, more acupuncture-oriented style of abdominal diagnosis based on the 56th Difficult Issue in the *Classic of Difficult Issues (Nan Jing)* where I am looking for accumulations (*shaku*), hardnesses, or areas of pressure pain. While I obviously place great overall emphasis on Akabane findings, I try not to be too rigid in the application of my diagnostic tools.

CASE FOUR

Jennifer B., a 36 year-old Caucasian female first presented on Feburary 9, 1996 with a chief complaint of severe cervical dysplasia first diagnosed on November 30, 1995. Five endocervical specimens were taken and the pathology report found severe squamous dysplasia with associated cellular changes due to of human papilloma, and focal endocervical squamous metaplasia with chronic inflammation on three of the specimens. Moderate imflammation was found on the other two. Vital signs were normal at the time of the original interview. She reported having a white milky leukorrhea, clotty menses, and slight acne. Otherwise, she was healthy.

Miki Shima's Approach

Her tongue was very damp with a thin white coat and tooth marks. Her pulse was deep, rapid and tense, particularly in the *chi* position. The patient's abdomen revealed epigastric and subcostal spasm, supraumbilical palpitation, spleen *shaku* and periumbilical moisture, stagnant stool, lateral abdominal spasm and weakness in the kidney reflect area.

The diagnosis was vacuity of the *chong* and *ren* vessels, and heart vacuity palpitation arising out of kidney vacuity.

TREATMENT:

1) Shima needled the first and second confluences, and the *yin qiao/ren* and *chong/yin wei* extraordinary vessel connections in the following manner.

He stimulated the second confluence because of the the trajectory of the liver channel through the

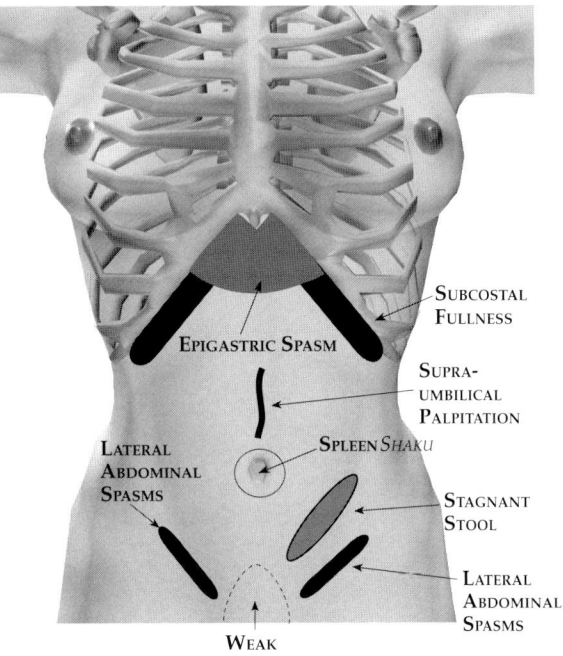

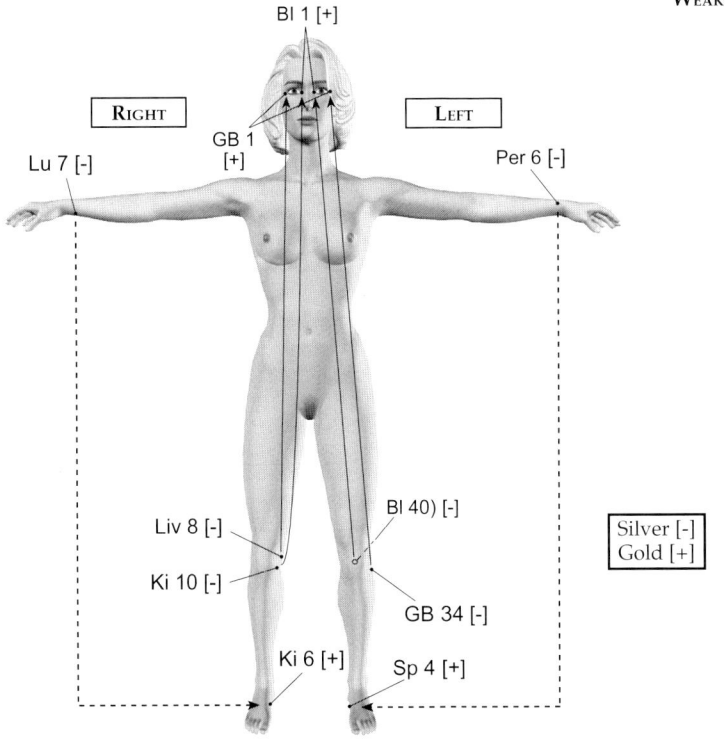

- Subcostal Fullness
- Epigastric Spasm
- Supra-umbilical Palpitation
- Lateral Abdominal Spasms
- Spleen *Shaku*
- Stagnant Stool
- Lateral Abdominal Spasms
- Weak

Bl 1 [+]
RIGHT   GB 1 [+]   LEFT
Lu 7 [-]   Per 6 [-]
Liv 8 [-]   Bl 40) [-]
Ki 10 [-]
GB 34 [-]
Ki 6 [+]   Sp 4 [+]

Silver [-]
Gold [+]

genital region. Shima emphasized the *yin qiao* connection because the *chi* pulses were more vacuous in the right *cun* pulse.

Shima prescribed the following herbal prescriptions for one month.

Gui Zhi Jia Lung Gu Mu Li Tang (Cinnamon Twig Decoction Plus Dragon Bone and Oyster Shell), two capsules, twice daily before meals.[30] This was administered to address the supraumbilical palpitations, and dysfunctional stress response.

Ban Xia Xie Xin Tang (Pinellia Heart-Draining Decoction), two capsules, twice daily before meals.[31] This was administered to address the epigastric spasms, supraumbilical palpitation, and to calm the spirit.

Liu Wei Di Huang Wan (Six Ingredient Rehmannia Pill), two capsules, twice daily after meals. This was administered to strengthen the kidneys.

Tao He Cheng Qi Tang (Peach Kernel Qi-Coordinating Decoction) two capsules, twice daily after meals.[32] This was administered to address the stagnant stool abdominal confirmation.

2ND TREATMENT

Ms. B. returned on Feburary 26, 1996, and reported that her menstruation on Feburary 10 had been normal as usual with no clotting and that she felt well. Vital signs were all normal.

Her pulse was deep and vacuous, however, her abdomen exhibited less epigastric spasm, the skin was drier, and the spleen *shaku* was more relaxed, yet there was more strength in her lower abdominal region overall.

Shima needled the same pattern.

THIRD TREATMENT

On March 11, 1996, Ms. B. reported that she was feeling good but rather stressed and that she no longer had leukorrhea. Her menstruation on March 5 had occurred on time and lasted 5 days. It had been heavy, with some clotting toward the end.

Ms. B. had been sleeping well, she was having two loose bowel movements per day, and nocturia twice at night. Vital signs were normal. Her pulse was wiry, tense and deep, presenting in a *ren* vessel pattern. Although her abdomen still exhibited some epigastric spasm, it was firmer and dryer overall.

Miki Shima's Approach

TREATMENT:

1) Shima needled the first and third confluences, and the *ren/yin qiao*, and *chong/yin wei* extraordinary vessel connections in the following manner.

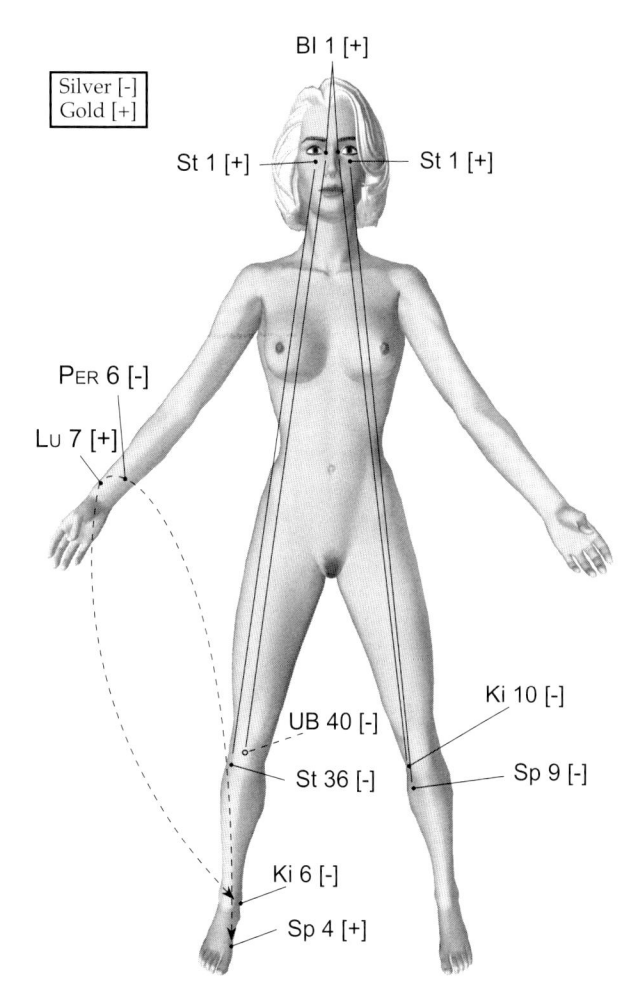

Bl 1 [+]
Silver [-]
Gold [+]
St 1 [+]   St 1 [+]
Per 6 [-]
Lu 7 [+]
Ki 10 [-]
UB 40 [-]
St 36 [-]   Sp 9 [-]
Ki 6 [-]
Sp 4 [+]

Shima chose the third confluence because the patient complained of loose stools. He based his extraordinary vessel treatment on the pulse presentation.

Shima prescribed the following herbal preparations for one month:

Ban Xia Hou Po Tang (Pinellia and Magnolia Bark Decoction) two capsules, twice daily before meals.[33] This was administered to calm the spirit and to address the increased abdominal tenderness.

Xiao Yao San (Free Wanderer Powder), two capsules, twice daily before meals.[34] This was administered because the pulse was especially tense and wiry and because of the stress the patient was experiencing.

4TH TREATMENT

Ms. B. returned on April 8, 1996 and reported that she had no pain or discharge. Her menstruation in April had been light and on time with no cramping. She complained of continuing stress. Her vital signs were all normal. Ms. B.'s pulse was *yin qiao* and her abdomen exhibited supraumbilical aortic palpitations.

TREATMENT:

1) Shima needled the second and fourth confluences, and the *yin qiao/ren*, and *chong/ yin wei* extraordinary vessel connections in the following manner.

Shima selected the fourth confluence based on the abdominal presentation of aortic palpitation. The extraordinary vessel connection was chosen based on the pulse presentation.

Silver [-]
Gold [+]

BI 1 [+]
GB 1 [+]
GB 1 [+]
Ht 3 [+]
Lu 7 [-]
Per 6 [-]
SI 8 [+]
Liv 8 [-]
GB 34 [-]
Ki 6 [+]
Sp 4 [+]

Note: Extraordinary vessel connections are administrated bilaterally.

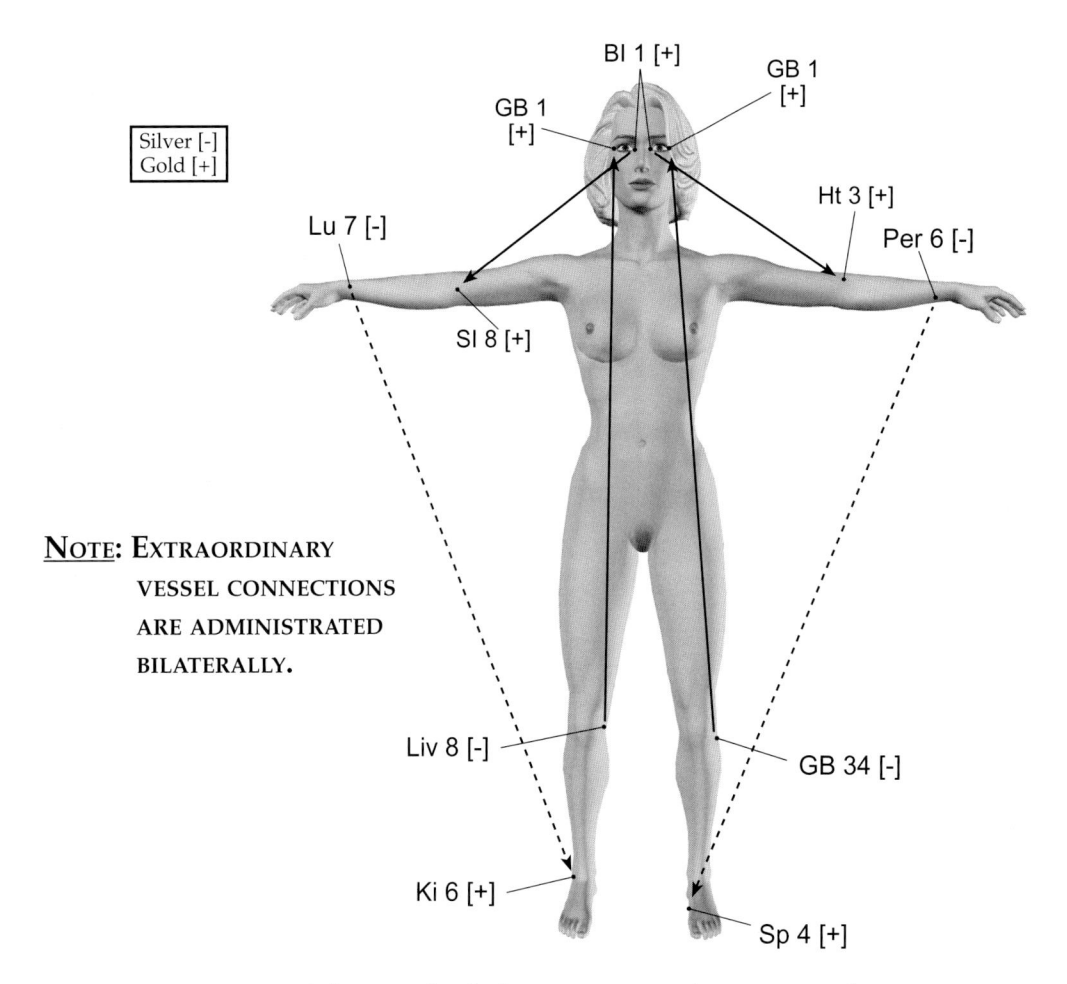

Shima prescribed the following herbal prescriptions for one month.

Gui Zhi Jia Lung Gu Mu Li Tang (Cinnamon Twig Decoction Plus Dragon Bone and Oyster Shell), two capsules, twice daily before meals. This was administered to address the supraumbilical palpitations.

Yi Gan Ji Jia Chen Pi Ban Xia Tang (Liver Repressing Decoction plus Orange Peel and Pinellia Decoction), two capsules, twice daily before meals.[35] This was administered to address the subcostal tension and liver qi stagnation due to stress.

Ban Xia Xie Xin Tang (Pinellia Heart-Draining Decoction) two capsules, twice daily before meals. This was administered to address the subcostal tension and epigastric spasm.

Tao He Cheng Qi Tang (Peach Kernal Qi-Coordinating Decoction) two capsules, twice daily before meals. This was administered to address the stool amassment in the lower abdomen.

5TH TREATMENT

Ms. B. returned on May 6, 1996, to report that she was experiencing some mild breakthrough bleeding and some cramping. She had no breast tenderness and her skin was clearing. Her vital signs were all normal. Her pulse was wiry, floating and replete. Her abdomen exhibited epigastric spasm, supra-umbilical palpitation, spleen *shaku*, and subumbilical weakness.

Shima needled the first and fourth confluences, and the *du/yang qiao* extraordinary vessel connections in the following manner.

Shima selected the first confluence to address the kidney vacuity evident in the abdomen. The fourth confluence addressed the supra-umbilical palpitations. His choice of extraordinary vessel connections was based on the pulse, which was essentially a *du* vessel pattern.

6TH TREATMENT

The patient returned on June 3, 1996. Her abdomen showed her usual epigastric spasm and a midline chopstick below the umbilicus.

TREATMENT:

1) Shima needled the first and third confluences, and the *yin qiao/ren*, and *chong/ yin wei* extraordinary vessel connections in the following manner.

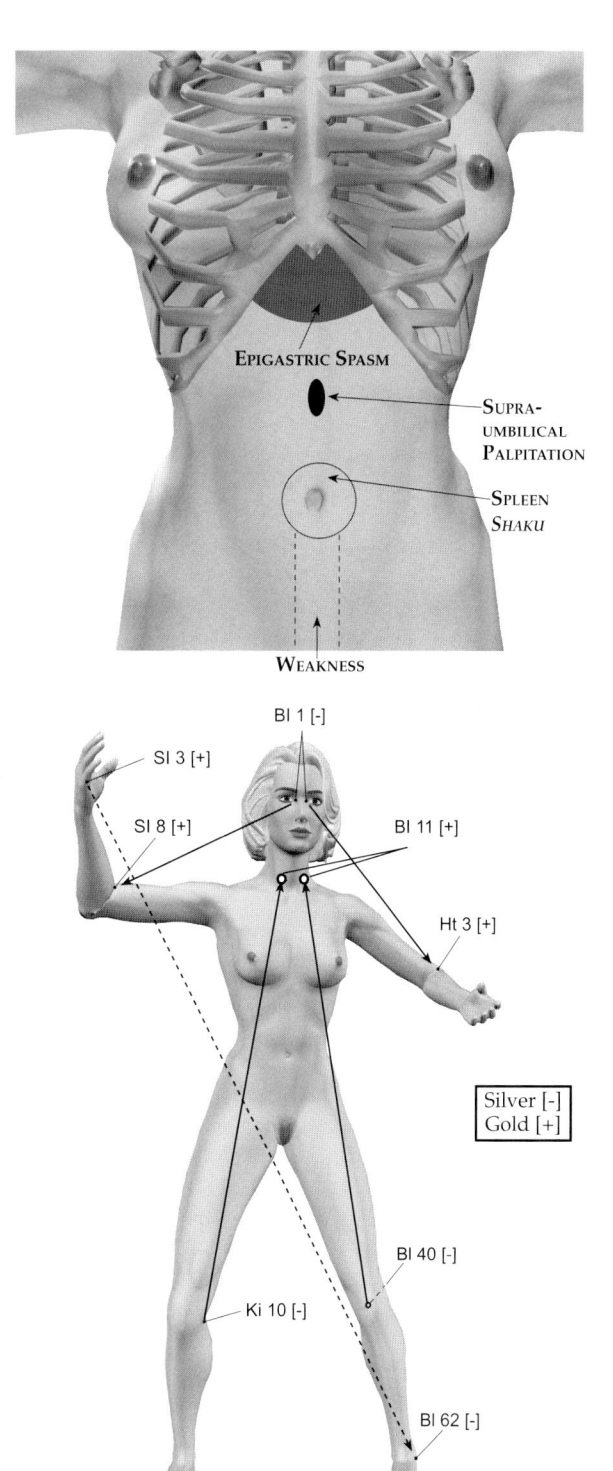

NOTE: EXTRAORDINARY VESSEL CONNECTIONS ARE ADMINISTRATED CONTRALATERALLY\BILATERALLY.

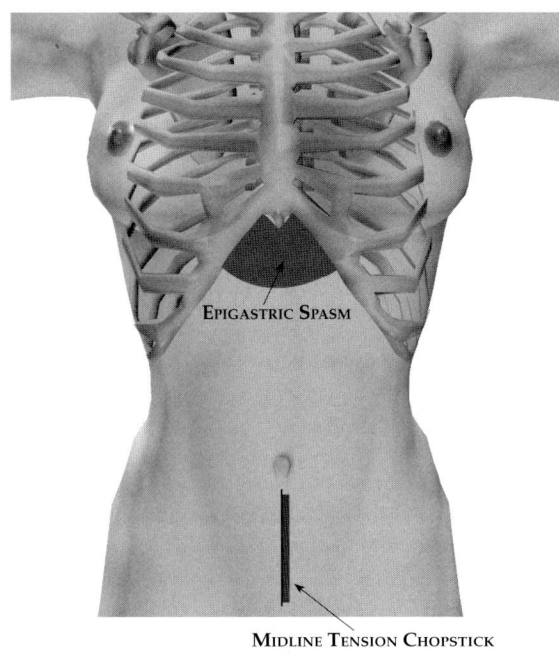

Shima prescribed the following herbal presriptions.

Ban Xia Xie Xin Tang (Pinellia Heart-Draining Decoction) 2 capsules, twice daily, before meals. This addressed the subcostal tension and supraumbilical palpitations.

Ba Wei Wan (Eight Ingredients Pills) 2 capsules, twice daily before meals.[36] This addressed the subumbilical chopstick.

Over the ensuing months Ms. B. had two more PAP smears. On June 25, 1996, pathology report showed epithelial cell abnormalitites, low grade squamous intraepithelial lesion and cellular changes associated with human papilloma virus. On October 1, 1996, the pathology report showed epithelial cell abnormalitites, atypical squamous cells of undetermined significance and a low grade intraepithelial lesion.

7TH TREATMENT

Shima again saw the patient on October 30, 1996 who reported that she was doing well. Vital signs were all normal.

Her pulse was rapid, tight and deep. The abdomen exhibited epigastric spasm and subcostal tension, supraumbilical palpitation, spleen *shaku* and some lower abdominal blood stasis.

EPIGASTRIC SPASM

MIDLINE TENSION CHOPSTICK

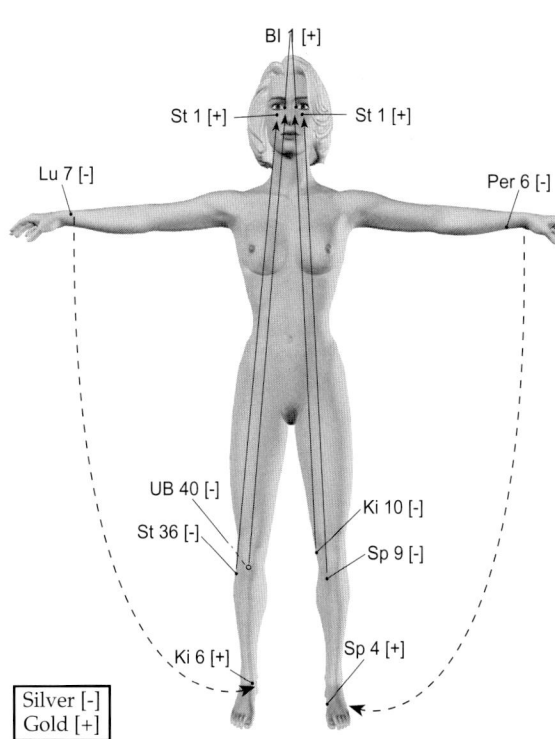

Bl 1 [+]
St 1 [+]   St 1 [+]
Lu 7 [-]   Per 6 [-]
UB 40 [-]   Ki 10 [-]
St 36 [-]   Sp 9 [-]
Ki 6 [+]   Sp 4 [+]

Silver [-]
Gold [+]

NOTE: EXTRAORDINARY VESSEL CONNECTIONS ARE ADMINISTRATED BILATERALLY.

Treatment:

1) Shima needled the second and fifth confluences, and the *ren/ yin qiao* and *chong/ yin wei* extraordinary vessel connections in the following manner.

Shima then prescribed the following herbal formulas for one month.

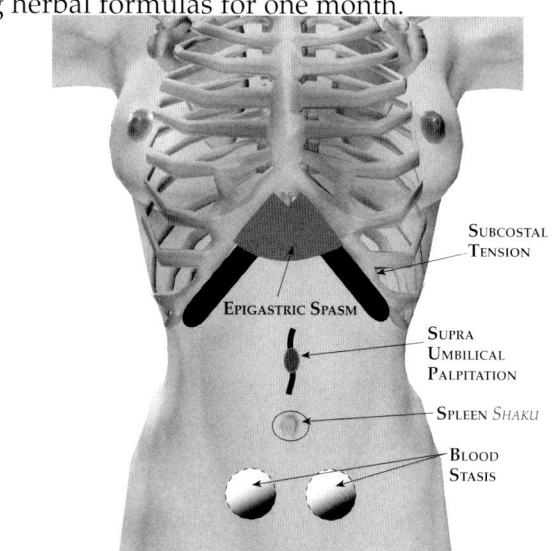

Ban Xia Hou Po Tang (Pinellia and Magnolia Bark Decoction), two capsules, twice daily before meals. This was administered to address the epigastric spasm and the gastrointestinal upset.[37]

Xiao Chai Hu Tang (Minor Bupleurum Decoction), two capsules, twice daily, before meals.[38]

This was administered because the subcostal tension was minor and the patient complained of an upset stomach.

Dang Gui Shao Yang San (*Tang Kuei* and Peony Powder), two capsules, twice daily, between meals.[39] This was administered to address blood stasis presenting the context of spleen and kidney *shaku*.

8th Treatment

Ms. B. returned on December 14, 1996. Her pulse was moderate, her abdomen was firmer overall, the palpitation and subcostal tension was gone, and the lower abdominal blood stasis was now limited to the left side.

Treatment:

1) Shima needled the third confluence and the *ren/yin qiao* vessel connection in the following manner.

Labels on figure:
- Subcostal Tension
- Epigastric Spasm
- Supra Umbilical Palpitation
- Spleen *Shaku*
- Blood Stasis

- GB 1 [+]
- GB 1 [+]
- GB 12 [-]
- GB 12 [-]
- Per 6 [-]
- Lu 7 [+]
- Per 3 [+]
- TB 10 [+]
- Silver [-]
- Gold [+]
- GB 34 [-]
- Liv 8 [-]
- Sp 4 [+]
- Ki 6 [-]

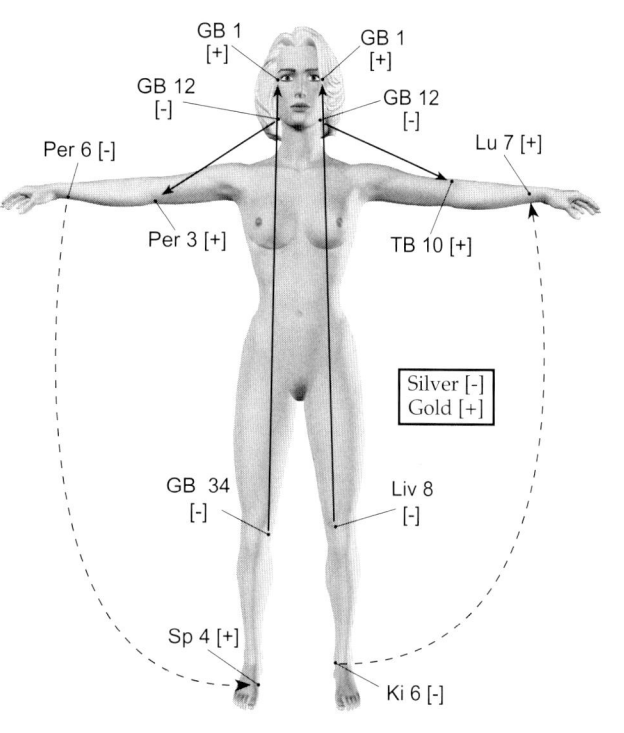

Note: Extraordinary Vessel connections are administrated bilaterally.

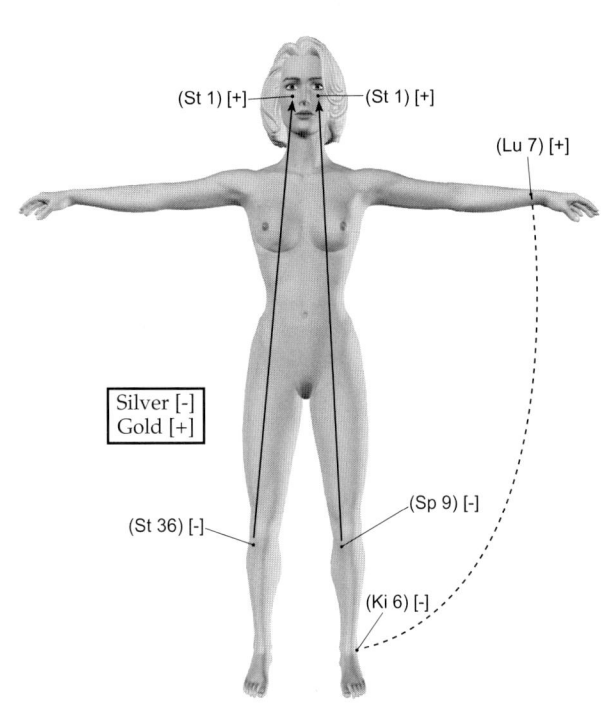

194 The Channel Divergences

(St 1) [+]
(St 1) [+]
(Lu 7) [+]
Silver [-]
Gold [+]
(St 36) [-]
(Sp 9) [-]
(Ki 6) [-]

NOTE: EXTRAORDINARY VESSEL CONNECTIONS ARE ADMINISTRATED BILATERALLY.

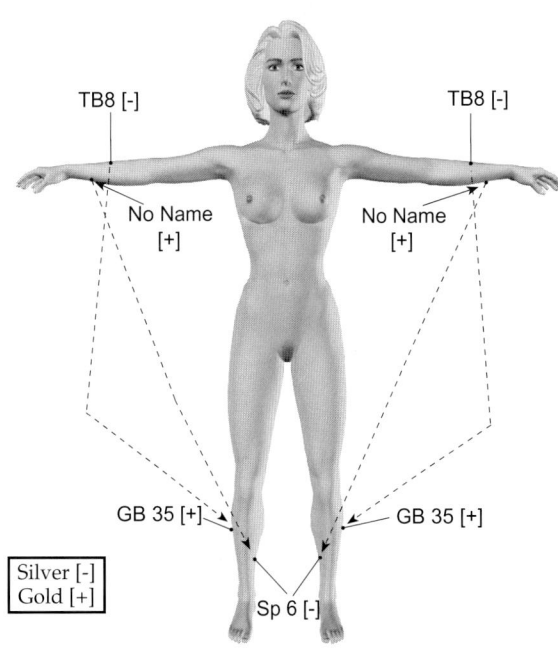

TB8 [-]
TB8 [-]
No Name [+]
No Name [+]
GB 35 [+]
GB 35 [+]
Silver [-]
Gold [+]
Sp 6 [-]

CONNECTION IS BILATERAL
(On back of arm) - T 8 [-] → GB 35 [+]
(On palmside of arm) - No name [+] → SP6 [-]

9th Treatment

On her final visit Ms. B. reported that her dysplasia was gone and her periods were no longer a problem. The pathology report was within normal limits. Vital signs were all normal. Her pulse was bilaterally mildly wiry; her abdomen strong with some residual blood stasis.

Shima administered the NIP Protocol #2 with gold and silver needles in the following manner to consolidate the therapeutic effect.

Shima prescribed the following:

Si Wu Tang (Four Agents Decoction), two capsules twice daily between meals, and *Bu Zhong Yi Qi Tang* (Center-Supplementing Qi-Boosting Decoction), two capsules twice daily before meals.[40,41] These were administered to supplement the qi and nourish liver blood to promote fertility because the patient expressed her desire to become pregnant.

CASE FIVE

Ms. Isabelle E., a 32 year-old female presented August 20, 1999 with a chief complaint of habitual miscarriage. She reported that she had suffered three miscarriages in the past five years and had tried in-vitro fertilization, and hormone therapy to no avail.

Ms. E. also reported that she frequently had poor digestion and complained of gas in her lower GI tract and loose stools. The patient reported that she had mild bronchial asthma but did not require inhalers. Her vital signs were all normal

Her pulse was deep, vacuous and fine and her abdomen exhibited epigastric spasm, spleen shaku, and extreme lower abdominal weakness.

The diagnosis was chronic severe spleen and kidney and lung vacuity.

TREATMENT:

1) Shima needled the first and sixth confluences, and the *ren/yin qiao*, and *chong/yin wei* extraordinary vessel connections in the following manner.

Shima selected the first confluence because of the obvious kidney vacuity, and the sixth confluence to address the lung involvement. Shima prescribed the following medicinals for one month.

Li Zhong Tang (Center-Rectifying Decoction), two capsules, twice daily between meals.[42]

This was administered to address the loose stools and generalized gastrointestinal distress in the context of spleen *shaku*.

Wen Jing Tang (Menses-Warming Decoction), two capsules, twice daily between meals. This was administered to address the *chong* and *ren* vacuity presenting in the context of spleen *shaku*.

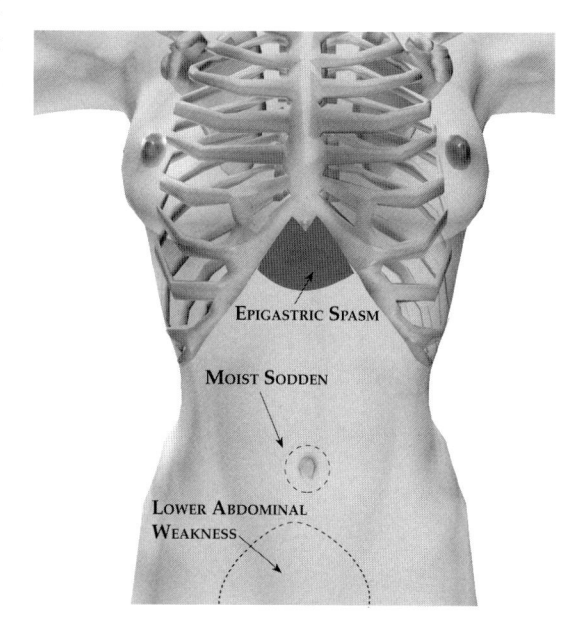

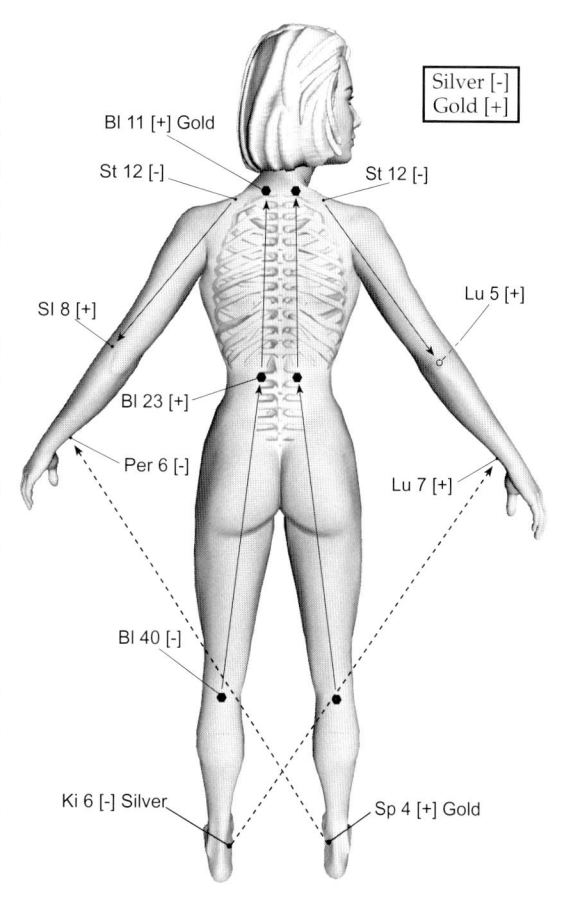

Zuo You Gui Tang (Left and Right Restoration Decoction), two capsules each, twice daily between meals was prescribed to address the kidney vacuity presenting as lower abdominal weakness.

2ND TREATMENT

Ms. E. returned on August 31, 1999. She reported that her menstruation had been normal with no cramping or clotting, and that her digestion had improved.

Her pulse was moderate and vacuous, and her abdomen was stronger with more tone.

Shima administered the same treatment.

3RD TREATMENT

Ms. E. returned on Sept. 16, 1999 with little new to report. Her pulse was moderate and mildly wiry and her abdomen was normal except for a slight weakness in the kidney reflex area.

Shima administered the same treatment.

4TH TREATMENT

On October 5, 1999 the patient reported that she was currently menstruating with a normal flow, no cramping or clotting. Her pulse was wiry and deep.

TREATMENT:

1) Shima administered the Kidney Return Protocol and supplemented the *ren/yin qiao*, and *chong/yin wei* extraordinary vessel connections in the following manner.

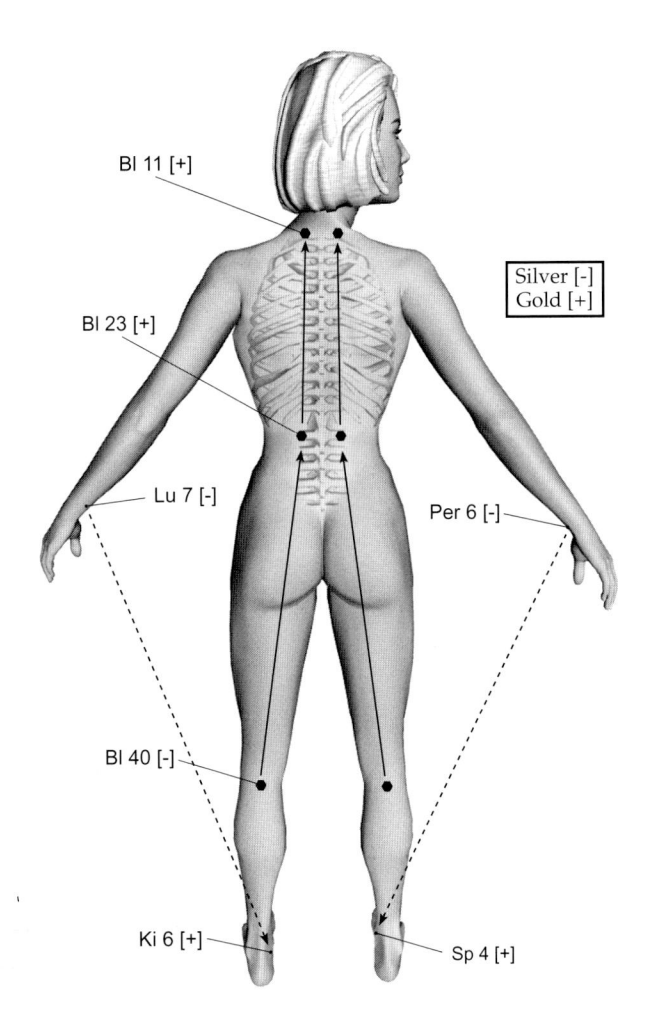

Bl 11 [+]
Bl 23 [+]
Lu 7 [-]
Per 6 [-]
Bl 40 [-]
Ki 6 [+]
Sp 4 [+]

Silver [-]
Gold [+]

5TH TREATMENT

On November 2, 1999, Ms. E. reported that she was pregnant and that she had gained 5 pounds. She was very happy but tired and nauseated.

All therapy suspended at this time. In June she delivered a healthy 5.8 pound baby boy one month prematurely.

CONCLUSION

The material contained in this book is not the final word on the channel divergences and our presentation of the range of approaches to channel divergence therapy is by no means exhaustive. Nevertheless, we have tried to present the reader with some of the tools that are necessary to conceptually evaluate any channel divergence therapy whether or not it appears in this book. As we have seen, the nature of the channel divergences can be extremely difficult to pin down. Moreover, not all of the current assumptions concerning the channel divergences are necessarily based on textual fact. Be that as it may, the channel divergences as a whole offer the potential for allowing us to interact with our patients in an efficacious manner.

We hope that we have presented a sufficient variety of perspectives on the channel divergences so that most acupuncturists will have found something that they can integrate into their practices. One of the most definitive things that can be said regarding the channel divergences is that our understanding of them is evolving and there is no one way to use them. We have found the channel divergences to be an extremely useful clinical tool and it is our hope that you will too.

ENDNOTES

[1] *Ido-no-Nippon-Sha* translates poorly into English. A rough translation would be Medicine Path Company of Japan. The publishing house has chosen an English title some what arbitrarily.
[2] Those familiar with Shima's videos on the channel divergences will note his extensive use of other methods of inducing a qi-bias, including IP cords and electricity. While he still teaches these methods, in his own practice, Shima prefers to use bi-metal needles and, to a lesser extent, electrical stimulation.
[3] See Oleson.
[4] Personal communication with Shoji Kobayashi.
[5] See, for example, Chapter 10, *Divine Pivot*.
[6] Irie, Seiji: 4
[7] The pinyin equivalent of *hie* is *leng*.

[8] See Appendix 9 for more information on this device.
[9] This is the principle upon which Li Dong-yuan's theory is based.
[10] One of the primary methods Shima uses for diagnosing the extraordinary vessels is the pulse. A further discussion of extraordinary vessel pulse diagnosis appears in Appendix 2.
[11] Kanari: 34-41.
[12] The *gan/yin wei* connection is Liv 4 and Per 6.
[13] The *wei/da chang* connection is St 40 and LI 5.
[14] The *xin/shen* connection is Ht 5 and Ki 6.
[15] The question of cure is an interesting one. When subjected to close scrutiny, it appears that true cures are actually rather rare, at least in conventional medicine. In the book *The Best Alternative Medicine* (Simon & Schuster, NY, 2000, p. 33), Kenneth R. Pelletier reports on an article that originally appeared in the Nov. 11, 1988 edition of the Journal of the American Medical Association. He states :

> Most recently a review by Jeanette Ezzo and Dr. Brian M. Berman of the University of Maryland was undertaken under the auspices of the international Cochrane Collaboration that focuses on "evidence-based medicine" for both conventional and alternative medicine. Based on 159 reviews of conventional medical practices, the reviewers found that only 20.8 percent evidenced a positive effect on the treated group over the control group. For the vast majority of the conventional medical practices, the evidence ranged from 6.9 percent demonstrating harm, to 24.5 percent resulting in no effect at all.

While two of the cases presented here do not purport to be cures, they nevertheless demonstrate a positive effect from the therapies administered.
[16] *Shaku* (Chinese: *pi ji*) is discussed in the 55th and 56th Difficult Issue of the *Nan Jing* (*Classic of Difficult Issues*). We adopt the Japanese term here because it has developed a specific meaning in the context of the *Kanpo* tradition. *Shaku* is defined as a blockage of qi and blood in the viscera and is experienced by the patient as tenderness upon deep palpation. *Shaku* differs from *ju*, which is a blockage of qi and blood in the bowels. *Ju* presents as tightness of the abdominal muscles felt upon light pressure. *Shaku* typcally occurs in a specific reflex area with visceral associations. For instance, spleen *shaku* occurs in the periumbilical region while kidney *shaku* occurs above the pubic bone.
[17] A further discussion of Omura's Thymus-regulating holes appears in Appendix 4.
[18] The *da chang/wei* connection also had a deviation of 37, however, Shima chose to disregard it.
[19] *You Gui Wan* (Right Restoring [Life-gate] Pills) contains: *Fu Zi* (Radix Lateralis Aconiti Charmichaeli Praepartae), *Rou Gui* (Cortex Cinnamomi), *Lu Jiao Jiao* (Colla Cornu Cervi), *Shu Di Huang* (Radix Rehmanniae Glutinosae Conquitae), *Shan Yu Zhu* (Fructus Corni Officianalis), *Shan Yao* (Radix Dioscoreae Oppositae), *Gou Qi Zi* (Fructus Lycii Chinensis), *Tu Su Zi* (Semen Cuscutae Chinensis), *Du Zhong* (Cortex Eucommiae Ulmoidis), and *Dang Gui*.
[20] *Zuo Gui Wan* (Left Restoring [Life-gate] Pills) contains: *Shu Di Huang* (Radix Rehmanniae Glutinosae Conquitae), *Shan Yu Zhu* (Fructus Corni Officianalis), *Shan Yao* (Radix Dioscoreae Oppositae), *Gou Qi Zi* (Fructus Lycii Chinensis), *Fu Ling* (Sclerotium Poria Cocos), and *Zhi Gan Cao*.
[21] The concentration ratio of all the desiccated extracts cited in the present work is 5:1
[22] Dr. Lai 's prescription contained *Ba Ji Tian* (Radix Morinda Officinalis) 4 *qian*, *Dang Gui* (Radix Angelicae Sinensis) 3 *qian*, *Yin Chai Hu* (Radix Stellariae Dictomae) 5 *qian*, *Xu Duan* (Radix Dipsacus Asperi) 3 *qian*, *Gu Sui Bu* (Rhizoma Drynariae) 4 *qian*, *Wei Ling Xian* (Rhizoma Clematwice Dailyis) 3 *qian*, *Bei Huang Qi* (Radix Astragalus Membrnacae) 3 *qian*, *Hu Luan Ling Zhi* (Sclertoium Lingzhi) 2 *qian*, *Ren Shen* (Radix Panacis Ginseng) 3 *qian*, *Zao Ren* (Prepared Semen zizyphi Spinosae) 3 *qian*. *Gao Ben* (Radix Ligustici Gaoben) 3 *qian*, *Shou Wu* (Radix Polygonum Multiflorum) 3 *qian*, *Bai Ji Li* (Fructus Tribuli Terrestris) 3 *qian*, *Yuan Zhi* (Radix Polygala Tenufolia) 3 *qian*, *Gan Cao* (Radix Glycyrrhizae Uralensis) 3 *qian*, *Xiao Hui Xiang* (Fructus Foeoniculi) 3 *qian*, *Zhu Feng* (Bambusae Concretio Silicae) 3 *qian*, *Chuan Shan Jia* (Squama Mantidis Pentadactylae) 2 *qian*, *E Jiao* (Corii Asini Gelatinum) 3 *qian*, *Ban Xia* (Rhizoma Pinelliae Ternatae) 3 *qian*, *Dang Shen* (Radix Codonopsis Pilosulae) 5 *qian*, and *Yu Jin* 's oncological therapies.
[23] *Ba Zhen Tang* (Eight Gem Decoction) contains: *Ren Shen* (Radix Panacis Ginseng), *Bai Zhu*

(Rhizoma Atractylodes Macrocephelae), *Fu Ling* (Sclerotium Poria Cocos), and *Zhi Gan Cao* (Honey-Fried Radix Glycyrrhizae Uralensis), *Shu Di Huang* (Radix Rehmaniae Glutinosae Conquitae), *Dang Gui* (Radix Angelicae Sinensis), *Bai Sha* (Radix Paeoniae Lactiflorae), and *Chuan Xiong* (Radix Ligustici Wallichi).

[24] We have omitted the second office visit simply because the patient had little to report and it was not terribly interesting.

[25] The terms concretions and conglomerations (*zheng jia*) are typically used in TCM parlance to denote abdominal masses, particularly uterine fibroids. In the Japanese *Kanpo* tradition, accumulation (*ji* in Chinese or *shaku* in Japanese), and is the preferred term. *Shaku* may involve any of the viscera and kidney *shaku* suggests a deep stagnation of qi and blood in the kidney reflex area of the lower abdomen below *Guan Yuan* (CV 4). Uterine fibroids correlate closely to kidney *shaku*, particularly its subcategory known as running piglet. While we often tend to think of running piglet as a subjective sensation on the part of the patient, it may also have a physical presence. The 56th Difficult Issue of the *Classic of Difficult Issues* states: "*Shaku* of the kidney is called running piglet and presents in the lower abdomen, ascending to below the heart. Like a piglet, it may move up and down unexpectantly. It lasts a long time without ending."

[26] *Wen Jing Tang* (Menses-Warming Decoction) contains: *Wu Zhu Yu* (Fructus Evodia Rutaecarpae), *Gui Zhi* (Ramulus Cinamomi Cassiae), *Dang Gui* (Radix Angelicae Sinensis), *Bai Shao* (Radix Paeoniae Lactiflorae), *Chuan Xiong* (Radix Ligustici Wallichi), *E Jiao* (Gelatinum Corii Asini), *Mai Men Dong* (Tuber Ophiopogonis Japonici), *Mu Dan Pi* (Cortex Mouton Radicis), *Ban Xia* (Rhizoma Pinelliae Ternatae), *Sheng Jiang* (Rhizoma Zingeberis Officianalis Recens), *Ren Shen* (Radix Panacis Ginseng), *Gan Cao* (Radix Glycyrrhizae Uralensis), and *Da Zao* (Fructus Zizyphi Jujube).

[27] *Yi Gan Ji Jia Chen Pi Ban Xia* (Liver Repressing Decoction plus Orange Peel and Pinellia) contains: *Dang Gui* (Radix Angelicae Sinensis), *Gou Teng* (Ramulus Uncaria Cum Uncis), *Chuan Xiong* (Radix Ligustici Wallichi), *Ban Xia* (Rhizoma Pinelliae Ternatae), *Chen Pi* (Pericarpium Citri Reticulatae), *Fu Ling* (Sclerotium Poriae Cocos), *Gan Cao* (Radix Glycyrrhizae Uralesis), *Chai Hu* (Radix Bupleurum Chinensis) and *Bai Zhu* (Rhizoma Atractylodes Macrocephelae).

[28] *Du Huo Sheng Qi Tang* (*Du Huo* and Mistletoe Decoction) contains: *Du Huo* (Radix Angelicae Pubescens), *Xi Xin* (Herba Asari Cum Radice), *Fang Feng* (Radix Ledeouriellae Sesloidis), *Qin Jiao* (Gentiana Qinjiao), *Sang Ji Sheng* (Ramulus Loranthus Sangjisheng), *Du Zhong* (Cortex Eucommiae Ulmoidis), *Niu Xi* (Radix Achyranthes Bidentatae), *Rou Gui* (Cortex Cinnamomi Cassiae), *Dang Gui* (Radix Angelicae Sinensis), *Chuan Xiong* (Radix Ligustici Wallichi), *Sheng Di Huang* (Radix Rehmanniae Glutinosae), *Bai Shao* (Radix Paeoniae Lactiflorae), *Ren Shen* (Radix Panacis Ginseng), *Fu Ling* (Sclerotium Poriae Cocos), and *Zhi Gan Cao* (mix-fried Radix Glycyrrhizae Uralensis).

[29] Miki Shima's use of the Ht 5/Ki 6 and Lu 7/Sp 4 pairs as "extra" extraordinary vessel pairs was suggested to him by Tadashi Irie. As we have seen in Chapter 6, there are a number of these adjunctive extraordinary vessel pairings extant in the literature. In addition to the orthodox extraordinary vessel pairings Shima prefers the pairs Per 6/ Liv 4, LI 5/St 40, Ht 7/Ki 6 and Lu 7/Sp 4 for a total of eight extraordinary vessel pairs.

[30] *Gui Zhi Jia Long Gu Mu Li Tang* (Cinnamon Twig Decoction Plus Dragon Bone and Oyster Shell) contains: *Gui Zhi* (Ramulus Cinnamomi Cassia), *Bai Shao* (Radix Paeoniae Lactiflorae), *Long Gu* (Os Draconis), *Mu Li* (Concha Ostrea), *Sheng Jiang* (Rhizoma Zingeberis Officianalis Recens), *Da Zao* (Fructus Zizyphi Jujubae) and *Gan Cao* (Radix Glycyrrhizae Uralensis).

[31] *Ban Xia Xie Xin Tang* (Pinellia Heart-Draining Decoction) contains: *Ban Xia* (Rhizoma Pinelliae Ternatae), *Gan Jiang* (Rhizoma Zingeberis Officianalis), *Huang Qin* (Radix Scutellariae Baicalensis), *Huang Lian* (Rhizoma Coptidis Chinensis), *Ren Shen* (Radix Panacis Ginseng), *Da Zao* (Fructus Zizyphi Jujubae) and *Gan Cao* (Mix-fried Radix Glycyrrhizae Uralensis).

[32] *Tao He Cheng Qi Tang* (Peach Kernel Qi Coordinating Decoction) contains: *Tao Ren* (Semen Pruni Persicae), *Da Huang* (Radix et Rhizoma Rhei), *Gui Zhi* (Ramulus Cinnamomi Cassiae, *Mang Xiao* (Miribilitum), *Zhi Gan Cao*

[33] *Ban Xia Hou Po Tang* (Pinellia and Magnolia Bark Decoction) contains: *Ban Xia* (Rhizoma Pinelliae Ternatae), *Hou Po* (Cortex Magnolia Officianals), *Fu Ling* (Sclerotium Poria Cocos), *Gan Jiang* (Rhizoma Zingeberis Officianalis), and *Zi Su Ye* (Folium Perillae Frutescentis).

[34] *Xiao Yao San* (Free Wanderer Powder) contains: *Chai Hu* (Radix Bupleuri), *Dang Gui* (Radix Angelica Sinensis), *Bai Shao* (Radix Paeoniae Lactiflorae), *Bai Zhu* (Rhizoma Atractylodes Macrocephe-

lae), *Fu Ling* (Sclerotium Poriae Cocos), *Zhi Gan Cao* (Mix-fried Radix Glycyrrhizae Uralensis).

[35] *Yi Gan Ji Jia Chen Pi Ban Xia Tang* (Liver Repressing Decoction plus Orange Peel and Pinellia Decoction) contains: *Dang Gui* (Radix Angelicae Sinensis), *Gou Teng* (Ramulus Uncaria Cum Uncis), *Chuan Xiong* (Radix Ligustici Wallichi), *Ban Xia* (Rhizoma Pinelliae Ternatae), *Chen Pi* (Pericarpium Citri Reticulatae), *Fu Ling* (Sclerotium Poriae Cocos), *Gan Cao* (Radix Glycyrrhizae Uralesis), *Chai Hu* (Radix Bupleurum Chinensis) and *Bai Zhu* (Rhizoma Atractylodes Macrocephelae).

[36] *Ba Wei Wan* (Eight Ingredients Pills) contains: *Gui Zhi* (Ramulus Cinnamomi Cassiae), *Fu Zi* (Radix Lateralis Aconiti Charmichaeli), *Shu Di Huang* (Radix Rehmanniae Glutinosae Conquitae), *Shan Yu Zhu* (Fructus Corni Officianalis), *Shan Yao* (Radix Dioscoreae Oppositae), *Fu Ling* (Sclerotium Poria Cocos), *Ze Xie* (Rhizoma Alismatis Orientalis), and *Mu Dan Pi* (Cortex Moutan Radicis).

[37] Each caspule contained 500 milligrams of herbal product.

[38] *Xiao Chai Hu Tang* (Minor Bupleurum Decoction) contains: *Chai Hu* (Radix Bupleuri), *Huang Qin* (Radix Scutellariae Baicalensis), *Ban Xia* (Rhizoma Pinelliae Ternatae), *Sheng Jiang* (Rhizoma Zingeberis Officianalis Recens), *Ren Shen* (Radix Panacis Ginseng), *Zhi Gan Cao* (Mix-fried Radix Glycyrrhizae Uralensis), and *Da Zao* (Fructus Zizyphi Jujube).

[39] *Dang Gui Shao Yang San* (Tang Kuei and Peony Powder) contains: *Dang Gui* (Radix Angelica Sinensis), *Bai Shao* (Radix Paeoniae Lactiflorae), *Bai Zhu* (Rhizoma Atractylodes Macrocephelae), *Fu Ling* (Sclerotium Poriae Cocos), *Zi Xie* (Rhizoma Alismatis Orientalis), and *Chuan Xiong* (Radix Ligustici Wallichi).

[40] *Si Wu Tang* (Four Agents Decoction) contains: *Shu Di Huang* (Radix Rehmanniae Glutinosae Conquitae), *Dang Gui* (Radix Angelicae Sinensis), *Bai Shao* (Radix Paeoniae Lactiflorae), and *Chuan Xiong* (Radix Ligustici Wallichi).

[41] *Bu Zhong Yi Qi Tang* (Center-Supplementing Qi-Boosting Decoction) contains: *Huang Qi* (Radix Astragali Membranacei), *Ren Shen* (Radix Panacis Ginseng), *Bai Zhu* (Radix Atractylodes Macrocephelae), *Zhi Gan Cao* (Mix-fried Radix Glycyrrhizae Uralensis), *Dang Gui* (Radix Angelicae Sinensis), *Chen Pi* (Pericarpium Citri Reticulatae), *Sheng Ma* (Rhizoma Cimicifugae) and *Chai Hu* (Radix Bupleuri).

[42] *Li Zhong Tang* (Center-Rectifying Decoction) contains: *Gan Jiang* (Rhizoma Zingeberis Officianalis), *Ren Shen* (Radix Panacis Ginseng), *Bai Zhu* (Radix Atractylodes Macrocephelae) and *Zhi Gan Cao* (Mix-fried Radix Glycyrrhizae Uralensis).

Appendix 1:
Integrated Treatment Strategies: A Treatment Formulary

As we have seen, there are many ways to use the channel divergences in clinical practice, and most channel divergences specialists use them in conjunction with other layers of the system of channels and network vessels. We encourage the reader to integrate the channel divergences into his or her own practice in whatever manner is most comfortable for them. We have also seen that the criteria for selecting a channel divergence runs the gamut from a purely symptomatic "best guess" to an entirely constitutional, Akabane-based methodology that is applied regardless of the presenting symptoms.

What follows is a collection of protocols often used by Shima in the treatment of common complaints. These further illustrate how an experienced clinician might integrate a channel divergence therapy into a broader clinical context. Most importantly, these protocols are not presented as set pieces. There is no "Shima's Asthma Treatment" *per se.* Such a "by the number" treatment plan would contradict Shima's fundamental approach to acupuncture. The reader must determine an appropriate methodology for him or herself based on the unique presentation of each patient during a given acupuncture session. We have presented the following protocols as starting places only. For instance, many, but not all, migraines are due to liver counterflow and, therefore, the use of the second confluence is usually indicated. However, if the reader is called upon to treat a migraineur with a profound spleen vacuity and phlegm turbidity, the treatment plan must be adjusted accordingly to achieve an optimal therapeutic outcome.

The reader will notice that Shima uses both the extraordinary vessels and the channel divergences in nearly every protocol and that he does so in an extremely fluid manner. He sometimes uses a yang confluence hole on the left and a yin confluence hole on the right. At other times, he treats a channel divergence on the left and an extraordinary vessel on the right. Sometimes the treatments are administered bilaterally and appear very symmetrical, but most often they are not. To continue with the migraine example, this illness will likely call for an asymmetrical needling pattern that reflects the unilateral nature of the condition, while a protocol for cystitis or prostatitis typically calls for a more symmetrical needling pattern.

Although the master holes on the head and the holes on the extremities remain the same throughout all of the following examples, the standard polarities are not infrequently reversed to accommodate energetic presentations that countermand our common assumptions concerning how things should be hooked up. Again, in the case of migraines, the counterflow may be so profound that it is necessary to unequivocally direct the qi away from the head by administering negative poles to all points in this region and positive poles to the access holes. Once again, the implication is that there is no one single protocol or methodology for utilizing the channel divergences.

The point pairings described below are generally drawn unilaterally for clarity. For acute conditions, however, the extraordinary vessel pairings are typically connected contralaterally. For an acute asthma attack right *Lie Que* (Lu 7) is connected to left *Zhao Hai* (Ki 6) and vice versa. However, when treating a chronic asthmatic condition, right Lu 7 is connected to right Ki 6 when treating the condition during remission. There are a number of exceptions to this rule, however, for instance, Shima uses crossing extraordinary vessel connections in the case of fibromyalgia. Channel divergences pairings are never applied contralaterally.

MIGRAINE

STEP 1. Vigorously needle *Feng Fu* (GB 20) on the affected side to induce local vasoconstriction.

STEP 2. Needle the second confluence as well as the *yang qiao* vessel and *dai* vessel meeting holes. For nausea, use the third confluence. Needle the following pattern using gold and silver needles or IP cords. Electrical stimulation is contraindicated with migraine patients. If IP cords are used, they should be connected contralaterally to enhance the therapeutic effect.

Note the polarity reversal in the channel divergence connection. In the case of migraines, the ascending counterflow is so profound that it is necessary to unequivocally downbear the qi.

Appendix 1   203

NOTE: EXTRAORDINARY VESSEL CONNECTIONS ARE CONTRALATERAL & BILATERAL. ONLY ONE SET OF CONNECTIONS IS REPRESENTED HERE FOR GRAPHIC CLARITY.   →

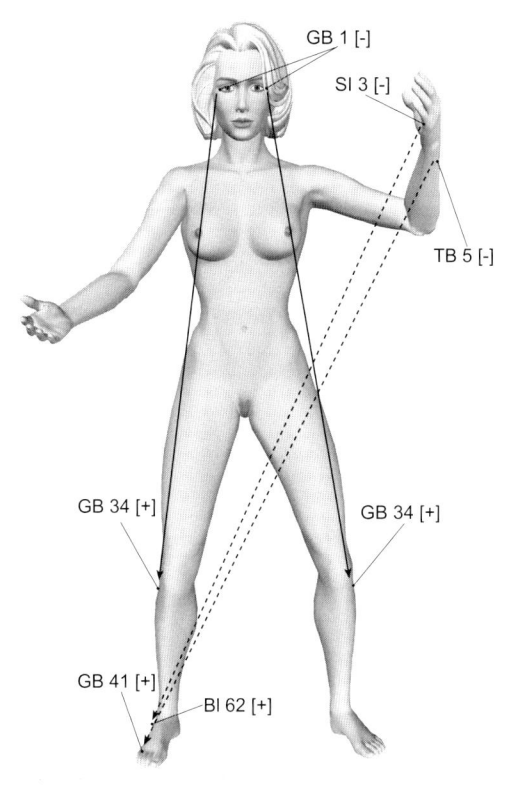

GB 1 [-]
SI 3 [-]
TB 5 [-]
GB 34 [+]
GB 34 [+]
GB 41 [+]
Bl 62 [+]

ALTERNATE NEEDLING PATTERN: →

AFFECTED SIDE   **UNAFFECTED SIDE**

In some cases, it is appropriate to bring the qi up in the channel divergence on the unaffected side and downbear it on the affected side.

GB 1 [-]
GB 1 [+]
SI 3 [-]
TB 5 [-]
GB 34 [+]
GB 34 [-]
GB 41 [+]
Bl 62 [+]

STEP 3. Auriculotherapy: Temples, Forehead, *Shen Men*, Sympathetic, Thalamus, Zero, Oscillation

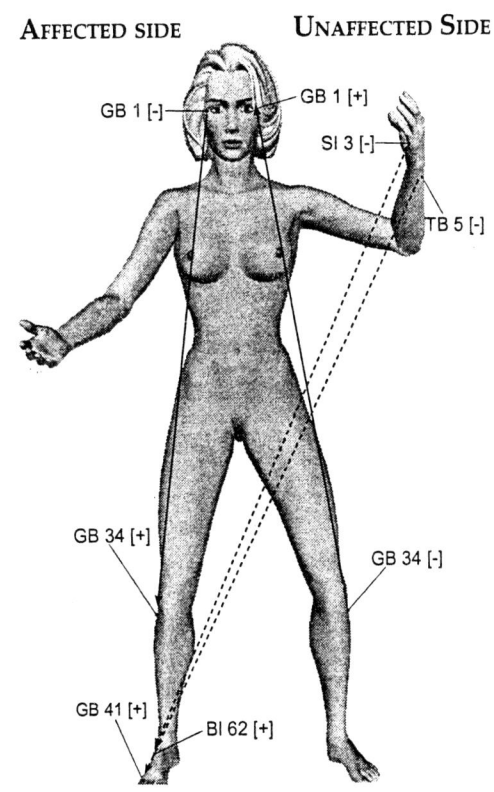

BRONCHIAL ASTHMA

During the acute phase of kidney vacuity pattern bronchial asthma with weak pulses in *chi* positions and weak *hara*, use: The Yin and Yang pairs of the first and sixth confluences and the *chong/yin wei* and *ren/yin qiao* connections.

⟶

NOTE: EXTRAORDINARY VESSEL CONNECTIONS ARE CONTRALATERAL & BILATERAL. ONLY ONE SET OF CONNECTIONS IS REPRESENTED HERE FOR GRAPHIC CLARITY.

Bl 1 [+]
Bl 1 [+]
St 12 [-]
St 12 [-]
LI 11 [+]
Lu 7 [-]
Lu 5 [+]
Per 6 [-]
Ki 10 [-]
UB 40 [-]
Ki 6 [+]
Sp 4 [+]

For chronic bronchial asthma or during remission with a liver pattern and a wiry pulse, use: The Yin and Yang pairs of the second and sixth confluences and the *ren/yin qiao* and *chong/yin wei* connections.

⟶

NOTE: EXTRAORDINARY VESSEL CONNECTIONS ARE BILATERAL & IPSILATERAL.

STEP 3. Auriculotherapy: Asthma, Antihistamine, Lung 1, Lung 2, Bronchi, Autonomic Point, Point Zero, *Shen Men*, Allergy Point, Adrenal Gland C, Master Cerebral, Psychosomatic Reactions 1

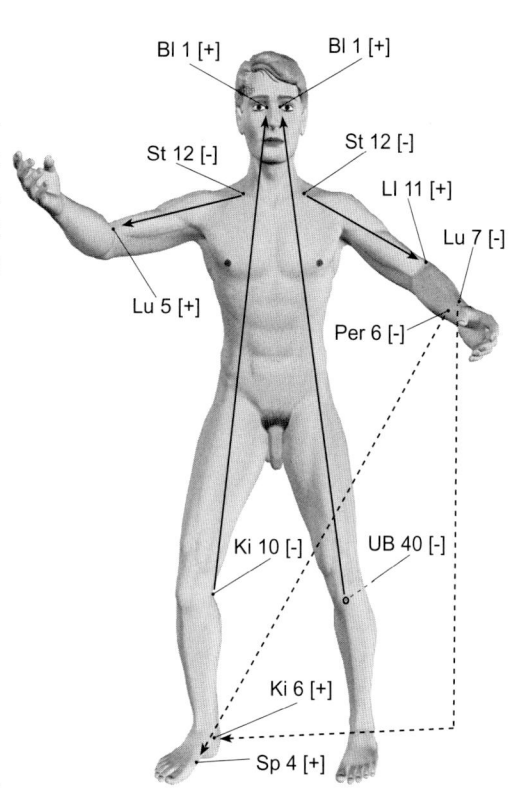

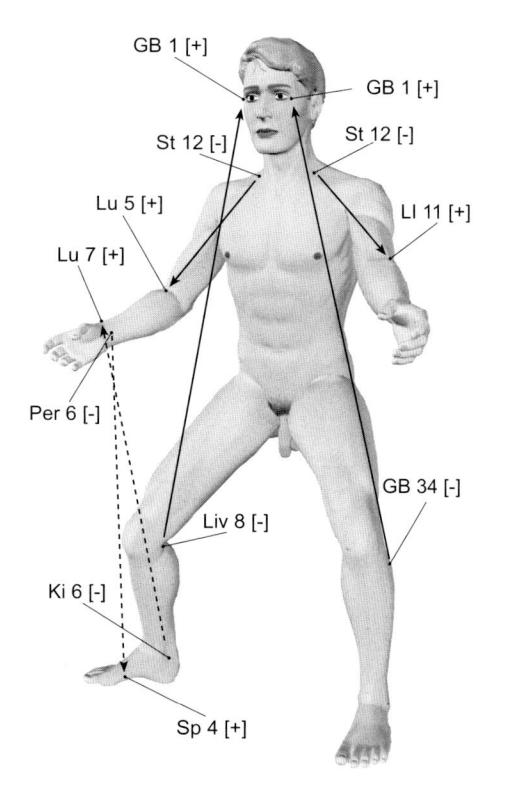

GB 1 [+]
GB 1 [+]
St 12 [-]
St 12 [-]
Lu 5 [+]
LI 11 [+]
Lu 7 [+]
Per 6 [-]
GB 34 [-]
Liv 8 [-]
Ki 6 [-]
Sp 4 [+]

Insomnia

Step 1. Bilateral Kidney Return.

First Confluence

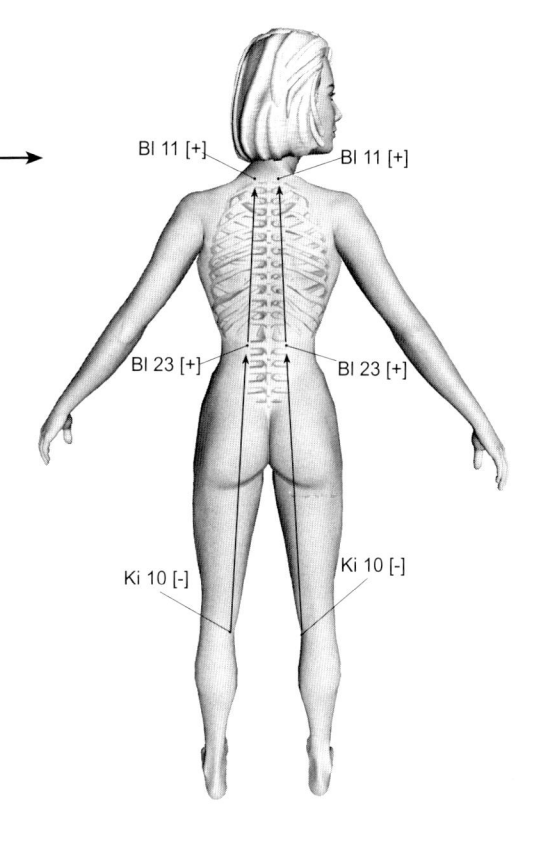

Step 2. Fourth confluence (yang pair left), *chong/yin wei* connection right & bypass treatment.

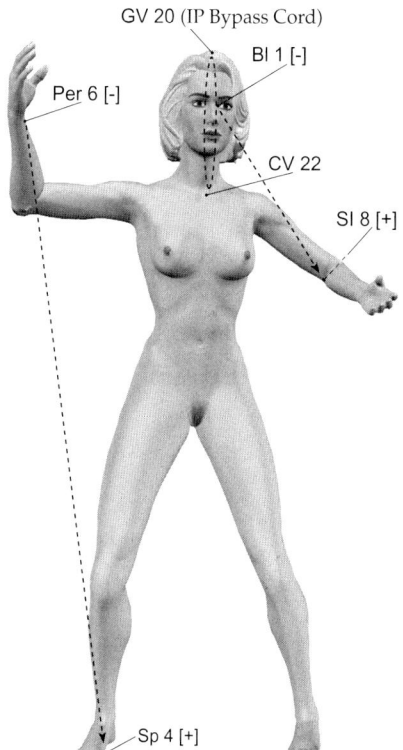

Step 3. Auriculotherapy: Insomnia 1, Insomnia 2, Pineal Gland, Master Cerebral, Point Zero, *Shen Men*, Thalamus, Forehead, Occuput, Brain, Heart C, and Kidney C

Hyper/hypothyroidism

Step 1. Fifth confluence, *du/yang qiao* & *ren/yin qiao* connections.

The following polarities are indicated for hypothyroidism where the fundamental intent is to upbear the qi. In the case of hyperthyroidism, the intent is to downbear the qi, so all polarities are reversed.

NOTE: EXTRAORDINARY VESSEL CONNECTIONS ARE BILATERAL & IPSILATERAL.

Step 2. General immunoregulation with *Shen Shu* (Bl 23), *Bai Hui* (GV 20), *San Yin Jiao* (Sp 6), *Zu San Li* (St 36), and *He Gu* (LI 4)

Step 3. Auriculotherapy: Thyroid Gland C, Thyroid Gland F, TSH, Point Zero, *Shen Men*, Endocrine, Brain

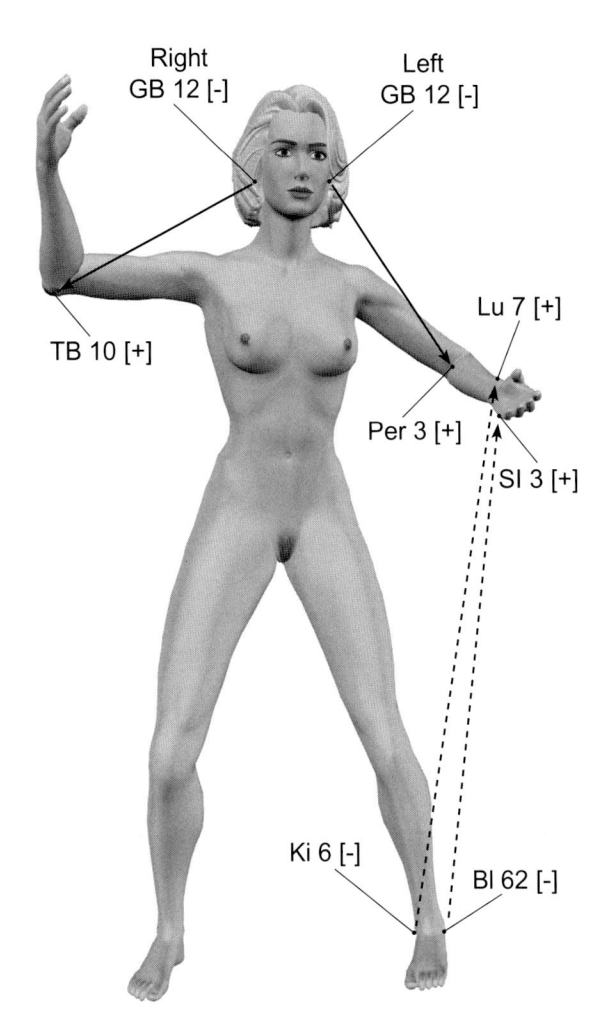

Right GB 12 [-]
Left GB 12 [-]
TB 10 [+]
Lu 7 [+]
Per 3 [+]
SI 3 [+]
Ki 6 [-]
Bl 62 [-]

Diabetes

Step 1. First confluence left and third confluence right with *yin wei/chong* right and *yang wei/dai* left. ⟶

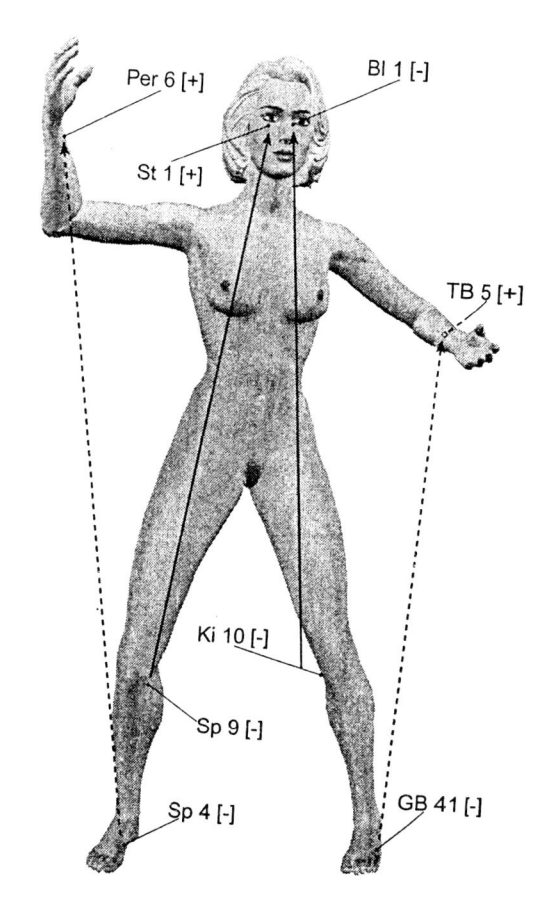

Step 2. The Fifth confluence is administrated to specifically address the endocrine system. ⟶

For false repletion patterns, use the triple burner yang confluence pair. For true vacuity patterns, use the pericardium yin confluence pair.

Step 3. Auriculotherapy: Pancreas, Pancreatitis, Point Zero, *Shen Men*, Endocrine Point, Liver

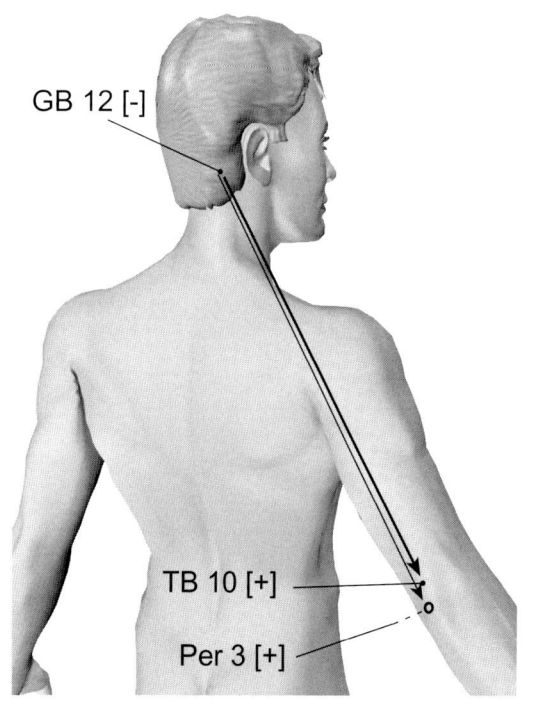

WILTING CONDITIONS (I.E., NEUROPATHIES & PARALYSIS)

STEP 1. For peripheral neuropathy, use auriculotherapy with the Hibiki method.

STEP 2. First confluence, *yang* and *yin qiao/ren* connections (for the lower extremities), or *du/yang qiao* and *ren* connections (for the upper extremities). For paralysis, conduct the qi to the area of weakness by putting the positive pole there. For example, in the case of paralysis of the lower extremities, all the holes needled on the leg should have a positive polarity.

STEP 3. Needle local points along the affected nerve trajectories on the affected extremity.

STEP 4. Auriculotherapy: Paralysis: Corresponding body area, Spinal Motor Neurons, Point Zero, *Shen Men*, Frontal Cortex, Cerebellum, Motor Neurons

Peripheral Neuralgia: Corresponding body area, Spinal Sensory Neurons, Point Zero, *Shen Men*, Thalamus, Brain Sympathetic, Adrenal C

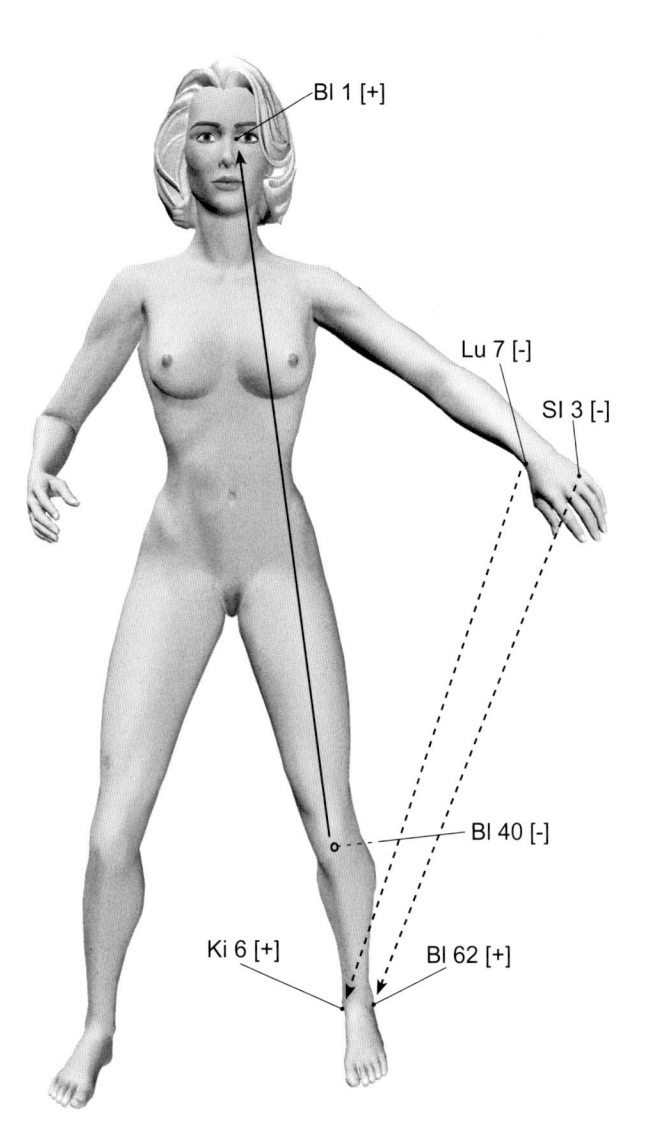

Bl 1 [+]
Lu 7 [-]
SI 3 [-]
Bl 40 [-]
Ki 6 [+]
Bl 62 [+]

<u>NOTE:</u> EXTRAORDINARY VESSEL CONNECTIONS ARE BILATERAL & IPSILATERAL.

Fibromyalgia

Step 1. Second confluence and *du/yang qiao* connection plus the *dai/yang wei* connection administered bilaterally. Despite the inherent chronic nature of this condition, the extraordinary vessel connection divergence is administered contralaterally.

Note: Extraordinary Vessel connections are bilateral & ipsilateral.

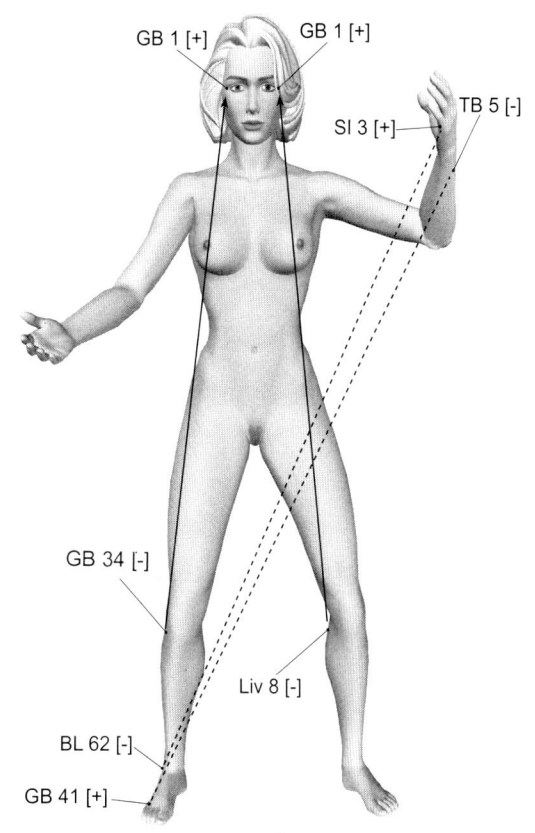

GB 1 [+]
GB 1 [+]
TB 5 [-]
SI 3 [+]
GB 34 [-]
Liv 8 [-]
BL 62 [-]
GB 41 [+]

Step 2. For sleep disturbance, treat the *du/yang qiao* connection contralaterally.

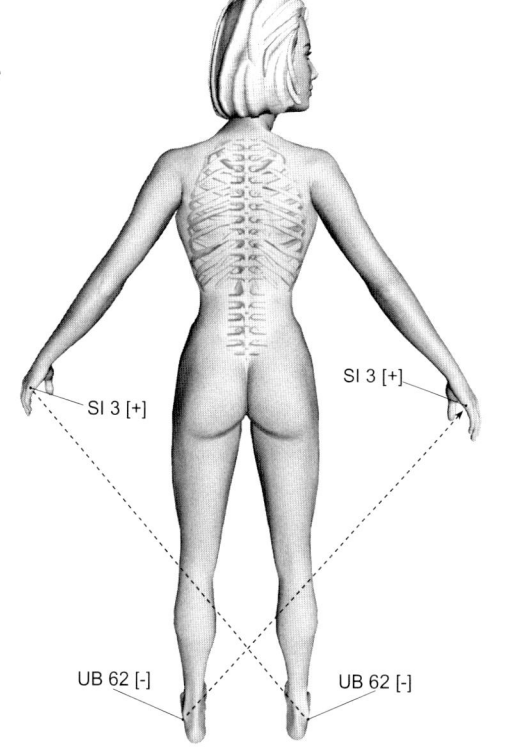

SI 3 [+]
SI 3 [+]
UB 62 [-]
UB 62 [-]

Step 3. Auriculotherapy: Thoracic Spine, Lumbosacral Spine, Point Zero, *Shen Men*, Thalamus, Abdomen, Kidney C, Sympathetic Chain, Antidepressant Point, Master Oscillation

Low Back Pain

Step 1. Hibiki Method

Locate and needle 5-10 *a shi* holes on the affected region of the back. This may include the thoracic region and the legs. Connect the negative lead of the Hibiki-7[1] device to the most caudal of the holes needled, then locate and stimulate a related point on the ear with the positive locator probe for 20-30 seconds. Move the negative lead to another needle on the back and repeat the process, stimulating all of the holes needled in this manner. The ear points may be needled subsequent to electrical stimulation with the Hibiki-7 device.

Auricular points may include: Thoracic Spine, Lumbosacral Spine, Buttocks, Sciatic Nerve, Lumbago, Point Zero, *Shen Men*, Thalamus, Sympathetic Chain, Bladder, Darwin's Point, Adrenal C, Muscle Relaxation

Alternate method: Step 1: Vigorous needling on local area.

Step 2. First confluence and *du/yang qiao and dai/yang wei* connections crossed bilaterally with electrical stimulation on the first confluence, 10Hz for 10 minutes.

Note: Extraordinary Vessel connections are bilateral & ipsilateral.

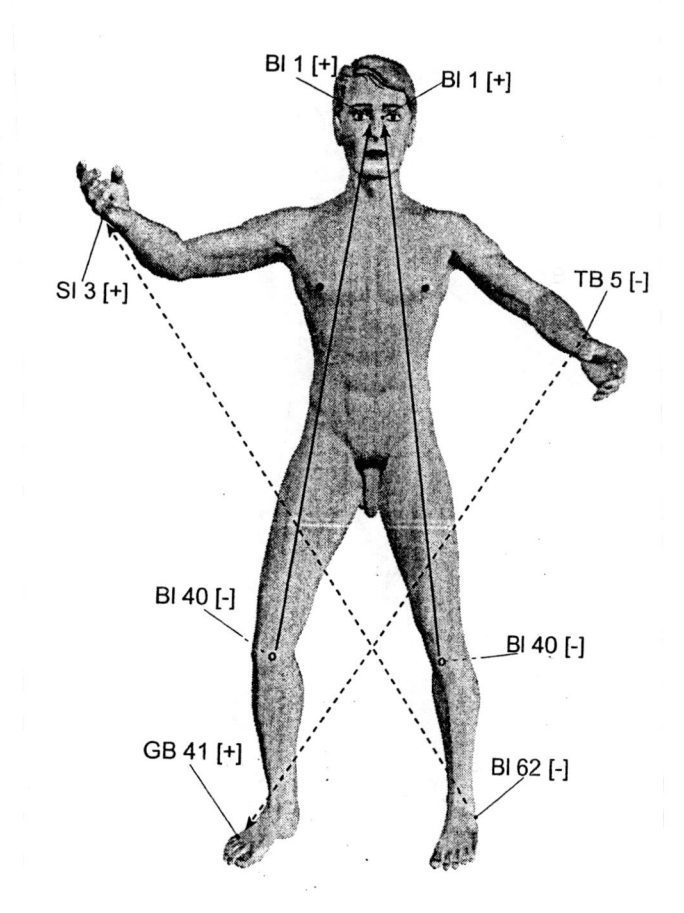

Bl 1 [+]
Bl 1 [+]
SI 3 [+]
TB 5 [-]
Bl 40 [-]
Bl 40 [-]
GB 41 [+]
Bl 62 [-]

ABDOMINAL PAIN

STEP 1. Third confluence, *chong/yin wei* connection & *da chang/wei* auxilliary extraordinary vessel connection.

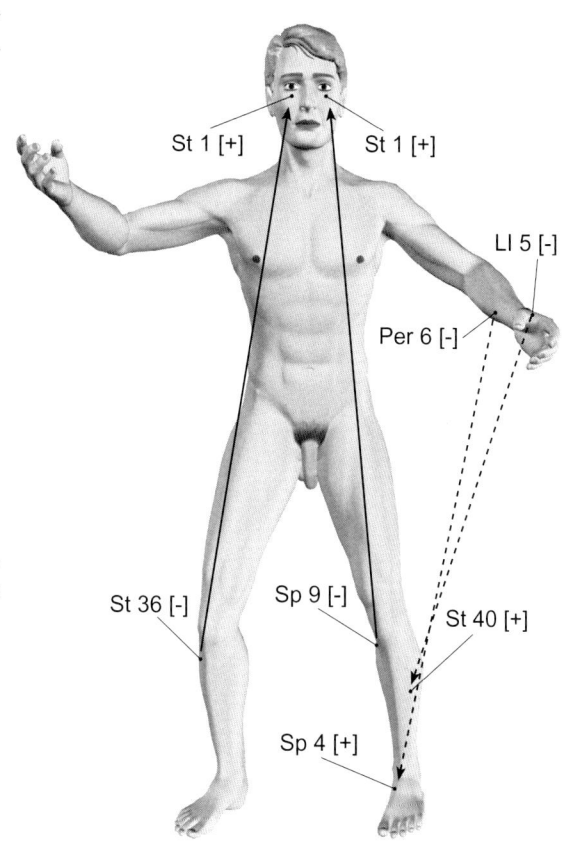

STEP: 2 Auriculotherapy: Abdomen, Pelvic Girdle, Autonomic Point, *Shen Men*, Point Zero

St 1 [+]
St 1 [+]
LI 5 [-]
Per 6 [-]
St 36 [-]
Sp 9 [-]
St 40 [+]
Sp 4 [+]

<u>NOTE</u>: EXTRAORDINARY VESSEL CONNECTIONS ARE BILATERAL & IPSILATERAL.

Intercostal Neuralgia

STEP 1. Needle the dorsal nerve root of the affected area on the painful side. Electrical stimulation should be applied at 1600Hz and 1-5 milliamperes for 3-9 minutes.

STEP 2. Second confluence and the *dai/yang wei* and *chong/yin wei*.

STEP 3. Auriculotherapy: Chest, Thoracic Spine, Point Zero, *Shen Men*, Occiput

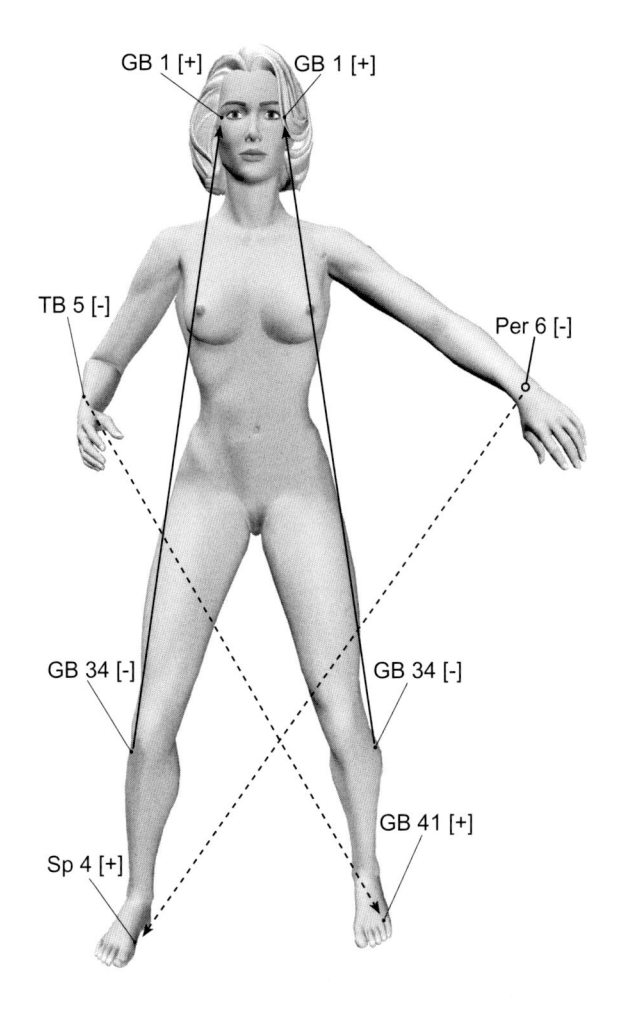

GB 1 [+]
GB 1 [+]
TB 5 [-]
Per 6 [-]
GB 34 [-]
GB 34 [-]
Sp 4 [+]
GB 41 [+]

NOTE: EXTRAORDINARY VESSEL CONNECTIONS ARE CONTRALATERAL & BILATERAL. ONLY ONE SET OF CONNECTIONS IS REPRESENTED HERE FOR GRAPHIC CLARITY.

Appendix 1

SINUSITIS

STEP 1. Sixth confluence & *du/yang qiao* vessel.

STEP 2. *Bai Hui* (GV 20), *Shen Ting* (GV 24), *Yin Tang*, *Ying Xiang* (LI 20)

STEP 3. Auriculotherapy: Inner Nose/ Oscillation Point, Frontal Sinus, Point Zero, *Shen Men*, Adrenal C, Antihistamine, Allergy Point

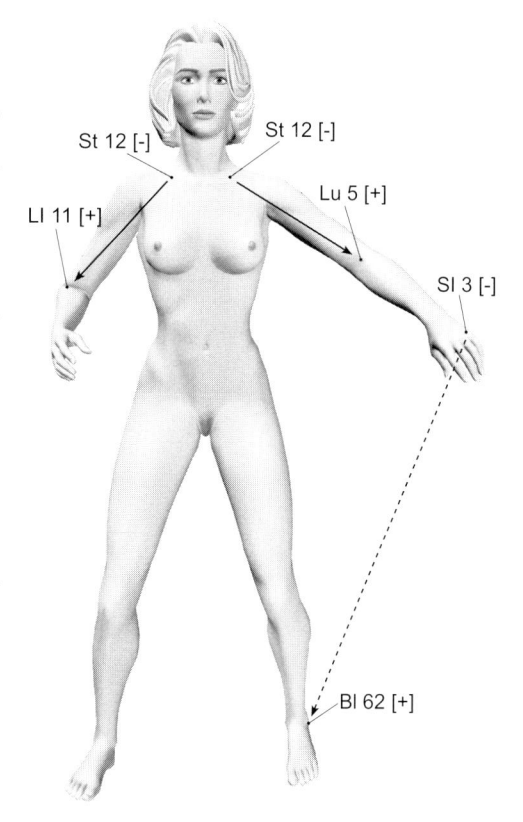

St 12 [-]   St 12 [-]
LI 11 [+]   Lu 5 [+]
SI 3 [-]
Bl 62 [+]

HYPERTENSION

STEP 1. Fifth and second confluences and the *chong/yin wei* vessel and *yin qiao/ren* connections.

STEP 2. Auriculotherapy: Hypertension 1, Hypertension 2, Hypertensive Groove, Heart C, Heart F, Marvelous Point, Tranquilizer, Autonomic Point Point Zero, *Shen Men*, Adrenal C, Kidney C, Apex of the Ear

<u>NOTE</u>: EXTRAORDINARY VESSEL CONNECTIONS ARE CONTRALATERAL & BILATERAL. ONLY ONE SET OF CONNECTIONS IS REPRESENTED HERE FOR GRAPHIC CLARITY.

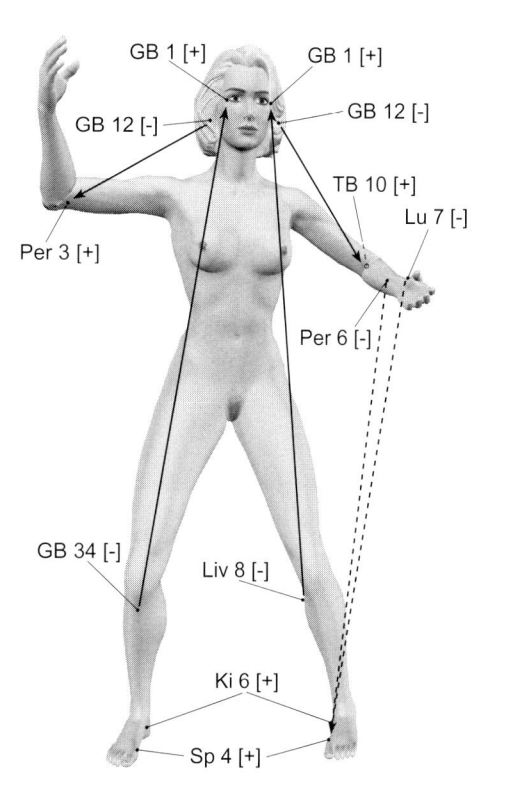

GB 1 [+]   GB 1 [+]
GB 12 [-]   GB 12 [-]
TB 10 [+]
Lu 7 [-]
Per 3 [+]
Per 6 [-]
GB 34 [-]   Liv 8 [-]
Ki 6 [+]
Sp 4 [+]

Post Cardiovascular Accident (CVA)

Acupuncture should be administered every other day for the first month, every two days for the second month, and twice a week for the following six months. For the first six months, acupuncture should be applied on the scalp on the unaffected side, while distal body points and ear points are applied on the affected side.

Step 1. Scalp acupuncture is applied first to the sensory-motor areas on the contralateral side.[2]

Step 2. Local areas of paralysis are then treated with acupuncture using low frequency mirco- or milli-current, 1-5Hz per second for 20-30 minutes.

Step 3. First and second confluences and the *du/yang qiao* and *dai/yang wei* connections.

Step 4. Auriculotherapy on the affected side with needles retained for 20 minutes: Corresponding body area, Brain, Adrenal Gland C, Adrenal Gland F, ACTH, *Shen Men*, Autonomic Master Cerebral, Endocrine Point

NOTE: EXTRAORDINARY VESSEL CONNECTIONS ARE CONTRALATERAL & BILATERAL. ONLY ONE SET OF CONNECTIONS IS REPRESENTED HERE FOR GRAPHIC CLARITY.

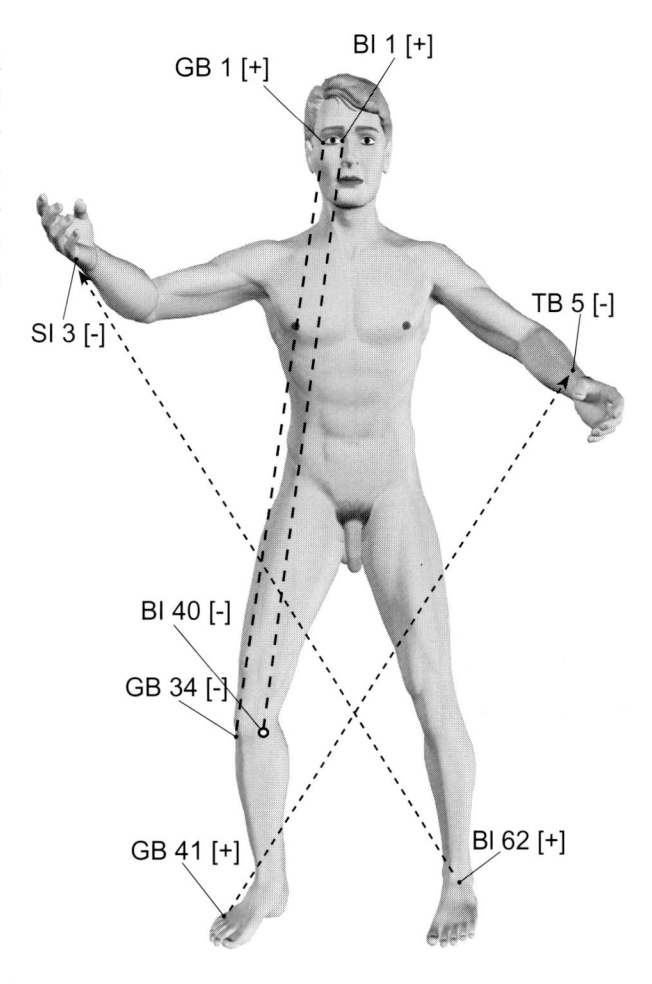

GB 1 [+]
Bl 1 [+]
SI 3 [-]
TB 5 [-]
Bl 40 [-]
GB 34 [-]
GB 41 [+]
Bl 62 [+]

Rheumatoid Arthritis

Step 1. First and second confluences, *chong/yin wei* and *ren/yin qiao* connections. ⟶

Step 2. Auriculotherapy: Corresponding body area, Point Zero, *Shen Men*, Thalamus, Endocrine, Allergy Point, Adrenal C, Master Oscillation, Kidney C, Omega 2

NOTE: EXTRAORDINARY VESSEL CONNECTIONS ARE CONTRALATERAL & BILATERAL. ONLY ONE SET OF CONNECTIONS IS REPRESENTED HERE FOR GRAPHIC CLARITY.

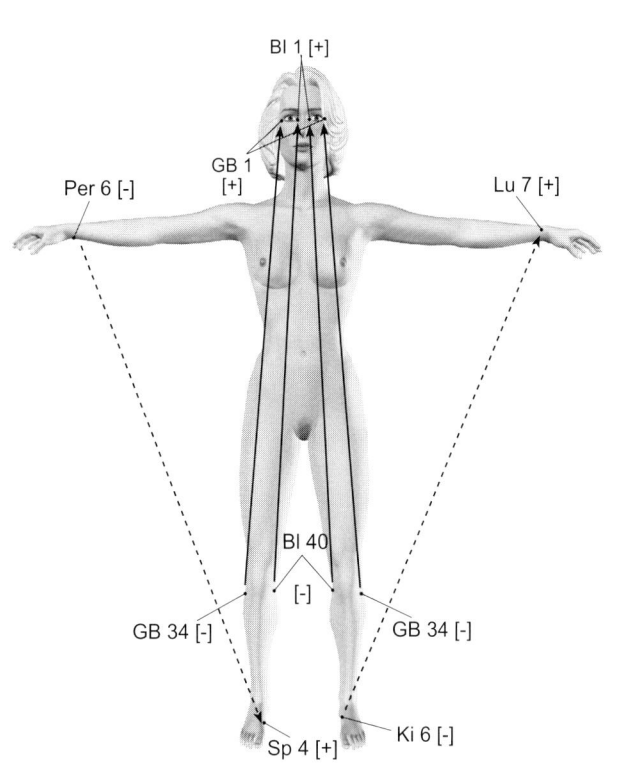

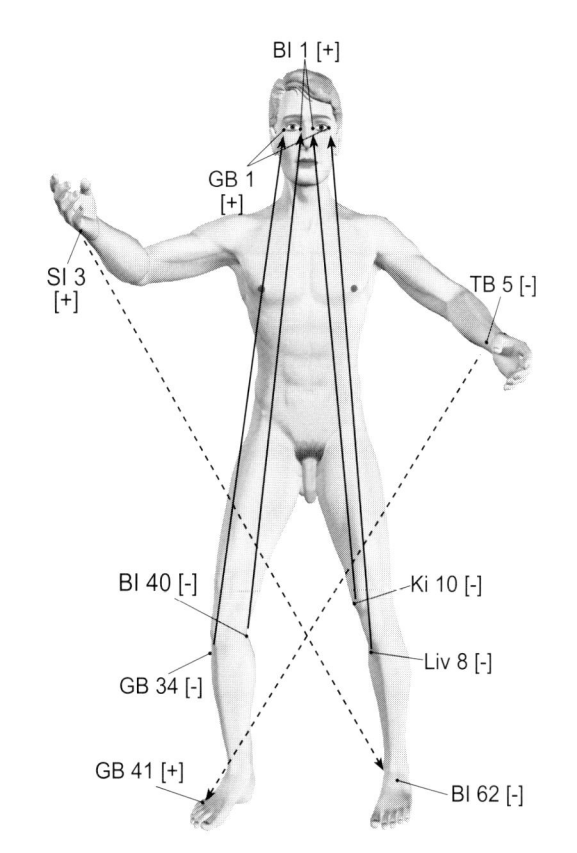

- Bl 1 [+]
- GB 1 [+]
- Per 6 [-]
- Lu 7 [+]
- Bl 40 [-]
- GB 34 [-]
- GB 34 [-]
- Sp 4 [+]
- Ki 6 [-]

Obsessive-compulsive Disorder

Step 1. First and second confluences, *du/yang qiao* and *dai/yang wei* connections. ⟶

NOTE: EXTRAORDINARY VESSEL CONNECTIONS ARE CONTRALATERAL & BILATERAL. ONLY ONE SET OF CONNECTIONS IS REPRESENTED HERE FOR GRAPHIC CLARITY.

- Bl 1 [+]
- GB 1 [+]
- SI 3 [+]
- TB 5 [-]
- Bl 40 [-]
- Ki 10 [-]
- GB 34 [-]
- Liv 8 [-]
- GB 41 [+]
- Bl 62 [-]

Or second and fourth confluences, *du/yang qiao* and *dai/yang wei* connections. ⟶

STEP 2. Auriculotherapy: Master Cerebral, Frontal Cortex, Point Zero, *Shen Men*, Thalamus, Heart C, Anterior & Posterior Hypothalamus.

The former needling pattern is indicated for individuals in whom anxiety and obsession are the predominant symptoms. The latter pattern is indicated for individuals who are predominantly compulsive.

NOTE: EXTRAORDINARY VESSEL CONNECTIONS ARE CONTRALATERAL & BILATERAL. ONLY ONE SET OF CONNECTIONS IS REPRESENTED HERE FOR GRAPHIC CLARITY.

Bl 1 [-]
GB 1 [+]
GB 1 [+]
SI 3 [+]
SI 8 [+]
TB 5 [-]
Ht 3 [+]
GB 34 [-]
Liv 8 [-]
GB 41 [+]
Bl 62 [-]

HYPOGLYCEMIA

Third and fifth confluences, *chong/yin wei* and *dai/yang wei* vessel connections. ⟶

STEP 2. Auriculotherapy: Pancreas, Stomach, Autonomic Point, Thalamus, Adrenal C, Kidney C, Liver, Point Zero, *Shen Men*, Heart C, Spleen F

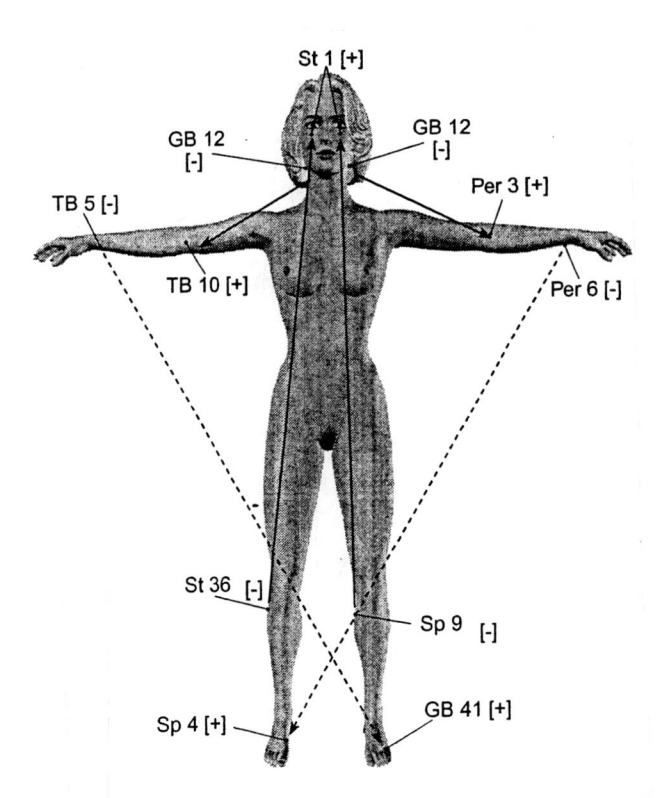

St 1 [+]
GB 12 [-]
GB 12 [-]
Per 3 [+]
TB 5 [-]
TB 10 [+]
Per 6 [-]
St 36 [-]
Sp 9 [-]
Sp 4 [+]
GB 41 [+]

Pain From Endometriosis

Step 1. First and second confluences, *chong/yin wei* vessel and *ren/yin qiao* connections. ⟶

NOTE: EXTRAORDINARY VESSEL CONNECTIONS ARE CONTRALATERAL & BILATERAL. ONLY ONE SET OF CONNECTIONS IS REPRESENTED HERE FOR GRAPHIC CLARITY.

Or first and fifth confluences, *chong/yin wei* vessel and *ren/yin qiao* connections. ⟶

Step 2. Auriculotherapy: Uterus C, Uterus F, Ovary C, Ovary F, *Shen Men*, Endocrine Point, Point Zero, Abdomen, Adrenal C, Adrenal F

The former needling pattern is indicated for endometriosis due to kidney-liver vacuity with no upward flaming of vacuity fire. The latter is indicated for more severe kidney vacuity with upward flaring of vacuity fire.

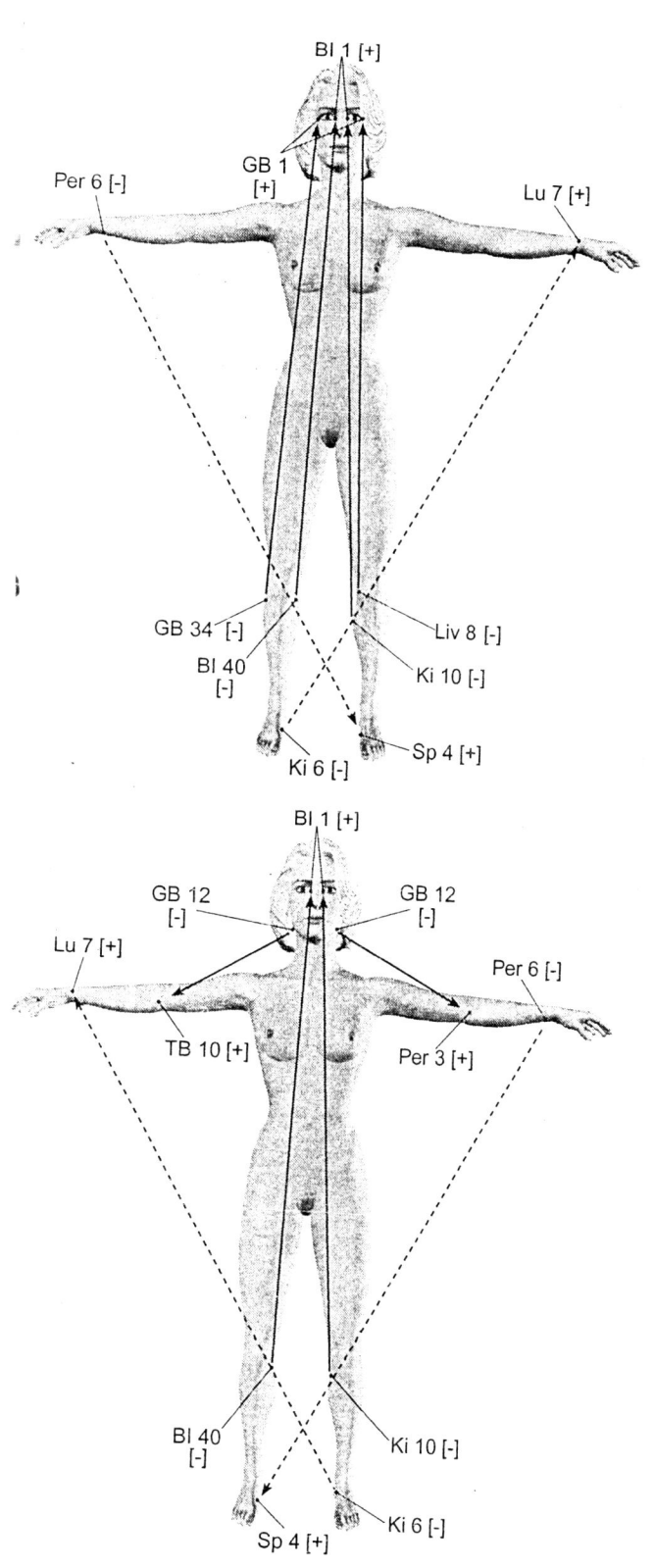

(Diagram 1 labels: Bl 1 [+], GB 1 [+], Per 6 [-], Lu 7 [+], GB 34 [-], Bl 40 [-], Liv 8 [-], Ki 10 [-], Ki 6 [-], Sp 4 [+])

(Diagram 2 labels: Bl 1 [+], GB 12 [-], GB 12 [-], Lu 7 [+], Per 6 [-], TB 10 [+], Per 3 [+], Bl 40 [-], Ki 10 [-], Sp 4 [+], Ki 6 [-])

LEUKOPENIA
(white cells less than 4000 per cubic centimeter)

STEP 1. Second confluence and *chong/yin wei* vessel connections

STEP 2. Auriculotherapy: Liver, Spleen C, Spleen F, Heart C, Kidney C, Adrenal C, Endocrine, *Shen Men*

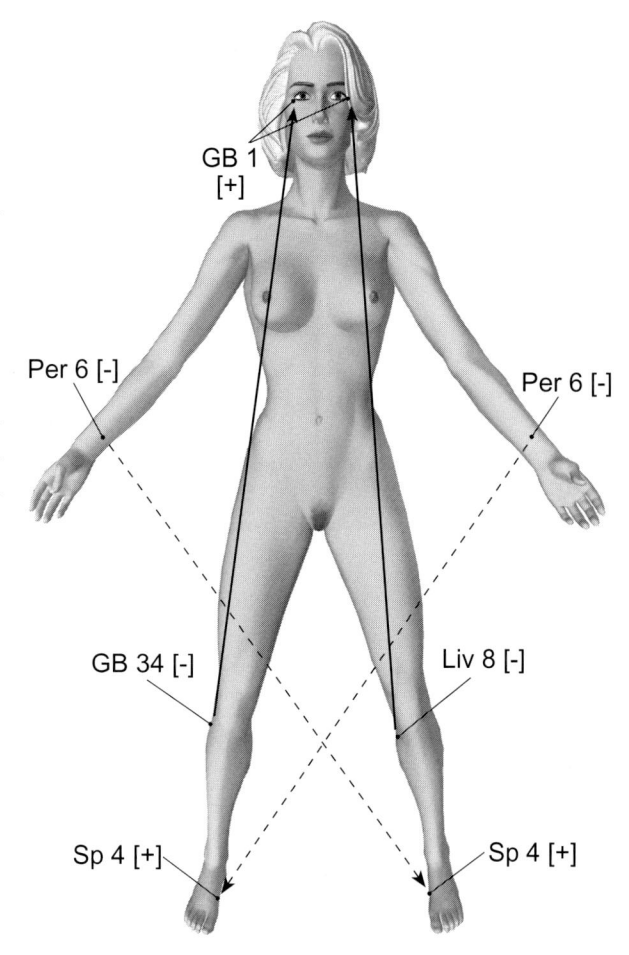

GB 1 [+]
Per 6 [-]
Per 6 [-]
GB 34 [-]
Liv 8 [-]
Sp 4 [+]
Sp 4 [+]

ENDNOTES

[1] See Appendix 5 for a discussion of the application of the Hibiki device.
[2] See Jiao and Yau

Appendix 2:
Extraordinary Vessel Pulses

The channels most commonly combined with channel divergences into an overall treatment strategy are the extraordinary vessels and Seki, Naomoto and Shima all combine these two facets of the channel system in their treatment style. As is evident from his case histories, it is most accurate to speak of Shima not as a channel divergence specialist but as a combined channel divergence and extraordinary vessel specialist since he rarely uses one without the other.

Historically, pulse diagnosis has held the position of the central diagnostic criteria in acupuncture practice. Nearly all styles of acupuncture practice employ some degree of pulse diagnosis and some rely almost exclusively on the pulse to guide diagnosis and treatment. It should come as no surprise then, that specific pulses have been associated with the extraordinary vessels going back at least as far as the first textbook on pulse diagnosis, *The Mai Jing (Pulse Classic)*, by Wang Shu-he written in 215 CE. Unfortunately, Wang's attributions of pulse images to the extraordinary vessels are often rather vague and tend to contradict one another. Li shi-zhen's *Qi Jing Ba Mai Kao (A Personal Critique of the Eight Vessels of the Extraordinary Channels)* written during the Ming dynasty in 1577, marks another milestone in the development of the pulse as a diagnostic criteria for the extraordinary vessels. However, while this text provides a more internally consistent description of the pulses pertaining to the extraordinary vessels, it is still rather difficult to make clinical use of. As is so often the case in the classical Chinese medical literature, we are left with intriguing information that we do not know how to use.

The well-known Ming dynasty physician, Li Zhong-zi, (1588-1655) was born 72 years after Li Shi-zhen. Li was a scholar of the classical medical literature and had a knack for communicating complex medical theories in simple terms. He was also a synthesist, drawing on the strengths of more orthodox theories to establish his own ideas, which lay equal emphasis on the spleen and kidney as the central vectors of pathodynamics. Li Zhong-zi made a number of contributions to medical literature including, *Nei Jing Zhi Yao (Essentials of the Inner Classic), Shi Cai San Shu (Shi Cai's Three Books), Lei Gong Pao Jiu Yao Xing Jie (Lei gong's Treatise on the Preparation of Materia Medica), Shan Han Kou Yao (The Gist of Cold Damage)* and the *Zheng Jia Zheng Yan (Correct Understanding for Diagnosticians)*. In this last work he left us with perhaps the most coherent presentation of extraordinary vessel pulse diagnosis extant in the literature and Li's discussion provides the basis for a modern extraordinary vessel pulse diagnosis developed by Katsuyasu Kido.

Li Zhong-zi's system of extraordinary vessel pulse diagnosis is similar enough to Li Shi-zhen's that he was in all probability significantly influenced by the *Qi Jing Ba Mai Kao*. While Li Zhong-zi's version of extraordinary vessel pulse diagnosis still requires a substantial amount of interpretation on the part of the modern reader, he makes a cogent presentation and his explanations give us a relatively clear sense of what he is trying to convey. Miki Shima has employed Li's pulse diagnosis for the past two decades and has found it to be an useful diagnostic tool, preferring it even to the various styles of abdominal diagnosis pertaining to the extraordinary vessels. What follows is a translation of Li Zhong-zi's description of the extraordinary vessel pulses accompanied by his explanations. This material is accompanied by a graphic representation of Li's extraordinary vessel pulse images by the modern extraordinary vessel specialist Katsuyasu Kido and finally by our own commentary.

Du Pulse

When the pulse image is one of beating straight up and down while still floating, this is the *du* [pulse].

Li's Explanation: When the pulse is strong and floating in the *cun*, *guan*, and *chi* positions, there is abnormality in the *du* vessel.

Du	Cun	Guan	Chi	
Superficial				Du Pulse
Middle				Normal Pulse
Deep				

Comment:
The *du* pulse is uniformly floating in all positions. It has strength and no pulse position is stronger than any other. From a *Shang Han* (Cold Damage) perspective, we might interpret this as a *tai yang* pulse.

Ren Pulse

When the pulse image is one of beating straight up and down while sinking, this is the *ren* [pulse].

Li's Explanation:
When the pulse is sunken and tense at the *cun*, *guan*, and *chi*, there is abnormality in the *ren* vessel.

Ren		*Cun*	*Guan*	*Chi*
	Superficial			
	Middle			
	Deep			

Comment:
The ren pulse is uniformly sinking in all positions and no more so in any one position than another. Li specifies that the *ren* pulse should also be tense, suggesting that this is not simply a deep and fine pulse. A tense pulse also has some width to it that a wiry pulse does not. Shima concurs that in his clinical experience the *ren* pulse must be uniformly deep and tense.

Chong Pulse

When the pulse image is one of beating straight up and down while confined, this is the *chong* [pulse].

Li's Explanation:
When the pulse is very hard at the *cun*, *guan* and *chi* positions, there is abnormality in the *chong* vessel.

Chong		*Cun*	*Guan*	*Chi*
	Superficial			
	Middle			
	Deep			

Comment:
The *chong* pulse is uniformly confined in all positions and no more so in any one position than another. A confined (*lao*) pulse is traditionally defined as forceful and sunken such that it feels "tied to the bone." More traditionally, such a pulse is typically associated with obstruction in general, particularly cold pain, and insufficiency of yang qi. Therefore, a *chong* pulse is not just a very deep pulse. It must also have some strength in all positions. Because of the depth implied by the term confined (*lao*), Kido interprets the *chong* pulse as being incrementally deeper than the *ren* pulse. It is Shima's opinion that in the context of the extraordinary vessels,

the forcefulness implied by a confined pulse is greater than the strength that must be present for a pulse to feel tense. Understood in this way, the *chong* pulse is not only deeper than the *ren* pulse, but it is also stronger.

DAI PULSE

When the pulse image is one of elastic hardness (*tan*) in the *guan* position on the right and left sides, this is the *dai* [pulse].

LI'S EXPLANATION:
When the *guan* pulse is felt as being especially strong on the right and left sides, there is abnormality in the *dai* vessel.

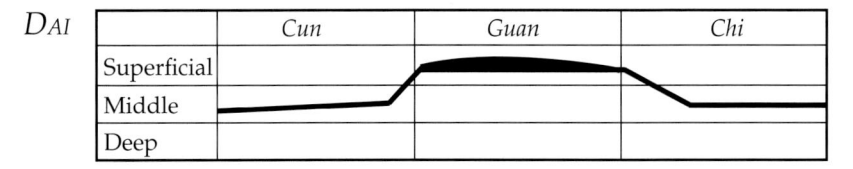

DAI	Cun	Guan	Chi
Superficial		▬▬▬	
Middle	▬▬		▬▬
Deep			

COMMENT:
The pulse of the *dai* or girdling vessel must be bilaterally strong, but only in the *guan* or middle positions. Since Li specifies that this pulse must be felt bilaterally, we may infer that a pulse that is strong in the *guan* position on one side and not the other is not a *dai* pulse. Shima, however, contends that this pulse may be felt unilaterally. Li's pulse description makes a certain amount of intuitive sense in that it is consistent with our understanding of the *dai* vessel as the only vessel with a horizontal trajectory which binds the other channels and vessels together like a belt. Given the anatomical location of this vessel, an imbalance in the *dai mai* would naturally be felt bilaterally, and in the middle position.

The use of the character *tan*, translated here as elastic hardness, is an interesting one. It means to play on a stringed instrument, and by extension, to rebound, or to press down. Read as *dan*, this character means a bullet pellet or pill. The *dai*, *yin qiao* and *yang qiao* pulses are all described as being *tan*. *Tan* not only conveys a sense of strength, but also a feeling of hardness, although this hardness may have some elastic or rebounding quality. However, it is not at all clear that *tan* is being used here in a technical sense with a highly specific meaning. Li simply interprets this pulse to mean strong.

The word *tan* is used in another pulse image, the flicking stone pulse (*tan shi mai*), which is one of the seven strange pulses (*qi guai mai*) signifying critical conditions. It is described as being sunken, replete, and feeling like flicking a stone with a finger.[2] It is not the stone that is rebounding but the finger that is rebounding off of the stone. Here again, we are presented with an image of hardness, however, this is a completely different pulse from the pulse of the *dai mai*, which is not sinking and is felt only in the *guan* position. In fact, Kido's graphic representation depicts a pulse that is felt strongly but only superficially.

YANG QIAO PULSE

When the pulse image is one of strength in the *cun* position on the right and left sides, this is the *yang qiao* [pulse].

LI'S EXPLANATION:
When the *cun* pulse is felt especially strong on the right and left sides, there is abnormality in the *yang qiao* vessel.

YANG QIAO	Cun	Guan	Chi
Superficial	■───		
Middle		───	───
Deep			

COMMENT:
Like the pulse of the *dai* vessel, the pulse of the *yang qiao* vessel must be felt bilaterally and it is also *tan*, with an elastic hardness that is felt particularly in the *cun* position closest to the wrist. Kido's graphic interpretation depicts a pulse in the *cun* position that is not only stronger than the pulses in the *guan* and *chi* positions but is also distinctly more superficial. It would seem that Kido interprets this notion of *tan* as conveying superficiality in addition to strength.

YIN QIAO PULSE

When the pulse image is one of strength in the *chi* position on the right and left sides, this is the *yin qiao* [pulse].

LI'S EXPLANATION:
When the *chi* pulse is felt especially strong on the right and left sides, there is abnormality in the *yin qiao/ren* vessel.

YIN QIAO	Cun	Guan	Chi
Superficial			───
Middle	───	───	
Deep			

COMMENT:
The *yin qiao* pulse is essentially a mirror image of the *yang qiao* pulse. Although, it too, must be palpated bilaterally, and has an elastic hardness. This pulse is felt in the *chi* position. This hardness may occasionally extend into the *guan* position. The

3ʳᴅ difficult issue in the *Nan Jing (Classic of Difficult Issues)* refers to this as *da guo*, or great excess. Nevertheless, the hard quality of this pulse will not extend into the *cun* position.

YANG WEI PULSE

When the pulse image is felt more medially in the *chi* position than in the *cun* position, this is the *yang wei* [pulse].

LI'S EXPLANATION:
When the *chi* pulse is felt more medially and the *cun* pulse is felt more laterally, deviating from the central line of the pulse, there is abnormality in the *yang wei* vessel.

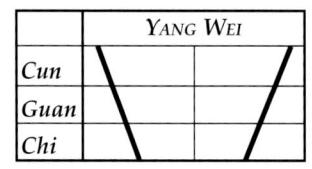

	YANG WEI	
Cun		
Guan		
Chi		

YIN WEI PULSE

When the pulse image is felt more laterally in the *chi* position than in the *cun* position, this is the *yin wei* [pulse].

LI'S EXPLANATION:
When the *chi* pulse is felt more laterally and the *cun* pulse is felt more medially, deviating from the central line of the pulse, there is abnormality in the *yin wei* vessel.

	YIN WEI	
Cun		
Guan		
Chi		

COMMENT:
The pulses of the *yang wei* and *yin wei* vessels are perhaps the most interesting extraordinary vessel pulses because they are palpated in three dimensions. They are determined not only by their length and depth along the three pulse positions, but also by their medial or lateral orientation on the wrist. They are part of the system of pulse diagnosis referred to as the *Nine Pulse Pathways of the wrist pulse (Qi Kou Jiu Dao Mai)*. A version of this diagnostic style first appears in Chapter 26 of the *Elementary Questions*, The Discourse on the Eight Facets of the Spirit Radiance, where it is part of the *san cai*, the pulses of heaven, humanity and earth referring to the facial, radial, and foot pulses.

This method divides three *cun*, *guan* and *chi* pulse positions laterally into medial, central and lateral aspects. This yields a total of nine pulse positions without taking pulse depth into account at all. For instance, a pulse felt in the lateral aspect of the *cun* position is interpreted differently than a pulse that is felt in the medial aspect of the *cun* position. It is essentially a different pulse. This system is to some degree, a refinement of more orthodox methods of pulse diagnosis. In the Nine Pulse Pathways system we would generally interpret most pulses as occurring in the central aspect of the *cun*, *guan*, and *chi* positions, regardless of the depth or quality of the pulse.

The *yang wei* and *yin wei* pulses are often ignored unless one knows to look for them, although one may occasionally feel a pulse that feels particularly lateral or medial in a particular position. Once one has a conceptual framework to make use of these pulse images, however, they are easily identified and remembered. Li defines them exclusively in terms of the relative laterality of the cun and chi positions. We must assume that the pulse beats "straight up and down" in all three positions. The *yang wei* is more lateral in the *cun* position just as the *yang qiao* is felt more strongly in the *yang* position.

ENDNOTES

[2] Wiseman and Feng: 527

Appendix 3:
Auxiliary Diagnostic Methods

Since any diagnostic method that yields a viscera-bowel correspondence may potentially be used as a criterion for constructing a channel divergences treatment, it is not surprising that a wide range of such approaches have been explored. Omura's bi-digital O-ring test will be discussed separately in Appendix 10. The following is an overview of a few of the other most important auxiliary methods of diagnosis employed by the channel divergences specialists discussed in the present work.

Man's Prognosis/Wrist Pulse Method (*Ren Ying/Cun Kou Fa*)

This method of pulse diagnosis is based on Chapter 48, "On Prohibitions for Study" of the *Divine Pivot*. This method is still commonly used in Japan. It involves a comparison of the Man's Prognosis (*ren ying*) pulse at the carotid artery on the throat with the Wrist Pulse (*cun kou*) of the radial artery at the styloid process on the ventral surface of the wrist.

In its most basic application, Man's Prognosis/Wrist Pulse diagnosis provides the evaluator with information about the severity and nature of the disease as opposed to guiding one to a specific disease diagnosis. The practitioner first palpates the carotid artery bilaterally and determines the strongest side. Next, the radial pulse at the wrist is palpated and the strongest side is determined. The radial and carotid pulses are then compared. If the two pulses are strongest on the same side, then the patient's condition is considered a straightforward one. If the two pulses are stronger on opposing sides, the prognosis is more guarded. In addition, the relative strengths between the radial and carotid are compared. This provides information on the overall depth of the disease and which of the three yang or three yin channels to treat.[3]

In Naomoto's use of this system, a Man's Prognosis pulse that is smaller than the Wrist Pulse indicates to use the fourth through the sixth confluences, while an Inch Mouth pulse that is smaller than the Man's Prognosis pulse indicates the use of the first through the third confluences.

TONAL DIAGNOSIS

Tonal diagnosis is among the most arcane of the diagnostic methods developed by the members of the Topological Acupuncture Society. Each of the tones of the Chinese pentatonic scale is assigned a five phase designation which also determines its resonance with a given viscus or bowel. The tone *Gong* at 440.0Hz/second (A) is an earth tone and, therefore, resonates with the spleen. *Wei*, at 392.0Hz/second (G), is a fire tone that resonates with the heart. The tone *Jie*, at 329.6Hz/second (E), is a wood tone and, therefore, resonates with the liver. *Shang*, at 293.6Hz/second (D), is a metal tone and, therefore, resonates with the lungs. *Gong*, at 261.6Hz/second (C), is a water tone that resonates with the kidneys.[4]

These sounds were originally made on bamboo pipes. However, the mode of production is largely irrelevant as evidenced by the fact that Naomoto often used a tuning fork and ultimately the human voice. Naomoto originally stimulated the patient's body directly with a tuning fork. With the tuning fork resonating at a given sound, he then muscle-tested the patient, looking for the weakest response to the five tones which, in turn, indicated the most imbalanced viscus. He later moved to simply having the patient vocalize each of the sounds and circle the character denoting each sound while he muscle-tested them.

Naomoto's tonal determination of the weakest or most imbalanced yin viscus weighed heavily in his overall diagnosis of which channel divergences confluence pair to treat. Because his channel divergences treatments are based on the channel relationships of the Chinese clock, he described the tonal correspondences as follows:

Tone	Phase	Pitch	Viscus	Antipode
Gong	Water	A	Kidneys	Large Intestine
Wei	Fire	G	Heart	Gallbladder
Jie	Wood	E	Liver	Small Intestine
Shang	Metal	D	Lungs	Urinary Bladder
Gong	Earth	C	Spleen	Triple Burner

HIRATA ZONES

One of the auxiliary methods of diagnosing the channel divergences favored by Irie early in his investigations was the Hirata Zones. These were first described in the 1930s by Kurakichi Hirata. He went to Kyoto City Medical College in 1920, but later on gave up on Western medicine and developed his own style of acupuncture. In 1982 Yoshio Manaka published a book profiling Hirata's work titled *Hirata Shiki Nesshin Shigeki Ryoho (Hirata's Heated Needle Stimulation Treatment)*. Although there are Hirata Zone correspondences throughout the entire body and they are typically evaluated by means of visual examination, Irie limited his use of this system to palpation for pressure pain on the zones on the medial aspect of the lower extremity. His findings based on the Hirata Zones on the legs were then cross-referenced with other diagnostic methods.

Each of the zones numbered below corresponds to the following areas:

1. Bronchials
2. Lungs
3. Heart
4. Liver
5. Gallbladder
6. Spleen (Pancreas)
7. Stomach
8. Kidney
9. Large Intestine
10. Small Intestine
11. Bladder
12. Reproductive Organs

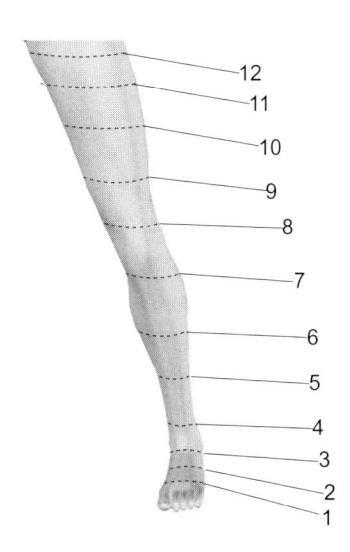

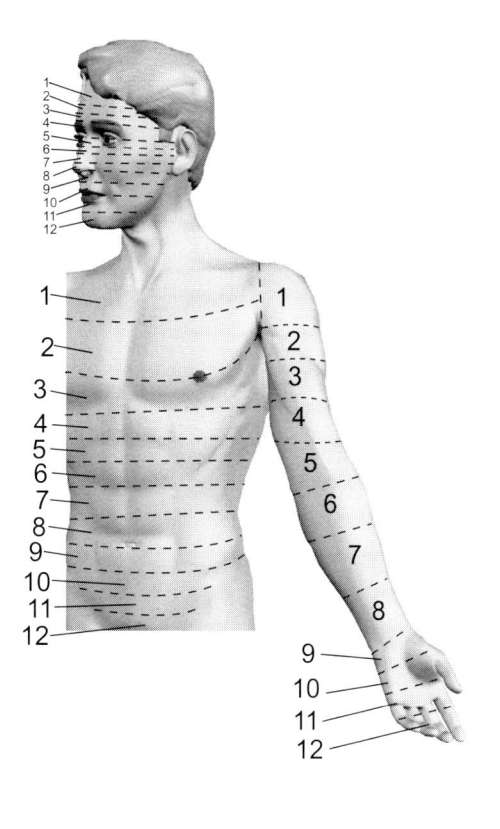

Mubun Oda's Facial Diagnosis

Another of the auxiliary methods of diagnosing the channel divergences favored by Irie was Mubun Oda's Facial Diagnosis. This method was first described in 1685 by Mubun Oda in his *Shindo Hiketsu Shu (A Collection of Secret Skills in the Art of Acupuncture)*.[5] Once again, Irie used this methodology in a very limited manner, palpating the reflex areas on the face for pressure pain as a means of confirming which channel divergence to use. His findings based on this method of facial diagnosis were then cross-referenced with other diagnostic methods.

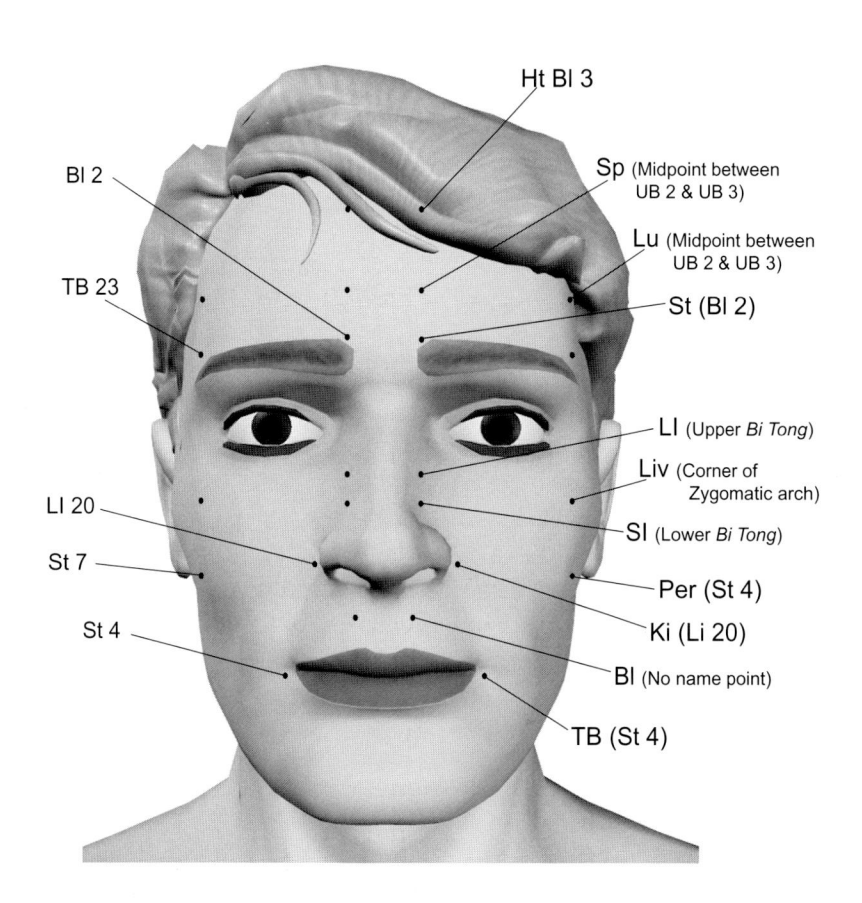

APPENDIX 4:
AUXILIARY TREATMENT METHODS

NORMAL [CHANNEL] ION PUMPING (NIP) PROTOCOLS

Seki's NIP protocols were used by many members of the Japanese Topological Acupuncture Society, including Yoshio Manaka himself. These are normal or primary channel IP protocols as opposed to extraordinary vessel IP protocols. Manaka's well-known *Tai Yi* treatment is essentially NIP Protocol #1. As is evident from his case histories, Seki limited his use of the NIP methodology primarily to the first and second protocols. In general, he used NIP Protocol #1 for vacuity pain and NIP Protocol #2 for replete pain. It is unclear just how Seki arrived at this clinical distinction. However, he appears to have been fairly consistent in his application of it. All of the NIP protocols are applied bilaterally. The *Mu Mei Ketsu* or No Name hole in Seki's NIP treatment is located five *cun* proximal to the wrist crease on the hand *shao yin* heart channel.

1	No Name	[+] ←	Sp 6	[-]	Produces General Supplementation
	TB 8	[-] →	GB 35	[+]	

2	No Name	[-] →	Sp 6	[+]	Produces General Drainage
	TB 8	[+] ←	GB 35	[-]	

232   The Channel Divergences

3	No Name	[+] →	TB 8	[-]	Rarely Used
	No Name	[+] →	TB 8	[-]	

4	No Name	[-] →	TB 8	[+]	Rarely Used
	No Name	[-] →	TB 8	[+]	

5	Sp 6	[-] →	GB 39	[+]	Rarely Used
	Sp 6	[-] →	GB 39	[+]	

6	Sp 6	← [+]	GB 39	[-]	Rarely Used
	Sp 6	← [+]	GB 39	[-]	

7	No Name	[-] ↘	Sp 6	[+]	Rarely Used
	TB 8	[-] ↗	GB 35	[+]	

8	No Name	[+] ↘	Sp 6	[-]	Rarely Used
	TB 8	[+] ↗	GB 35	[-]	

9	No Name	[+] ↘	Sp 6	[+]	Rarely Used
	TB 8	[-] ↗	GB 35	[-]	

10	No Name	[-] ↘	Sp 6	[-]	Rarely Used
	TB 8	[+] ↗	GB 35	[+]	

11	No Name	[-] →	Sp 6	[+]	Drains the Yin Supplements the Yang
	TB 8	[-] →	GB 35	[+]	

12	No Name	[-] ←	Sp 6	[+]	Drains the Yang Supplements the Yin
	TB 8	[-] ←	GB 35	[+]	

LEFT-RIGHT IP #1

L	TB 8	[-]		R	GB 35	[+]
	No Name	[+]			Sp 6	[-]

L	TB 8	[-]		R	GB 35	[+]
	No Name	[+]			Sp 6	[-]

YOSHIAKI OMURA'S THYMUS-REGULATING HOLES

Omura's thymus-regulating holes are *Xuan Ji* (CV 21) and any tender points inferior and bilateral. Independent of Omura's bi-digital O-ring testing, Miki Shima needles them on patients suffering from immunodeficiency diseases, such as cancer. They are contraindicated in cases of hyperactive immune responses, such as allergies and autoimmune disorders.

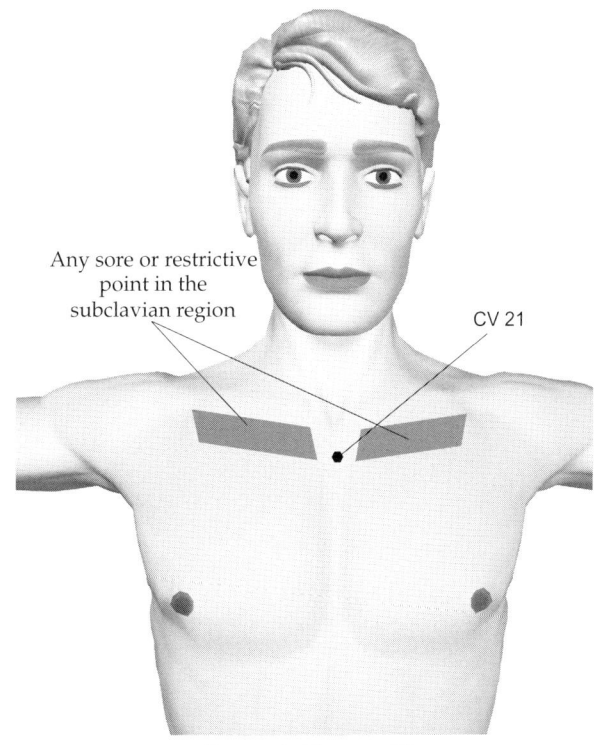

Any sore or restrictive point in the subclavian region

CV 21

OMURA'S THYMUS HOLES

Endnotes

[3] The *Jin Gei Myaku I Kai* (Renying Cunkou Pulse Medical Society) was founded by Domei Ogura. Members of this society strictly practice acupuncture based on the pulse diagnosis presented in the *Divine Pivot*.

[4] Jeans: p. 22

[5] This man's correct name was Mubusai Oda, however he was generally called Mubun Oda.

Appendix 5:
Ear Acupuncture Strategies:
The Hibiki Method

The channel divergences are a primary means by which Chinese medical theory explains how auriculotherapy influences the body as a whole. The channel divergence system ensures that every element of the channel and network vessel system has some means of communication with the head and, by extension, the ear regardless of whether the channel is yin or yang or is located on the hands or feet. It is not surprising then that the integration of auriculotherapy with a channel divergence strategy can yield a potent combination and this relationship has been exploited by a number of channel divergence specialists. Miki Shima has found the Hibiki method to be a particularly effective modality when used in conjunction with a channel divergence strategy.

The Hibiki-7 Point Location Device was first conceived by Yoshio Manaka and built by Shigeji Naomoto at the Asahi Research Institute in Kyoto, Japan. This device was originally designed as a dual point-location and treatment device. As with most location devices, the Hibiki-7 measures electrical impedance on the skin. The patient holds a grounding probe in his or her hand while the practitioner uses the locator probe connected to the other end of the circuit to locate and treat points on the ear. Shima considers this to be one of the better location methods currently available, and he uses it extensively for this function.[6]

It was Naomoto who developed the technique of using the Hibiki-7 device to treat pain. Rather than having the patient hold the ground in their hand, he attached that lead directly to a local point in a painful area. He would then locate and timulate the related points on the ear with the locator probe attached to the positive lead. Each of the ear points is stimulated with the locator probe for a period of 20-30 seconds. During this process, the patient experiences the electrical stimuli primarily in the ear and only secondarily at the point on the affected area. This technique has proved very effective in producing rapid pain relief, and Shima has used it extensively as an adjunctive treatment to an overall channel divergence strategy.[7]

At the time of this writing, the Hibiki-7 device has limited availability in the United States. However, a number of comparable machines are available through Oriental Medical Supply. Foremost among these are the ITO-4107, the Pointer F-2, and the AWQ-104. Miki Shima has applied the Hibiki technique to good effect using all of these machines and they are easily substituted for the Hibiki device. A further discussion of the specifications for each of these machines appears in Appendix 9.

Naomoto's Hibiki-7 Auriculotherapy Method[8]

In addition to applying the Hibiki-7 device to the treatment of pain, Naomoto also developed a method for integrating the extraordinary vessels into this technique. A relevant extraordinary vessel connection is first activated using a typical ion pumping cord arrangement. The negative lead of the Hibiki-7 device is connected to the master hole of a related extraordinary vessel.

Finally, the positive lead of the Hibiki-7 device is used to stimulate the associated posterior auricular master hole for the area one desires to treat. Naomoto's use of the posterior auricle is interesting in light of the phased system of auriculotherapy developed in the West. The points he designates on the posterior auricle are Noigier's phase IV points, which are typically indicated for chronic problems, particularly those characterized by stiffness.

Example of Naomoto's Hibiki Methodology

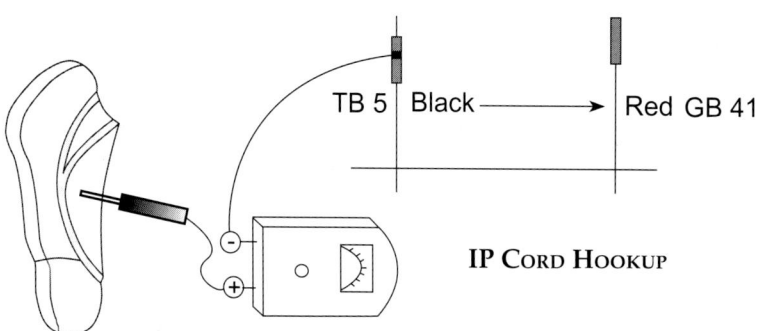

TB 5 | Black ⟶ | Red GB 41

IP Cord Hookup

Associated Ear Point

1. Waist and lower extremity
2. Shoulder and upper extremity
3. Shoulder motor points
4. Neck and face
5. Occiput and head

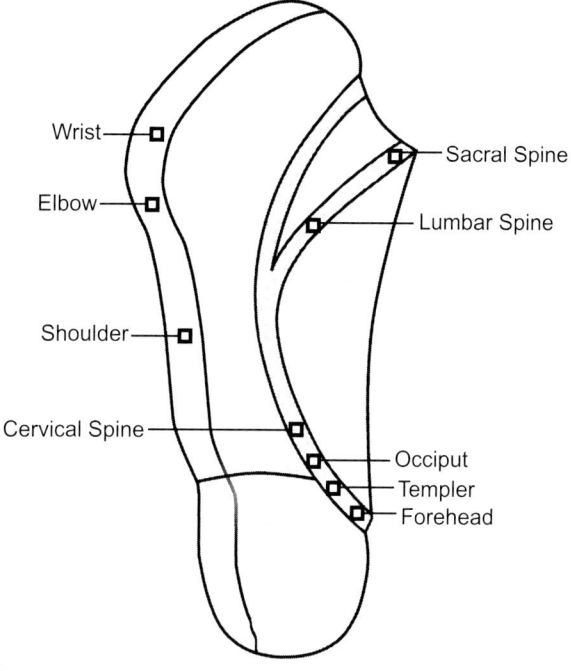

SHIMA'S CHANNEL DIVERGENCES ADAPTATION OF NAOMOTO'S HIBIKI METHOD

Miki Shima has adapted Naomoto's Hibiki technique to the channel divergences in a manner similar to the connections used for the extraordinary vessels. When used with the channel divergences, the negative lead of the Hibiki-7 device is attached to the access hole of the relevant channel divergence pairing. The positive lead is used to stimulate relevant points on the ear. Rather than limiting himself to Naomoto's associated ear points, Shima avails himself of the full range of options afforded by French and Chinese systems of auriculotherapy. This technique is particularly indicated for pain of visceral or bowel origin, such as pain due to malignancies.

EXAMPLE 1

Relevant Ear Hole   Channel Divergence IP Connection [Second Confluence]

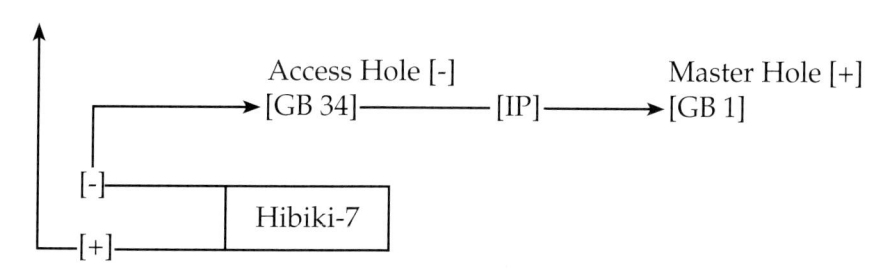

                    Access Hole [-]   Master Hole [+]
                    → [GB 34] ———— [IP] ———— → [GB 1]

           [-]
           [+]   Hibiki-7

Example 2

Associated Ear Hole   Channel Divergence IP Connection [Fifth Confluence]

```
                    Access Hole [-]                  Master Hole [+]
         ┌─────────→ [GB 12]─────────── [IP] ──────→ [Per 3]
         │
         │  [-]┐
         │     │   Hibiki-7
         └─[+]─┘
```

STEP 1. The associated auricular hole is generally a local viscera or bowel point, such as the liver point for pain due to a liver cancer. Other functional points may be stimulated as a given situation dictates.

STEP 2. Each auricular hole is stimulated for 10-30 seconds each.

STEP 3. Channel divergences connections are established using ion pumping cords or electrical stimulation at 1Hz and 10-40 microamps and 9 volts at a constant current for 10 minutes.

STEP 4. The above treatment strategy is easily integrated with auriculotherapy protocols that address laterality disturbances.

Endnotes

[6] As with any electro-acupuncture measurement device, there is some question as to exactly what is being measured. Acupuncture measuring devices often measure changes in impedance that they create themselves in the process of measurement. Birch and Felt, 1999; 170-171, have reviewed many of the difficulties inherent in the electrical measurement of acupuncture holes. Shima has nevertheless found the Hibiki machine to be a useful clinical tool in spite of the fact that he is aware of these technical issues.

[7] Naomoto, 1985: 21-25

[8] Naomoto, 1985-A: 21-25

Appendix 6:
Tadashi Irie's Confluence-based Herbal Formulas

Tadashi Irie's approach to the channel divergences is perhaps best characterized by his thoroughness and he went to great lengths to identify channel divergence imbalances at many different levels. In addition, he was unique among the channel divergence investigators of the Topological Acupuncture Society in that he incorporated herbal medicine into his treatment plans. In fact, he was trained as an herbalist prior to being trained as an acupuncturist. Irie's correlation of Chinese herbal formulas to the various confluences of the channel divergences reflects a rather iconoclastic approach to Chinese herbal medicine.

Because Chinese herbal medicine has tended to focus most heavily on the yin viscera, one might simply assume that any herbal formula that influences a given viscus must then influence the associated confluence. For instance, *Liu Wei Di Huang Wan* (Six Flavor Rehmannia Pills) is a classic prescription for kidney vacuity. Therefore, it is reasonable to surmise that it influences the first confluence of the urinary bladder and kidneys. Approached in this manner, the attribution of herbal formulas to the confluence pairs of the channel divergences is pretty straightforward but not very enlightening. However, Irie brought his own methodology for diagnosing the channel divergences to bear on this question and arrived at some channel divergences correlations that often differ radically from what one might expect. According to Irie's system, for instance, *Liu Wei Di Huang Wan* is a third confluence formula.

It is clear that Irie's herbal assignments are the product of his elaborate methods of empirical testing and, as such, he made no effort to reconcile them with any theoretical understanding of Chinese herbal medicine. While it may be tempting to just shrug our shoulders at many of the connections he makes between herbal prescriptions and the channel divergences, they, nevertheless, bear some reflection. One way to make greater sense of Irie's correlations is to view the prescriptions in terms of their influence on the yang channel of each confluence pair. It is useful to remember that many channel divergences investigators consider the yang channel of a confluence pair to be the dominant channel. Viewed in this way, Irie's herbal assignments for each of the confluence pairs makes a great deal more sense. For instance, *Ge Gen Tang* (Pueraria Decoction), *Gui Zhi Tang Jia Bai Zhu* (Cinnamon Twig Decoction Plus Atractylodes), and *Yue Bi Jia Zhu Tang* (Maidservant from Yue Decoction Plus Atractylodes) are easily understood as primarily influencing the *tai yang* aspect and, therefore, correspond to the first confluence. *Zhu Ling Tang* (Polyporus Decoction) and *Wu Ling San* (Five [Ingredients] Poria Powder) correspond to the first confluence by virtue of their influence on the urinary bladder. *Da Huang Gan Cao Wan* (Rhubarb & Licorice Decoction), *Ma Zi Ren Wan* (Cannabis Seed Pills), and *Da Huang Mu Dan Tang* (Rhubarb & Moutan Decoction) also make sense as fourth confluence formulas if we consider their influence on the small intestine.

This is not to say that the yin viscus is ignored entirely. *Zhen Wu Tang* (Genuine Warrior Decoction) and *Shi Quan Da Bu Tang* (Ten [Ingredients] Completely & Greatly Supplementing Decoction) are easily understood as first confluence formulas by virtue of their influence on the original qi in general and the kidneys in particular. Similarly, *Jia Wei Xiao Yao San* (Added Flavors Rambling Powder) is an obvious choice for a second confluence prescription given its resonance with the liver, and *Si Wu Tang* (Four Materials Decoction) reflects the role of the liver in blood storage.

All of this is, of course, purely conjecture occurring after the fact. Irie simply applied his magnetic and bi-digital O-ring or friction testing methodology for the channel divergences to Chinese herbal formulas and let the chips fall where they may. Many of Irie's formula correlations are difficult to rationalize even when employing the most athletic of theoretical gymnastics. Be that as it may, if we are willing to accept the proposition that Irie's methodology actually reflects resonances on the level of the channel divergences, then we are faced with the possibility that we may need to revisit some of our assumptions concerning the scope of influence of these formulas.

The First Confluence:
Urinary Bladder & Kidney Channel Divergences

Ge Gen Tang (Pueraria Decoction)
Ge Gen Jia Bai Zhu Tang (Pueraria Plus Atractylodes Decoction)
Ge Gen Jia Bai Zhu Fu Tang (Pueraria Plus Atractylodes & Aconite Decoction)
Gui Zhi Jia Bai Zhu Tang (Cinnamon Twig Plus Atractylodes Decoction)
Gui Zhi Jia Long Gu Mu Li Tang (Cinnamon Twig Plus Dragon Bone & Oyster Shell Decoction)
Gui Zhi Jia Shao Yao Tang (Cinnamon Twig Plus Peony Decoction)
Gui Zhi Jia Gui Tang (Cinnamon Twig Plus Cinnamon Decoction)
Gui Zhi Qu Zhi Jia Fu Ling Bai Zhu Tang (Cinnamon Twig Minus Cinnamon Plus Poria & Atractylodes Salvaging Decoction)
Dang Qi Jian Zhong Tang (Dang Gui & Astragalus Fortify the Center Decoction)
Yue Bi Jia Zhu Tang (Maidservant from Yue Plus Atractylodes Decoction)
Yue Bi Jia Zhu Fu Tang (Maidservant from Yue Plus Atractylodes & Aconite Decoction)
Fang Ji Huang Qi Tang (Stephania & Astragalus Decoction)
Ling Gui Zhu Gan Tang (Poria, Cinnamon, Atractylodes & Licorice Decoction)
Ling Gan Jiang Wei Xi Ban Ren Tang (Poria, Licorice, Ginger, Schizandra & Asarum Decoction)
Zhen Wu Tang (Genuine Warrior Decoction)
Si Ni Tang (Four Counterflows Decoction)
Ba Wei Wan (Eight Flavors Pills)
Shao Yao Gan Cao Tang (Peony & Licorice Decoction)
Zhu Ling Tang (Polyporus Decoction)
Wu Lin San (Five [Ingredients] Poria Powder)
Qing Xin Lian Zi Yin (Clearing the Heart Lotus Seed Beverage)
Shi Quan Da Bu Tang (Ten [Ingredients] Completely & Greatly Supplementing Decoction)
Sheng Ma Ge Gen Tang (Cimicifuga & Pueraria Decoction)
Chai Ge Jie Ji Tang (Bupleurum & Pueraria Resolve the Muscles Decoction)
Chai Hu Gui Zhi Gan Jiang Tang (Bupleurum, Cinnamon Twig & Dry Ginger Decoction)
Huang Tu Tang (Yellow Earth Decoction)
Xiong Gui Tiao Xue Yin (Ligusticum & Dang Gui Blood-regulating Beverage)

The Second Confluence:
Gallbladder & Liver Channel Divergences

Da Chai Hu Tang (Major Bupleurum Decoction)
Xiao Chai Hu Tang (Minor Bupleurum Decoction)
Chai Hu Jia Long Gu Mu Li Tang (Bupleurum Plus Dragon Bone & Oyster Shell Decoction)

Chai Hu Gui Zhi Tang (Bupleurum & Cinnamon Twig Decoction)
Ban Xia Xie Xin Tang (Pinellia Drain the Heart Decoction)
Yin Chen Hao Tang (Artemesia Capillaris Decoction)
Chai Hu Qing Gan San (Bupleurum Clear the Liver Powder)
Jia Wei Xiao Yao San (Added Flavors Rambling Powder)
Chai Hu Shu Gan Tang (Bupleurum Course the Liver Decoction)
Long Dan Xie Gan Tang (Gentiana Drain the Liver Decoction)
Yi Gan San Jia Chen Pi Ban Xia (Restrain the Liver Powder Plus Orange Peel & Pinellia)
Si Wu Tang (Four Materials Decoction)
Tong Dao San (Freeing & Abducting Powder)
Dang Gui Shao Yao San (Dang Gui & Peony Powder)
Gui Zhi Fu Ling Wan Jia Huang Qin Hong Hua (Cinnamon Twig and Poria Pills Plus Scutellaria & Carthamus)
Jing Jie Lian Qiao Tang (Schizonepeta & Forsythia Decoction)
Xiong Gui E Jiao Tang (Ligusticum, Dang Gui & Donkey Skin Glue Decoction)
Dang Gui Jian Zhong Tang (Dang Gui Fortify the Center Decoction)
Chai Xian Tang (Bupleurum Downward Fall Decoction)
Qing Yan Li Ge Tang (Throat-clearing Diaphragm-disinhibiting Decoction)
Chai Shao Liu Jun Zi Tang (Bupleurum & Peony Six Gentlemen Decoction)
Xiang Xiong Tang (Cyperus & Ligusticum Decoction)
Fang Feng Tong San (Ledebouriella Sagely Freeing Powder)
Qing Shu Yi Qi Tang (Clear Summerheat & Boost the Qi Decoction)

The Third Confluence:
Stomach & Spleen Channel Divergences

Gui Zhi Ge Gen Tang (Cinnamon Twig & Pueraria Decoction)
Ge Gen Tang Jia Xing Ren (Pueraria Decoction Plus Armeniaca)
Ge Gen Tang Jia Shi Gao (Pueraria Decoction Plus Gypsum)
Ma Huang Tang (Ephedra Decoction)
Ma Xing Yi Gan Tang (Ephedra, Armeniaca, Coix & Licorice Decoction)
Ma Xing Gan Shi Tang (Ephedra, Armeniaca, Licorice & Gypsum Decoction)
Gan Cao Xie Xin Tang (Licorice Drain the Heart Decoction)
Ren Shen Tang (Ginseng Decoction)
Fu Ling Tang (Poria Decoction)
Gui Zhi Ren Shen Tang (Cinnamon Twig & Ginseng Decoction)
Huang Qin Tang (Scutellaria Decoction)
Tiao Wei Cheng Qi Tang (Regulate the Stomach & Order the Qi Decoction)
San Huang Xie Xin Tang (Three Yellows Drain the Heart Decoction)
Bai Hu Jia Ren Shen Tang (White Tiger Plus Ginseng Decoction)
Xiao Jian Zhong Tang (Minor Fortify the Center Decoction)
Wen Jing Tang (Warm the Menses Decoction)
Dang Gui Si Ni Jia Wu Zhu Yi Sheng Jiang Tang (Dang Gui Four Counterflows Plus

Evodia & Uncooked Ginger Decoction)
Gui Zhi Fu Ling Wan Jia Hong Hua (Cinnamon Twig & Poria Pills Plus Carthamus)
Wu Ling San (Five [Ingredients] Poria Powder)
Ping Wei San (Calm the Stomach Powder)
Er Chen Tang (Two Aged [Ingredients] Decoction)
An Zhong San (Quiet the Middle Powder)
Zhi Bai Ba Wei Wan (Anemarrhena & Phellodendron Eight Flavors Pills)
Liu Wei Wan (Six Flavors Pills)
Dang Gui Yin Zi (Dang Gui Beverage)
Mai Men Dong Yin Zi (Ophiopogon Beverage)
Jiu Wei Bing Lang Tang (Nine Flavors Areca Decoction)
Huo Xiang Zheng Qi San (Agastaches Correct the Qi Powder)
Qing Shu Yi Qi Tang (Clear Summerheat & Boost the Qi Decoction)
Shi Wei Bai Du Tang (Ten Flavors Overcome Toxins Decoction)
Qing Shang Fang Feng Tang (Clear the Upper [Body] Ledebouriella Decoction)
Bai Zhi Sheng Ma Tang (Angelica, Dahurica & Cimicifuga Decoction)
Shu Jing Huo Xue Tang (Soothe the Channels & Quicken the Blood Decoction)
Yi Yi Ren Tang (Coix Decoction)
Wen Qing Yin (Warming & Clearing Decoction)
Zhu Ye Shi Gao Tang (Bamboo Leaf & Gypsum Decoction)
Gui Zhi Shao Yao Zhi Mu Tang (Cinnamon Twig, Peony & Anemarrhena Decoction)
Nei Tuo San (Internal Out-thrusting Powder)

THE FOURTH CONFLUENCE:
SMALL INTESTINE & HEART CHANNEL DIVERGENCES

Ban Xia Hou Po Tang (Pinellia & Magnolia Decoction)
Mai Men Dong Tang (Ophiopogon Decoction)
Da Huang Gan Cao Wan (Rhubarb & Licorice Decoction)
Ma Zi Ren Wan (Cannabis Seed Pills)
Xiang Su San (Cyperus & Perilla Powder)
Yin Qiao San (Lonicera & Forsythia Powder)
Gui Pi Tang (Restore the Spleen Decoction)
Su Zi Jiang Qi Tang (Perilla Fruit Downbear the Qi Decoction)
Sheng Mai San (Engender the Pulse Powder)
Chuan Xiong Cha Tiao San (Ligusticum & Tea Mixed Powder)
Gui Zhi Gan Cao Long Gu Mu Li Tang (Cinnamon Twig, Licorice, Dragon Bone & Oyster Shell Decoction)
Da Huang Mu Dan Tang (Rhubarb & Moutan Decoction)

THE FIFTH CONFLUENCE:
TRIPLE BURNER & PERICARDIUM CHANNEL DIVERGENCES

Gui Zhi Tang (Cinnamon Twig Decoction)
Xiao Qing Long Tang (Minor Blue-green Dragon Decoction)
Gui Zhi Er Yue Bi Tang (Cinnamon Twig Two Part [to One Part] Maidservant from Yue Decoction)
Tao He Cheng Qi Tang (Persica Order the Qi Decoction)
San Wu Huang Qin Tang (Three Materials Scutellaria Decoction)
Huang Lian Tang (Coptis Decoction)
Da Cheng Qi Tang (Major Order the Qi Decoction)
Bu Zhong Yi Qi Tang (Supplement the Middle & Boost the Qi Decoction)
Liu Jun Zi Tang (Six Gentlemen Decoction)
Si Jun Si Tang (Four Gentlemen Decoction)
Gou Teng San (Uncaria Powder)
Ban Xia Bai Zhu Tian Ma Tang (Pinellia, Atractylodes & Gastrodia Decoction)
Xiao Feng San (Disperse Wind Powder)
Jing Fang Bai Du San (Schizonepeta & Ledebouriella Overcome Toxins Powder)
Huang Lian Jie Du San (Coptis Resolve Toxins Powder)
Gan Mai Da Zao Tang (Licorice, Ophiopogon & Red Date Decoction)

THE SIXTH CONFLUENCE:
LARGE INTESTINE & LUNGS CHANNEL DIVERGENCES

Gan Cao Gan Jiang Tang (Licorice & Dry Ginger Decoction)
Zhi Gan Cao Tang (Mix-fried Licorice Decoction)
Ma Huang Fu Zi Gan Cao Tang (Ephedra, Aconite & Licorice Decoction)
Gui Zhi Fu Ling Wan (Cinnamon Twig & Poria Decoction)
Ge Gen Jia Ban Xia Tang (Pueraria Plus Pinellia Decoction)
Dang Gui Si Ni Tang (Dang Gui Four Counterflows Decoction)
Xie Bai San (Drain the White Powder)
Wu Ji San (Five Accumulations Powder)
Qian Jin Dang Gui Tang (Thousand [Pieces of] Gold Dang Gui Decoction)
Xing Su San (Armeniaca & Perilla Powder)
Fen Xin Qi Yin (Separate the Heart Qi Drink)

APPENDIX 7:
CHANNEL DIVERGENCE HOLE PAIRINGS

As we have seen, there is a great deal of variety in how various clinicians go about accessing the channel divergences. The following table summarizes the basic strategies used by the acupuncturists discussed in the present work.

Assumed Place of Divergence	Master Holes	Acupuncturist
Source/Network	Irie Master Holes	Irie
Network/Cleft	No Master Holes	Irie
Source/Network	Irie Master Holes	Seki
Source/Network	Bypass Holes	Seki
Network/Confluence	*Liu zhu* source w/Yin Channel	Naomoto
Confluence	Irie Master Holes	Shima
Variable	Variable Master Holes	Helms

Appendix 8:
Tadashi Irie's Magnet Specifications

Tadashi Irie created some rather unique magnetic devices in the course of refining his diagnostic process for the channel divergences. When contrasted with electro-acupuncture machines or even ion pumping cords, however, Irie's tools are decidedly low-tech. The materials required are readily available and they are easily assembled.

Materials:
One 800 gauss PIP magnet[9]
One 2 inch section of drinking straw
Two Q-tips
Superglue

Irie's Cylinder Magnet

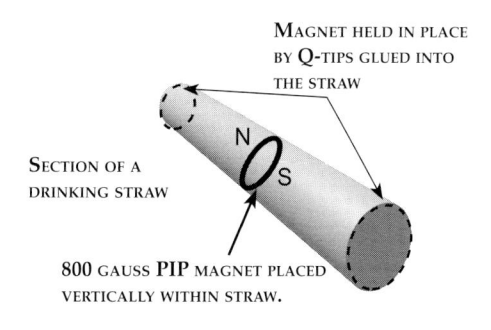

Magnet held in place by Q-tips glued into the straw

Section of a drinking straw

800 gauss PIP magnet placed vertically within straw.

The purpose of the cylinder magnet assembly is to orient an 800 gauss discoid PIP magnet at a right angle to the surface of the skin. The magnet is placed vertically in the center of the section of drinking straw. The cotton ends of the Q-tips are broken off, glue is applied to them and they are inserted into either end of the straw as a means of securing the magnet in an upright or vertical position. When Irie refers to the use of a cylinder magnet, he is referring specifically to this device.

Irie's Bar Magnet

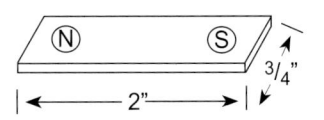

800 gauss PIP magnet glued on a piece of plastic

Materials:
One 800 gauss PIP magnet
One piece of plastic 2 inches X 3/4 inch X 1/8 inch
Superglue

The purpose of the bar magnet assembly is to orient two 800 gauss discoid PIP magnets with opposing polarities on the surface of the skin. A magnet is glued on either end of the strip of plastic with their poles reversed. When Irie refers to the use of a bar magnet, he is referring specifically to this device.

PIP magnets are no longer available through Oriental Medical Supply, however they do offer a number of viable substitutes. There has been some confusion concerning the polarity designations of therapeutic magnets. OMS uses the designations bionorth (-) and biosouth (+) in referring to therapeutic magnets. The bionorth pole of a magnet will swing to point toward the geographic south pole of the Earth while the biosouth pole of a magnet will swing to point toward the geographic north pole. Irie uses the terms north (+) and south (-) in this way.

Endnotes

[9] PIP is a brand name. It is Japanese onomatopoeia for "peeling off of a plaster."

Appendix 9:
Electro-acupuncture Devices

Electrostimulator 8/C
The primary electrical acupuncture device Miki Shima uses for channel divergence and extraordianry vessel therapy is the Electrostimulator 8/C produced by Pantheon Research. This machine combines four channels of microcurrent and four channels of milliampere current capability in a single unit. All eight outputs can be used simultaneously. The four microcurrent channels utilize a bi-polar square wave of 10 volts from 0-600 microamperes. There are two selectable waveforms with four milliampere channels for electro-acupuncture and trans-cutaneous electrical nerve stimulation (TENS). The frequency range is from 0.5-1500Hz. The machine has continuous, mixed, and discontinuous modes of operation with an adjustable mixed frequency to 200Hz.

Hibiki-7
Shima prefers the Hibiki-7 for auriculotherapy and somato-auricular therapy. The Hibiki-7 is a portable electro-acupuncture measurement and treatment device with two output channels and a fixed frequency of 50 Hz has a volt and current setting of 0-3 volts, and 0-6 milliamperes. Maximum voltage is 60 volts with a 100 kohm load. The pulse width is 400 microseconds and the pulse shape is a bi-phasic spike with a continuous pulse mode. Hole detection is registered by both meter and sound. The power source is a 9 volt battery.

The Hibiki-7 is not the only machine suitable for use when administering the techniques profiled in Appendix 4. The ITO-4107, Pointer F-2 and AWQ-104 machines may all be used for combination auricular-channel divergence therapy. These machines are available through Oriental Medical Supply.

The ITO-4107 machine

The ITO-4107 machine is a four output electro-acupuncture device. Two frequency ranges are available, 1-150 or 10-1,500 Hz. There is a low volt and current setting of 0-16 volts, 0-32 milliamperes and a high volt and current setting of 0-24 volts and 0-38 milliamperes. Maximum voltage is 38 or 62 volts with a 100 kohm load. The pulse width is 50 microseconds and the pulse shape is a bi-phasic square with negative spike. The pulse mode is continuous, intermittent or rate modulated. Hole detection is registered by both meter and sound. Six standard AA batteries provide the power source.

The Pointer F-2 machine

The Pointer F-2 machine is a two output electro-acupuncture device. The frequency ranges from 1-100 Hz. The voltage ranges from 0-30 volts and the current ranges from 0-60 milliamperes. The pulse width ranges from 250-50 microseconds and the pulse shape is a bi-phasic square with negative spike. Maximum voltage is 125 volts with a 100 kohm load. The pulse mode is continuous, intermittent or rate modulated. Both meter and sound register hole detection. Probe frequency and voltage is 1-100 Hz and 0-2.5 volts. Six standard 1.5 volt size C batteries provide the power source.

The AWQ-104 Bio-Tech machine

The AWQ-104 Bio-Tech machine is a four output electro-acupuncture device. Two frequency ranges are available, 0-100 or 0-1000 Hz. There is a low volt and current setting of 0-4 volts, 0-8 milliamperes, and a high volt and current setting of 0-30 volts and 0-60 milliamperes. Maximum voltage is 7 or 50 volts with a 100 kohm load. The pulse width is 400 microseconds or 40 microseconds and the pulse shape is a bi-phasic square with negative spike. The pulse mode is continuous, intermittent or rate modulated. Both light and sound register hole detection. One 9 volt battery provides the power source.

Appendix 10:
Omura's bi-digital O-ring test

Kinesiological testing in the context of acupuncture practice has been the topic of a great deal of recent debate. The chiropractic blending of Applied Kinesiology and acupuncture, and the growing popularity of the Nambudripad Allergy Elimination Technique (NAET) and its variants has brought muscle testing into mainstream acupuncture practice. In purporting to bypass the subjective responses of the patient, muscle testing has great appeal because it promises diagnostic objectivity without recourse to more technologically sophisticated electrical testing devices or laboratory assessments. However, the validity of all kinds of muscle testing, and the O-ring test developed by Dr. Yoshiaki Omura, M.D. in particular, has been called into question by a number of prominent thinkers in the field of Asian medicine.

Whatever the final verdict on the bi-digital O-ring test will be, it is a matter of historical fact that it has figured prominently in the historical development of channel divergence therapeutics. In light of this, it behooves the present authors to describe the technique in some detail. We readily concede that muscle testing is a fundamentally subjective enterprise, providing information that is ultimately no more objective than pulse, tongue or abdominal diagnosis. While neither of the present authors makes extensive use of the technique in our own clinical practice, we are of the opinion that Omura's bi-digital O-ring test remains a viable clinical tool on par with the other more venerable diagnostic methods we have just mentioned.

The bi-digital O-ring test is one of the simplest kinesiological tests currently used by acupuncturists, dentists and medical doctors today, and it is particularly popular in Japan. It is performed as follows: The examinee should first remove all objects with electric or magnetic fields (e.g. TV sets, computers, batteries, magnetic cards, etc.) from the room as well as chemicals, drugs, foods, drinks, tobacco, etc. from her body. Accessories and things in pockets should be set aside. The examinee is asked to form a fairly perfect circle (an O-Ring) by touching the tips of the thumb and one finger (e.g. the index finger) of one hand. The other hand should be made into a fist and held away from the trunk of the body.

The examiner then inserts a pair of her fingers (e.g. the index fingers) into the examinee's O-Ring, and joins them to his thumbs to make circles around the examinee's O-Ring. Then he pulls the examinee's O-Ring outward from both sides with his finger-circles, trying to open the O-Ring, while the examinee resists it.

The examiner must test for the correct combination of fingers which fulfills the following three necessary conditions for the bi-digital O-Ring Test: (1) the examinee's O-Ring cannot be opened when the examiner pulls the O-Ring apart with his finger-circles; (2) the O-Ring can be too easily opened to a fairly full extent when the examiner uses a pair of additional fingers (e.g. the middle fingers) and pulls. When the examinee's force is stronger than the examiner's, another weaker O-Ring (e.g. using the thumb and the middle finger, the thumb and the third finger, or the thumb and the little finger) may be tried. When the examinee's force is weaker than the examiner's, the examiner may try other weaker finger-circles (e.g. formed with the thumbs and the middle fingers). If no good match is found, the examinee's other hand may be tried. If a good match is found, the third condition should be tested: (3) the examinee is instructed to change the position of her head in four different directions (*i.e.,* head downward, head backward, and head rotated to the right and to the left) during which time the examiner pulls the O-Ring with a pair of fingers forming the circles as in the first condition. The force of the O-Ring should not change at all. A correct match of fingers is able to give a reliable bi-digital O-Ring test, if it satisfies all three conditions.

If there is a dysfunction in a certain organ, the O-Ring will open when it is pulled apart as the corresponding organ representation point (on the body surface) is stimulated, because the muscle force is weakened through a brain response, which decreases the muscle tone of the whole body.

An in-depth discussion of the validity of the bi-digital O-ring test is beyond the scope of the present work. For one of the most lucid and concise arguments for the validity of the O-ring test, we refer the reader to an article written by M.M. Van Benschoten that appeared in Volume 27, 1999, issue of the *American Journal of Acupuncture* (AJA). It appeared in that journal as a response to some of the key criticisms leveled against the O-ring test. In addition, a paper by Chifuyu Takashige titled "Involvement of the Pineal Body", is arguably the most scientific evaluation of the bi-digital O-ring test to appear in the literature. Dr. Takeshige is a neurologist who is professor emeritus of Showa Medical College. After becoming interested in Omura's work he formed a panel of investigators in Tokyo whose research demonstrated that the O-ring test influenced cerebral microcirculation. The article originally appeared in the *Journal of Acupuncture Electronics*, 1998; 13 (1): 41-4 and may be reviewed on-line at www.kisc.co.jp/o-ring/index/html.

More information on Omura's bi-digital O-ring test is available at the following locations.

800 Riverside Drive, 6-J, New York, NY, 10032
Phone (212) 781-6262.

Websites:

Dr. Omura - Publications
(http://www.home.netcom.com/~mareev/O.pubs.html)

Profile of Prof. Yoshiaki OMURA
(http://www.baobab.or.jp/~oring/omura.shtml)

The Formation and Basis of the Bi-Digital O-Ring Test
(http://www.baobab.or.jp/
)

O-Ring Center (English Version)
(http://www.baobab.or.jp/~oring/e_index.shtml)

Bibliography

Chinese Language Sources

淮南子
Huai Nan Zi (Master Huai Nan), Yanshan Press, Beijing, 1995

黄帝内经素文校释
Huang Di Nei Jing Su Wen Jiao Shi (*Annotated Huang Di's Inner Classic: Elementary Questions*), People's Health & Hygiene Press, Beijing, 1980

黄帝内经灵枢校释
Huang Di Nei Jing Ling Shu Jiao Shi (*Annotated Huang Di's Inner Classic: Divine Pivot*), People's Health & Hygiene Press, Beijing, 1980

邓良月, 中国经络文献通鉴
Deng Liang-yue *et al.*, *Zhong Guo Jing Luo Wen Ti Tong Lin*, (*Categorized Collection of Literatures on Chinese Channels & Network Vessels*), Qingdao Press, Qingdao, 1993

高武, 针灸聚英
Gao Wu, *Zhen Jiu Ju Ying*, (*The Gathering of the Blossoms of Acupuncture*), Shanghai Science & Technology Press, Shanghai, 1987

皇甫谧, 针灸甲乙经
Huang-fu Mi, *Zhen Jiu Jia Yi Jing* (*The Systematic Classic of Acupuncture & Moxibustion,*) People's Health & Hygiene Press, Beijing, 1981

黄寿祺 & 张善文, 周易译注
Huang Shou-qi, & Zhang Shan-wen, *Zhou Yi Yi Zhu*, (*The Changes of Zhou Explained*), Shanghai Ancient Authors Press, Shanghai, 1990

李东垣, 东垣医集
Li Dong-yuan, *Dong Yuan Yi Ji* (*The Collected Medical Works of Dong-yuan*), People's Health & Hygiene Press, Beijing, 1981

杨继洲, 针灸大成校释
Yang Ji-zhou, *Zhen Jiu Da Cheng Jiao Shi*, (*The Annotated Great Compendium of Acupuncture & Moxibustion*) People's Health & Hygiene Press, Beijing, 1981

王叔和, 脉经校释
Wang Shu-he, *Mai Jing Jiao Shi*, (*The Annotated Pulse Classic*), People's Health & Hygiene Press, Beijing 1981

张吉, et. al., 各家针灸医籍适
Zhang Ji, et. al., *Ge Jia Zhen Jiu Yi Ji Shi*, (*An Explanation of Acupuncture & Moxibustion Records of the Major Sects*), Chinese National Chinese Medical Press, Beijing, 1993

张介宾, 类经
Zhang Jie-bin, *Lei Jing*, (*The Categorized Classic*), People's Health & Hygiene Press, Beijing 1964

张隐庵, 帝内径素文集注, 中国医学大成
Zhang Yi-nan: *Huang Di Nei Jing Su Wen Ji Zhu* (*The Annotated Huang Di's Inner Classic: Elementary Questions*) in the anthology: *Zhong Guo Yi Xue Da Cheng* (*The Great Compendium Of Chinese Medical Studies*), Vol. 1, Shanghai Science & Technology Press, Shanghai, 1988

JAPANESE LANGUAGE SOURCES

赤羽幸兵卫皮内针法
Akabane, Kobei, *Hinaishin Ho* (*The Method of Hinaishin*), Ido-no-Nippon-Sha Ltd., Yokosuka, 1950

入江晴二灸法
Irie, Seiji, *Zusetsu Fukaya Kyuho* (*Illustrated Fukaya Moxibustion Methods*), Shizensha Publishing Co., Tokyo, 1980

入江正经别, 经筋, 奇经疗法
Irie, Tadashi, *Keibetsu, Keikin, Kikei Ryoho* (*Treatment of Channel Divergences, Channel Sinews & Extraordinary Vessels*), Ido-no-Nippon-Sha,Ltd., Yokosuka, 1979

入江正 经别, 经筋, 奇经疗法
Irie, Tadashi, Keibetsu, Keikin, Kikei Ryoho (Treatment of Channel Divergences, Channel Sinews & Extraordinary Vessels), revised edition, Ido-no-Nippon-Sha,Ltd., Yokosuka, 1982

入江正サンフランシスゴ讲义ノオト
Irie, Tadashi, Lecture Notes, San Francisco, 1986

入江正东洋医学原论
Irie Tadash*i, Toyo Igaku Genron* (*Principles of Oriental Medicine*), self-published, Osaka, 1989

板谷和子赤羽知热感度测定法私见补遗
Itaya, Kazuko, "*Akabaneshi Chinetsu Kando Sokuteiho Chiken Hoyi* (Supplementaty Observations on Thermal Sensitivity Testing by Mr. Akabane)," *Ion-pumping Medical Point*, Vol. 1, Jan. 3, Asahi Research Institute, Kyoto, 1979

金成彦一经络方向刺激法
Kanari, Hikoichi L.Ac., *Keiraku Hoko Shigekiho* (*Directional Stimulation Method of Acupuncture Channels*), Kanagawa, Wakeido, 1994

城户胜康, 奇经治疗
Kido, Katsuyasu, *Kikei Chiryo Extraordinary-Channel Treatment*, Kikei Chiryo Kenkyu Kai (Society for Researches on Extra-Channel Treatemnt, Osaka, 1978

木下晴都, 针灸学原论
Kinoshita, Hiruto, M.D., *Shinkyugaku Gen Ron* (*Principles of Acupuncture & Moxibustion*), Ido-no-Nippon-Sha Ltd., Yokosuka, 1976

间中喜雄平田式热针刺激疗法
Manaka, Yoshio, M.D. Ph.D."*Hirata Shiki Nesshin Shigeki Ryoho* (*Hirata's Heated Needle Stimulation Treatment*", Ido-no-Nippon-sha,Ltd., Yokosuka, Japan, 1982).

间中喜雄针灸の理论と考え方
Manaka, Yoshio, M.D., Ph.D, *Shinkyu No Riron To Kangaekata* (*Acupunture Theory & Concepts*), Sogensha, Osaka, 1983

直本茂司五行的音阶と音调テスト, 针灸トポロジ论文集
Naomoto, Shigeji, L.Ac. "*Gogyoteki Onkai to Oncho Testo* (Five Phase Scale & Tonal Diagnostic Testing)," *Shinku Toporoji Ronbunshu* (*Miscellaneous Papers on Topological Acupuncture*), Vol. 4, Asahi Research Institute, Kyoto, 1986

直本茂司弱电思考编针灸トポロジ论文集
Naomoto, Shigeji, "*Jaku Den Shiko Hen* (A Treatise on Weak Electrical Force)," *Shinkyu Toporoji Ronbunshu* (*Miscellaneous Papers on Topological Acupuncture*), Vol 4, Dec. 15, Asahi Research Institute, Kyoto, 1985-A

直本茂司三点结合と特功穴针灸トポロジ论文集
Naomoto, Shigeji, "*Santen Ketsugo to Tokkeketu* (Three Point Connections & Especially Effective Acu-points)," *Shinkyu Toporoji Ronbunshu* (*Miscellaneous Papers on Topological Acupuncture*), Vol 2, Asahi Research Institute, Kyoto, 1985-B

直本茂司弱电思考编针灸トポロジ论文集
Naomoto, Shigeji, "*Jaku Den Shiko Hen* (A Treatise on Weak Electrical Force)," *Shinkyu Toporoji Ronbunshu* (*Miscellaneous Papers on Topological Acupuncture*), Vol 3. Jun. 15, Asahi Research Institute, Kyoto, 1984

关行道针治疗及び磁疗针の Q&A
Seki, Kodo, M.D., "*Hari Chiryo Oyobi Jiryo no Q & A* (Questions & Answers on Acupuncture Treatment & Magnetic Treatment)," *Shinkyu Toporoji Ronbunshu* (*Miscellaneous Papers on Topological Acupuncture*), Vol. 4., Asahi Research Institute, Kyoto, 1986

关关行道现代电气针治疗学
Seki, Kodo, M.D., *Gendai Denkishin Chiryogaku* (*Modern Electro-acupuncture Therapeutics*), Shizen-sha Ltd., Tokyo, 1982

柴崎保三针灸医学体系
Shibazaki, Yasuzo, *Shinkyu Igaku Taikei, Kou Tei Dai Kei Rei Su* (*The Great Classic of Acupuncture Medicine*), Vol. 16, Yukon-sha, Kyoto, 1979

ENGLISH LANGUAGE SOURCES

Ames, Roger T. , *Wandering at Ease in the Zhuangzi*, State University of New York Press, Albany, 1998

Birch, Steven J. & Felt, Robert, *Understanding Acupuncture*, Churchill Livingston, London, 1999
Ellis, Andrew, Wiseman, Nigel & Boss, Ken, *Fundamental of Chinese Acupuncture,* Paradigm Publications, Brookline, MA, 1988

Fukishima, Kodo, *Meridian Therapy, A Hands-on Text on Traditional Japanese Hari Based on Pulse Diagnosis, Parts 1 &2,* Toyo Hari Medical Association, Tokyo, 1991

Graham, A.C., *Disputers of the Tao: Philosophical Argument in Ancient China*, Open Court Press, Chicago, 1989

Graham, A.C., *Chuang-Tzu, The Seven Inner Chapters and other witings from the book of Chuang-Tzu,* George Allen and Unwin, London, 1981

Hall, David, L. & Ames, Roger T., *Thinking from the Han: Self Truth & Transcendence in Chinese & Western Culture,* State University of New York Press, Albany, 1998

Hellige, Joseph B., *Hemispheric Asymmetry: What's Right and What's Left,* Harvard University Press. Cambridge, MA, 1993

Helms, Joseph M., M.D., *Acupuncture Energetics: A Clinical Approach for Physicians,* Medical Acupuncture Publishers, Berkeley, CA, 1995

Huang-fu Mi, *The Systematic Classic of Acupuncture and Moxibustion* (*A Translation of the Zhen Jiu Jia Yi Jing*), trans. by Yang Shou-zhong & Charles Chace, Blue Poppy Press, Boulder, CO, 1994

Jeans, Sir James, *Science & Music*, Dover Publications Inc., New York, NY, 1964

Jiao, Shunfa, *Scalp Acupuncture and Clinical Cases*, Foreign Language Press, Beijing, 1997

Jullien, Francois, *The Propensity of Things-Toward a History of Efficacy in China*, trans. by Janet Lloyd, Zone Books, New York, NY, 1995

Kenkusha's English-Japanese Dictionary, 5th Edition, Kenkyusha, Tokyo, 1980

Li Dong-yuan*, The Treatise on the Spleen & Stomach* (*A Translation of the Pi Wei Lun*), trans. by Yang Shou-zhong & Li Jian-yong, Blue Poppy Press, Boulder, CO, 1993

Low, Royston, *Secondary Vessels of Acupuncture*, Thorson's Publishers, Wellingborough, 1983

Manaka, Yoshio, Itaya, Kazuko & Birch, Steven, *Chasing the Dragon's Tail,* Paradigm Publications, Brookline, MA, 1995

Matsumoto, Kiiko & Birch, Steven, *Extraordinary Vessels,* Paradigm Publications, Brookline, MA, 1986

Matsumoto, Kiiko & Birch, Steven, *Hara Diagnosis: Reflections on the Sea,* Paradigm Publications, Brookline, MA, 1988

Mautner, Thomas, *The Penguin Dictionary of Philosophy*, Penguin Books, London, 1996

Miyawaki, Kazuto, *Extraordinary Vessel Treatment Manual,* trans. by Masayuki Hamazaki, self-published, (Ontario Canada), 1997

Ni, Yi-tian, *Navigating the Channels*, self-published, San Diego, 1996

Omura, Yoshiaki, "Bi-digital O-ring Test Molecular Identification & Localization Method and Its Application in Imaging of Internal Organs & Malignant Tumors as Well as Identification & Localization of Neurotransmitters & Micro-Organisms, Part 1," *International Journal of Acupuncture & Electro-Therapeutics Research,* Vol.11, 1986

Oleson, Terry, Ph.D., *Auriculotherapy Manual: Chinese & Western Systems of Ear Acupuncture*, 2nd edition, Health Care Alternatives, Los Angeles, CA, 1996

Pirog, John, E., *The Practical Application of Meridian Style Acupuncture*, Pacific View Press, Berkeley, CA, 1996

Seem, Mark, *Acupuncture Physical Medicine*, Blue Poppy Press, Boulder, CO, 1999

Shima, Miki, *The Medical I Ching, Oracle of the Healer Within,* Blue Poppy Press, Boulder, CO, 1991

Springer, Sally P. & Deutsch, George, *Left Brain Right Brain,* revised edition, W.H. Freeman & Co., New York, NY, 1981

Yau, P.S., *Scalp Needling Therapy*, Mayfair, Hong Kong, 1998

Xu Da-chun, *Forgotten Traditions of Ancient Chinese Medicine: A Chinese View from the Eighteenth Century*, trans. by Paul U. Unschuld, Paradigm Publications, Brookline, MA, 1990

Nan Jing, The Classic of Difficult Issues, trans. by Paul U. Unschuld, University of California Press, Berkeley, CA, 1986

Unschuld, Paul, *Medicine In China, A History of Ideas,* University of California Press, Berkeley, CA, 1985

FRENCH LANGUAGE SOURCES

Duron, A., Laville-Mery, Ch., & Borsarello, J., *Bioenergetic et Medicine Chinoise,* Maisonneuve, France, 1982

Kespi, Jean Marc, *Acupuncture*, Moulins les Metz, Maisonneuve, France, 1982

Nogier, Paul, M.D. & Nogier, Raphael, *Traite d'Ariculotherapie*, Moulin les Metz, France, 1969

Nogier, Raphael, M.D. *Introduction Practique, a l'auriculomedecine, La Photoperception Cutanee*, Haug International, Belgium, 1993

TRANSLATION RESOURCES

Matthews, R. H., *Matthew's Chinese English Dictionary*, Harvard University Press, Cambridge, MA, 1979

Todo, Yoshiaki, *Gakken Kanwa Jiten* (*Gakken Chinese-Japanese Dictionary*), Gakken Publications Inc., Tokyo

Wang Huan, *Chinese-English Dictionary of Function Words*, Sinolingua, Beijing, 1992

Wiseman, Nigel, *A Practical Dictionary of Chinese Medicine*, Paradigm Press, Brookline, MA, 1998

Wiseman, Nigel, *English-Chinese, Chinese English Dictionary of Chinese Medicine.* Hunan Science & Technology Press, Changsha, 1995

Wu Jing-rong, *The Pinyin Chinese-English Dictionary,* Commercial Press, Hong Kong, 1979

Zhang Shang-wen, *Zhou Yi Ci Dian*, (*A Dictionary of The Changes of Zhou*), Shanghai Ancient Authors Press, Shanghai, 1990

Index

A

a shi holes, 121, 210
abdominal diagnosis, 55-59, 94, 97, 101, 126, 131, 139, 155-156, 167, 186, 220, 251
abdominal pain, 80, 211
abdominal reflex holes, 95
abdominal skin, moist, 180
abdominal tenderness, 189
access holes, 66, 69, 79, 99, 102, 130, 138-139, 146, 148, 153, 202
Achilles tendinitis, 173
acne, 187
Acupuncture, A Comprehensive Text, 8, 49
Acupuncture Energetics, 68, 70
acute conditions, 151, 166, 202
Akabane, Kobei, 59
Akabane testing, 57, 61-62, 142-143, 149-150, 174
allergies, 233
alternate master holes, 140
American Journal of Acupuncture, 252
Ames, Roger, 35
ancestral qi, 50-53, 100, 147
anemia, 155
appetite excessive, 179
arthritis of the sternum, 155
asthma, 56, 98-100, 155, 195, 201-202, 204
atony, 71, 102
auriculotherapy, 97, 138, 145, 151, 158, 173, 181, 183, 185, 203-209, 211-218, 235-238, 249
AWQ-104 Bio-Tech Machine, 250

B

Ba Zhen Tang, 170, 199
Ba Wei Wan, 192, 200, 241, 243
back pain, 119, 121, 164, 210
bamboo pipes, 38, 228
Ban Xia Hou Po Tang, 189, 193, 200, 243
Ban Xia Xie Xin Tang, 188, 191-192, 200, 242
ben tun, 180
Bensky, Dan and O'Connor, John, 8
bi-digital O-ring test, 64, 78, 93, 100, 138, 227, 251-253
bi-metal needle techniques, 148
bi-metal needles, 87, 128, 146, 152, 198
biorhythmic treatments, 127-128
blood pressure, 145
Borsarello, J. 44
bowel movements, loose, 189
bowel movements resemble rabbit stools, 98
breast pain, 184, 186
bronchial asthma, 98, 195, 204
bruised easily, 179
Bu Zhong Yi Qi Tang, 194, 200, 244
burn, third-degree, 121

C

cancer, throat, 154, 166, 168-169
cardiovascular accident, 214
cervical dysplasia, 154, 186
chaotic conditions, 47, 49
chest pain, 155
Chinese musicology, 125
Chinese pentatonic scale, 228
Chinese clock, 20, 99, 125-127, 228
chocolate, cravings for, 169
cholecystitis, 56

chronic problems, 69, 169, 236
Ci Yuan (Sea of Words), 41
Classic of Difficult Issues, 57-58, 139, 157, 186, 198-199, 224
clotting, 170, 179, 188, 196-197
clotty menses, 187
colon cancer, 179
concentration and memory were poor, 155
confluence holes, 13, 138-139
constipation, 56
constitutional weaknesses, 149
cough, 177
cramps, 177
cross-needling, 46-48, 50, 52-53, 70, 73
CVA, 214

D

Da Huang Gan Cao Wan, 240, 243
Da Huang Mu Dan Tang, 240, 243
Daoist canon, 35
deep palpation, 157, 198
diabetes, 154, 169, 179, 207
diabetes mellitus, insulin dependent, 169
diagnostic parameters, 101, 125, 155
disease management, 154
disease diagnosis, 227
distinct meridians, 46, 68
Divine Pivot, 2-4, 6-7, 11, 13-14, 17, 20, 22-23, 36, 38, 41, 43-44, 46-51, 65-66, 73, 126, 198, 227, 234
dizziness, 80
dorsal nerve root, 212
Du Huo Sheng Qi Tang, 199
Duron, A, 44, 52
dysmenorrhea, 169-170, 179
dysplasia, 154, 186, 194

E

ear acupuncture, 138, 235
electrical impedance, 235
electrical stimulation therapy, 107
electrical measurement of acupuncture holes, 238

electro-acupuncture device, 146, 250
electrocardiogram, 155
Electrostimulator 8/C, 249
Elementary Questions, 43, 45-46, 73, 224
emotionally sensitive, 168
endocervical squamous metaplasia, 186
endometriosis, 217
epigastric area, pain in the upper, 133
epigastric spasm, 161, 180, 188-189, 191-193, 195
extraordinary vessel pairings, 143, 166, 199, 202
extraordinary vessel therapies, 53, 152
extraordinary vessel combinations, 149, 152
eyes, bags under her, 179

F

face was flushed, 97
facial diagnosis, 125, 230
fatigue, 155, 169
fibroids, 154, 179, 181, 186, 199
fibromyalgia, 202, 209
fukushin, 186

G

gallbladder disease, 56
gasp for air during sleep, 166
gastrointestinal upset, 193
Ge Gen Tang, 240-242
geographic north pole, 248
glucose levels, 173, 177
gold needle, 116, 147, 150, 158, 163, 166, 175, 177
gold and silver needle technique, 158
Gui Zhi Tang Jia Bai Zhu, 240-241
Gui Zhi Fu Ling Tang, 170, 181, 241
Gui Zhi Jia Lung Gu Mu Li Tang, 188, 190, 199
gynecological problems, 3

H

Hara Diagnosis: Reflections on the Sea, 59

headache, 80, 119
headaches, left-sided, 133
headaches, low-grade, 169, 173
headaches, occipital, 119, 155
heart disease, 142, 179
heat sensations at night, 155
Helms, Joseph, 68-69
hemorrhoidal pain, 98
hepatitis, 56, 69, 131, 155
hepatitis, acute, 69
Hibiki-7, 210, 235-237, 249
hie, 142, 198
hip pain, 155
Hirata, Kurakichi, 229
Hirata Zones, 100-101, 123, 229
Hirata Shiki Nesshin Shigeki Ryoho, 229
hormone therapy, 195
hot flashes, 155
Huai Nan Zi, 42, 52
human papilloma virus, 192
hyper/hypothyroidism, 206
hypertension, 141, 213
hypoglycemia, 216

I
IDDM1, 169
Ido-No-Nippon-Sha, 138, 198
in-vitro fertilization, 195
Inch Mouth pulse, 228
insomnia, 130, 169, 205
intercostal neuralgia, 212
intersection holes, 108
intraepithelial lesion, 192
intestines, achy 155
ion pumping cords, 87, 100, 107-108, 112, 116, 128, 131, 146, 152, 238, 247
Irie Master Holes, 79
Irie, Tadashi, 6-7, 10, 17, 29, 58, 62, 77-79, 87, 95, 97, 138, 152, 199, 239, 247
Irie's Confluence-based herbal formulas, 239
Itaya, Kazuko, 61
ITO-4107 Machine, 250

J
Japanese styles of practice, 155
Jin Gei Myaku I Kai, 234
Jin Gui Yao Lue (Essentials from the Golden Cabinet), 100
jing well holes, 46, 50, 52-53, 59-62, 70, 143, 182

K
kanpo yaku, 78, 100
Kawai, 130, 135
Kazuto Miyawaki, 110
Kespi, Jean Marc, 4
kidney function, 177
kidney return protocol, 146, 152-153, 197
Kidney channel divergence, 18, 87, 123
knee pain, 117-118
Kobayashi, Shoji, 139, 198
kori, 149
Kyoto City Medical College, 229

L
laterality disturbances, 238
left-right imbalances, 157, 163
Lei Jing: (The Categorization of the Classic), 24, 39, 51, 53
leukopenia, 218
leukorrhea, 187-188
Li Shi-zhen, 52, 219-220
Li Zhong Tang, 196, 200
Ling Shu (Divine Pivot), 2, 14
Ling Shu Ji Jiao Shi (Annotated Divine Pivot), 38
Liu Wei Di Huang Wan, 99, 188, 239
localized areas of stagnation, 149
Low Royston, 44-46, 50, 68, 72
low back pain, 164, 210
lower back pain, 164
lower abdominal flaccidity, 156, 161
lower abdominal blood stasis, 156, 193-194
lower abdominal weakness, 195-196
lump glomus, 181

M

macrocosmic influences, 29
magnet therapy, 149
magnet specifications, 247
Man's Prognosis pulse, 126, 227-228
Manaka, Yoshio, 42, 59, 61, 77, 111, 125, 128, 229, 231, 235
master-couple hole pairs, 150
Matsumoto, Kiiko, 42, 135
Meniere's disease, 133
menses, clotty, 187
menstrual discomfort, 186
menstruation, irregular, 169
microcosmic orbit, 112
midday-midnight needling method, 126
middle burner weakness, 157
migraine, 148, 202
miscarriage, 195
Misonou, Isai, 59
Mizuno, Tsuneo, 138
Modern Electro-Acupuncture Therapeutics, 101, 123
abdominal skin, moist, 180
mu alarm holes, 58, 126
Mu Mei Ketsu, 231
Mubun Oda, 230, 234
Mubun Oda's facial diagnosis, 230
muscle spasms, 122
muscle testing, 251

N

NAET, 251
Nakamura, Shoji 138
Nambudripad Allergy Elimination Technique, 251
Naomoto, Shigeji, 125, 130, 235
Nan Jing, 139, 186, 198, 224
Naomoto's Hibiki Method, 237
Naomoto's biorhythmic dual confluence pairings, 128-129
nausea, 202
Navigating the Channels of Traditional Chinese Medicine, 8, 67
neck pain, 119, 169
neck, nape of the, 7, 17, 20, 30
nenshin needle twirling technique, 120-121
neuropathies, 208
Ni, Yi-tian, 67
night sweats, 155
NIP/channel divergence protocol, 121-122
NIP protocol, 117-122, 132-133, 185-186, 194, 231
No Name hole, 135, 231
nocturia, 189
numbness, 102, 121, 131

O

obsessive-compulsive disorder, 215
Occidental Institute of Chinese Studies, 72, 75
Ogura, Domei, 234
Omura, Yoshiaki, 138, 233, 251
Omura's Thymus holes, 158
optic nerve, damage to, 133
optic nerve, trauma to, 133
Oriental Medical Supply, 236, 248, 250

P

pain relief, 236
palpatory findings, 99, 143
palpitation, 58, 187-188, 190-191, 193-194
Pantheon Research, 146, 249
paralysis, 208, 214
paresthesias, 102
pedunculated fibroid, 179
pelvic exam, 186
photophobia, 133
PIP magnet, 247-248
Pointer F-2 Machine, 250
points to earth, 23-25
points to heaven, 23, 25, 29
popliteal fossa, 6-7, 12, 16-18, 66
posterior auricular master hole, 236
postoperative atonic illness, 71
premenstrual syndrome, 169, 179
pressure pain reactivity, 80, 127

pressure pain, 59, 80, 95, 97-101, 119, 127, 131, 186, 229-230
primordial pathogen, 142

Q
Qi Jing Ba Mai Kao (A Personal Critique of the Eight Vessels of the Extraordinary Channels), 52, 219
qigong, 112

R
range of motion tests, 134-135
rectal problems, 3
ren ying-cun kou, 126
Renying Cunkou Pulse Medical Society, 234
rheumatoid arthritis, 215
running piglet, 180-181, 199

S
sciatica, 130
Seki bypass protocol, 116
Seki bypass strategy, 130
Seki's Electro-acupuncture Protocol, 102
Seki, Kodo, 77-78, 95, 101, 111
sesshokushin, 157, 173
shaku, 161, 164, 180-182, 186-188, 191, 193, 195-196, 198-199
Shang Han Lun (Treatise on Damage [Due to] Cold), 100
Shi Quan Da Bu Tang, 240-241
Shindo Hiketsu Shu, 230
Si Wu Tang, 170, 194, 200, 240, 242
side effects, unwanted, 149
sinusitis, 213
sleep, disturbed, 155
slow repolarization phase, 81
So, James Tin-yao, 59
solar plexus, 4-5
somato-auricular therapy, 138, 249
spasms, subcostal, 180
spleen *shaku*, 161, 164, 180, 182, 187-188, 191, 193, 195-196, 198
squamous intraepithelial, lesion low grade, 192
sternum, trauma to, 155
stomach pain, 97
stool stagnation, 180
stools, loose, 189, 195-196
stress, 188-190
stress response, dysfunctional, 188
subcostal tension, 156, 170-171, 190-194
subordinate channel divergence, 93-95
Suihara sound diagnosis, 135
supraumbilical aortic palpitations, 189
sweats, night, 155

T
tai ji quan, 33
Tai Yi treatment, 231
Tao Hong Si Wu Tang, 170
TENS, 249
The Hibiki Method, 208, 235
The Journal of Japanese Acupuncture, 138
The Twelve Officials, 53
thirsty, 98
throat cancer, 154, 166, 168-169
tonal diagnosis, 228
Topological Acupuncture Society, 55, 61, 101, 125-126, 130, 228, 231, 239
treatment formulary, 201
treatment methods, auxiliary, 231
tuning fork, 125, 228

U
universal access holes, 139
uterine bleeding, dysfunctional, 179
uterine fibroids, 154, 179, 181, 199

V
Van Benschoten, M. M., 252
vertigo, 133, 153
vital signs, 169, 179, 187-189, 191, 193-195

W
Wen Jing Tang, 182, 196, 199, 242

whiplash injury, 119
wilting conditions, 208
window of the sky hole, 7
Wiseman, Nigel 20, 38-39, 53, 64, 225
Worsley, J. R., 59
Wrist pulse, 126, 224, 227-228

X
Xiao Chai Hu Tang, 193, 200, 241
Xiao Yao San, 189, 200, 240, 242
Xuan Ji (CV 21), 158, 233

Y
Yi Gan Ji, 182, 190, 199-200
Yi Gan Ji Jia Chen Pi Ban Xia Tang, 190, 200
You Gui Wan, 168, 170, 198
Yu Dai Xin Yong (New Poems From the Jade Dynasty), 42
Yue Bi Jia Zhu Tang, 240-241

Z
Zhang Dong-sun, 34, 36, 39
Zhang Zhong-jing, 100
Zhang Jie-bin, 24, 51
Zhen Jiu Jia Yi Jing (Systematic Classic of Acupuncture & Moxibustion), 13
Zhen Wu Tang, 240-241
Zhong Guo Zhen Jiu Da Quan (A Comprehensive Encyclopedia of Chinese Acupuncture and Moxibustion), 8
Zhu Ling Tang, 240-241
Zhuang-Zi, 35-36, 39, 41
zi wu liu zhu liao fa, 126
Zuo Gui Wan, 166, 168, 170, 198

OTHER BOOKS ON CHINESE MEDICINE AVAILABLE FROM:
BLUE POPPY PRESS
5441 Western, Suite 2, Boulder, CO 80301
For ordering 1-800-487-9296 PH. 303\447-8372 FAX 303\245-8362
Email: info@bluepoppy.com Website: www.bluepoppy.com

A NEW AMERICAN ACUPUNCTURE
By Mark Seem
ISBN 0-936185-44-9

ACUPOINT POCKET REFERENCE
by Bob Flaws
ISBN 0-936185-93-7

ACUPUNCTURE AND MOXIBUSTION
FORMULAS & TREATMENTS
by Cheng Dan-an, trans. by Wu Ming
ISBN 0-936185-68-6

ACUPUNCTURE PHYSICAL MEDICINE:
An Acupuncture Touchpoint Approach to
the Treatment of Chronic Pain, Fatigue,
and Stress Disorders
by Mark Seem
ISBN 1-891845-13-6

AGING & BLOOD STASIS: A New
Approach to TCM Geriatrics
by Yan De-xin
ISBN 0-936185-63-5

BETTER BREAST HEALTH NATURALLY
with CHINESE MEDICINE
by Honora Lee Wolfe & Bob Flaws
ISBN 0-936185-90-2

THE BOOK OF JOOK: Chinese Medicinal
Porridges
by Bob Flaws
ISBN 0-936185-60-0

CHINESE MEDICAL PALMISTRY:
Your Health in Your Hand
by Zong Xiao-fan & Gary Liscum
ISBN 0-936185-64-3

CHINESE MEDICINAL TEAS: Simple,
Proven, Folk Formulas for Common
Diseases & Promoting Health
by Zong Xiao-fan & Gary Liscum
ISBN 0-936185-76-7

CHINESE MEDICINAL WINES
& ELIXIRS
by Bob Flaws
ISBN 0-936185-58-9

CHINESE PEDIATRIC MASSAGE
THERAPY: A Parent's & Practitioner's
Guide to the Prevention & Treatment of
Childhood Illness
by Fan Ya-li
ISBN 0-936185-54-6

CHINESE SELF-MASSAGE THERAPY:
The Easy Way to Health
by Fan Ya-li
ISBN 0-936185-74-0

THE CLASSIC OF DIFFICULTIES:
A Translation of the *Nan Jing*
translation by Bob Flaws
ISBN 1-891845-07-1

CURING ARTHRITIS NATURALLY
WITH CHINESE MEDICINE
by Douglas Frank & Bob Flaws
ISBN 0-936185-87-2

CURING DEPRESSION NATURALLY
WITH CHINESE MEDICINE
by Rosa Schnyer & Bob Flaws
ISBN 0-936185-94-5

CURING FIBROMYALGIA NATURALLY
WITH CHINESE MEDICINE
by Bob Flaws
ISBN 1-891845-08-9

CURING HAY FEVER NATURALLY
WITH CHINESE MEDICINE
by Bob Flaws
ISBN 0-936185-91-0

CURING HEADACHES NATURALLY
WITH CHINESE MEDICINE
by Bob Flaws
ISBN 0-936185-95-3-X

CURING IBS NATURALLY WITH
CHINESE MEDICINE
by Jane Bean Oberski
ISBN 1-891845-11-X

CURING INSOMNIA NATURALLY
WITH CHINESE MEDICINE
by Bob Flaws
ISBN 0-936185-85-6

CURING PMS NATURALLY WITH
CHINESE MEDICINE
by Bob Flaws
ISBN 0-936185-85-6

A STUDY OF DAOIST ACUPUNCTURE
& MOXIBUSTION
by Liu Zheng-cai
ISBN 1-891845-08-X

THE DIVINE FARMER'S MATERIA
MEDICA
A Translation of the *Shen Nong Ben Cao*
translation by Yang Shouz-zhong
ISBN 0-936185-96-1

THE DIVINELY RESPONDING CLASSIC:
A Translation of the *Shen Ying Jing* from
Zhen Jiu Da Cheng
trans. by Yang Shou-zhong & Liu
Feng-ting
ISBN 0-936185-55-4

DUI YAO: THE ART OF COMBINING
CHINESE HERBAL MEDICINALS
by Philippe Sionneau
ISBN 0-936185-81-3

ENDOMETRIOSIS, INFERTILITY AND
TRADITIONAL CHINESE MEDICINE:
A Laywoman's Guide
by Bob Flaws
ISBN 0-936185-14-7

THE ESSENCE OF LIU FENG-WU'S
GYNECOLOGY
by Liu Feng-wu, translated by Yang
Shou-zhong
ISBN 0-936185-88-0

EXTRA TREATISES BASED ON
INVESTIGATION & INQUIRY:
A Translation of Zhu Dan-xi's *Ge Zhi
Yu Lun*
translation by Yang Shou-zhong
ISBN 0-936185-53-8

FIRE IN THE VALLEY: TCM Diagnosis
& Treatment of Vaginal Diseases
by Bob Flaws
ISBN 0-936185-25-2

FU QING-ZHU'S GYNECOLOGY
trans. by Yang Shou-zhong and Liu
Da-wei
ISBN 0-936185-35-X

FULFILLING THE ESSENCE: A
Handbook of Traditional & Contemporary
Treatments for Female Infertility
by Bob Flaws
ISBN 0-936185-48-1

GOLDEN NEEDLE WANG LE-TING:
A 20th Century Master's Approach to
Acupuncture
by Yu Hui-chan and Han Fu-ru, trans. by
Shuai Xue-zhong
ISBN 0-936185-78-3

A GUIDE TO GYNECOLOGY
by Ye Heng-yin,
trans. by Bob Flaws and Shuai Xue-zhong
ISBN 1-891845-19-5

A HANDBOOK OF TCM PATTERNS
& TREATMENTS
by Bob Flaws & Daniel Finney
ISBN 0-936185-70-8

A HANDBOOK OF TRADITIONAL
CHINESE DERMATOLOGY
by Liang Jian-hui, trans. by Zhang
Ting-liang & Bob Flaws
ISBN 0-936185-07-4

A HANDBOOK OF TRADITIONAL
CHINESE GYNECOLOGY
by Zhejiang College of TCM, trans. by
Zhang Ting-liang & Bob Flaws
ISBN 0-936185-06-6 (4th edit.)

A HANDBOOK OF CHINESE
HEMATOLOGY
by Simon Becker
ISBN 1-891845-16-0

A HANDBOOK OF MENSTRUAL
DISEASES IN CHINESE MEDICINE
by Bob Flaws
ISBN 0-936185-82-1

A HANDBOOK of TCM PEDIATRICS
by Bob Flaws
ISBN 0-936185-72-4

A HANDBOOK OF TCM UROLOGY
& MALE SEXUAL DYSFUNCTION
by Anna Lin, OMD
ISBN 0-936185-36-8

THE HEART & ESSENCE OF DAN-XI'S
METHODS OF TREATMENT
by Xu Dan-xi, trans. by Yang Shou-zhong
ISBN 0-926185-49-X

THE HEART TRANSMISSION OF
MEDICINE
by Liu Yi-ren, trans. by Yang Shou-zhong
ISBN 0-936185-83-X

HIGHLIGHTS OF ANCIENT
ACUPUNCTURE PRESCRIPTIONS
trans. by Honora Lee Wolfe & Rose
Crescenz
ISBN 0-936185-23-6

IMPERIAL SECRETS OF HEALTH
& LONGEVITY
by Bob Flaws
ISBN 0-936185-51-1

KEEPING YOUR CHILD HEALTHY
WITH CHINESE MEDICINE
by Bob Flaws
ISBN 0-936185-71-6

THE LAKESIDE MASTER'S STUDY OF
THE PULSE
by Li Shi-zhen, trans. by Bob Flaws
ISBN 1-891845-01-2

Li Dong-yuan's TREATISE ON THE
SPLEEN & STOMACH,
A Translation of the *Pi Wei Lun*
trans. by Yang Shou-zhong
ISBN 0-936185-41-4

MASTER HUA'S CLASSIC OF THE
CENTRAL VISCERA
by Hua Tuo, trans. by Yang Shou-zhong
ISBN 0-936185-43-0

MASTER TONG'S ACUPUNCTURE
by Miriam Lee
ISBN 0-926185-37-6

THE MEDICAL I CHING: Oracle of the
Healer Within
by Miki Shima
ISBN 0-936185-38-4

MANAGING MENOPAUSE
NATURALLY with Chinese Medicine
by Honora Lee Wolfe
ISBN 0-936185-98-8

PAO ZHI: Introduction to Processing
Chinese Medicinals to Enhance Their
Therapeutic Effect
by Philippe Sionneau
ISBN 0-936185-62-1

PATH OF PREGNANCY, VOL. I,
Gestational Disorders
by Bob Flaws
ISBN 0-936185-39-2

PATH OF PREGNANCY, Vol. II,
Postpartum Diseases
by Bob Flaws
ISBN 0-936185-42-2

THE PULSE CLASSIC: A Translation
of the *Mai Jing*
by Wang Shu-he, trans. by Yang Shou-zhong
ISBN 0-936185-75-9

SEVENTY ESSENTIAL CHINESE
HERBAL FORMULAS
by Bob Flaws
ISBN 0-936185-59-7

SHAOLIN SECRET FORMULAS for
Treatment of External Injuries
by De Chan, trans. by Zhang Ting-liang
& Bob Flaws
ISBN 0-936185-08-2

STATEMENTS OF FACT IN
TRADITIONAL CHINESE MEDICINE
by Bob Flaws
ISBN 0-936185-52-X

STICKING TO THE POINT 1: A Rational
Methodology for the Step by Step
Formulation & Administration of an
Acupuncture Treatment
by Bob Flaws
ISBN 0-936185-17-1

STICKING TO THE POINT 2: A Study
of Acupuncture & Moxibustion Formulas
and Strategies
by Bob Flaws
ISBN 0-936185-97-X

A STUDY OF DAOIST ACUPUNCTURE
by Liu Zheng-cai
ISBN 1-891845-08-X

TEACH YOURSELF TO READ MODERN
MEDICAL CHINESE
by Bob Flaws
ISBN 0-936185-99-6

THE SYSTEMATIC CLASSIC OF
ACUPUNCTURE & MOXIBUSTION
A translation of the *Jia Yi Jing*
by Huang-fu Mi, trans. by Yang Shou-
zhong & Charles Chace
ISBN 0-936185-29-5

THE TAO OF HEALTHY EATING
ACCORDING TO CHINESE MEDICINE
by Bob Flaws
ISBN 0-936185-92-9

THE TREATMENT OF DISEASE IN TCM,
Vol I: Diseases of the Head & Face
Including Mental/Emotional Disorders
by Philippe Sionneau & Lü Gang
ISBN 0-936185-69-4

THE TREATMENT OF DISEASE IN TCM,
Vol. II: Diseases of the Eyes, Ears, Nose, &
Throat
by Sionneau & Lü
ISBN 0-936185-69-4

THE TREATMENT OF DISEASE, Vol. III:
Diseases of the Mouth, Lips, Tongue, Teeth
& Gums
by Sionneau & Lü
ISBN 0-936185-79-1

THE TREATMENT OF DISEASE, Vol IV:
Diseases of the Neck, Shoulders, Back, &
Limbs
by Philippe Sionneau & Lü Gang
ISBN 0-936185-89-9

THE TREATMENT OF DISEASE, Vol V:
Diseases of the Chest & Abdomen
by Philippe Sionneau & Lü Gang
ISBN 1-891845-02-0

THE TREATMENT OF DISEASE, Vol VI:
Diseases of the Urogential System
& Proctology
by Philippe Sionneau & Lü Gang
ISBN 1-891845-05-5

THE TREATMENT OF DISEASE, Vol VII:
General Symptoms
by Philippe Sionneau & Lü Gang
ISBN 1-891845-14-4

THE TREATMENT OF EXTERNAL
DISEASES WITH ACUPUNCTURE
& MOXIBUSTION
by Yan Cui-lan and Zhu Yun-long, trans.
by Yang Shou-zhong
ISBN 0-936185-80-5

THE TREATMENT OF DIABETES
MELLITUS WITH CHINESE MEDICINE
by Bob Flaws, Lynn Kuchinski &
Robert Casañas, MD
ISBN 1-891845-21-7

THE TREATMENT OF MODERN
WESTERN MEDICAL DISEASES WITH
CHINESE MEDICINE
by Bob Flaws & Philippe Sionneau
ISBN 1-891845-20-9

160 ESSENTIAL CHINESE HERBAL
PATENT MEDICINES
by Bob Flaws
ISBN 1-891945-12-8

630 QUESTIONS & ANSWERS ABOUT
CHINESE HERBAL MEDICINE:
A Workbook & Study Guide
by Bob Flaws
ISBN 1-891845-04-7

230 ESSENTIAL CHINESE MEDICINALS
by Bob Flaws
ISBN 1-891845-03-9